BSAVA M
Canine and Feline
Ultrasonography

T0266791

Editors:

Frances Barr
MA VetMB PhD DVR DipECVDI MRCVS
Department of Clinical Veterinary Science, University of Bristol, Langford
House, Langford, Bristol BS40 5DU, UK

and

Lorrie Gaschen
PhD Dr.habil DVM DrMedVet DipECVDI
School of Veterinary Medicine, Louisiana State University, Skip Bertman Drive,
Baton Rouge, Louisiana, LA 70803, USA

Published by:

British Small Animal Veterinary Association
Woodrow House, 1 Telford Way, Waterwells
Business Park, Quedgeley, Gloucester GL2 2AB

A Company Limited by Guarantee in England.
Registered Company No. 2837793.
Registered as a Charity.

First edition 2011
Reprinted 2012, 2016, 2018, 2019, 2022, 2024

ISBN   978 1 905319 30 5

The publishers, editors and contributors cannot take responsibility for information provided on
dosages and methods of application of drugs mentioned or referred to in this publication. Details of
this kind must be verified in each case by individual users from up to date literature published by the
manufacturers or suppliers of those drugs. Veterinary surgeons are reminded that in each case they
must follow all appropriate national legislation and regulations (for example, in the United Kingdom,
the prescribing cascade) from time to time in force.

Printed in the UK by Hobbs the Printers Ltd, Totton SO40 3WX
Printed on ECF paper made from sustainable forests

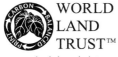

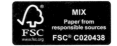

Titles in the BSAVA Manuals series:

For further information on these and all BSAVA publications, please visit our website: **www.bsava.com**

Contents

Video access
Previous printings of this edition included a DVD containing videos, but as most computers no longer have a DVD drive the videos are now available via the BSAVA Library. The videos can be accessed via the link or QR code provided at the end of the relevant chapters. All references to the DVD within this manual relate to the videos that are now available via the BSAVA Library.

Videos available from the BSAVA Library

See relevant chapters for details of how to access the videos

Equipment
Applying the 'image optimizer'
Changing acoustic power
Changing gain
Changing the number of focal zones
Time–gain compensation controls

Thorax
Fine-needle aspiration of a pulmonary mass
Lung lobe torsion
Normal lung
Pleural fluid
Pulmonary mass (1)
Pulmonary mass (2)

Heart
Atrial septal defect
Bubble study
Endocarditis (1)
Endocarditis (2)
Heart base mass
Hypertrophic cardiomyopathy (1)
Hypertrophic cardiomyopathy (2)
Left cranial view of the right atrium
Mitral valve regurgitation (1)
Mitral valve regurgitation (2)
Mitral valve regurgitation (3)
Patent ductus arteriosus
Patent ductus arteriosus viewed from a
    transoesophageal approach
Patent ductus arteriosus viewed from the left
    cranial window
Pericardial effusion
Pulmonic stenosis (1)
Pulmonic stenosis (2)
Right atrial mass
Subaortic stenosis (1)
Subaortic stenosis (2)
Subaortic stenosis (3)
Subaortic stenosis (4)
Systolic anterior motion of the chordae
Systolic anterior motion of the mitral valve
Tricuspid valve dysplasia (1)
Tricuspid valve dysplasia (2)
Tricuspid valve prolapse
Tricuspid valve regurgitation
Ventricular septal defect (1)
Ventricular septal defect (2)

Abdomen
Changes to the mesentery
Enlarged abdominal lymph nodes (1)
Enlarged abdominal lymph nodes (2)
Normal mesentery
Peritoneal effusion
Postsurgical hernia
Retroperitoneal effusion
'Smoke' in the caudal vena cava
Splenic thrombi

Liver
Hepatic venous congestion
Hepatocellular carcinoma with contrast
Hepatopathy with contrast
Obstructive cholestasis
Portosystemic shunt

Spleen
Normal spleen in a cat
Normal spleen in a dog
Splenic infarction (1)
Splenic infarction (2)
Splenic infarction (3)

Kidneys and proximal ureters
Chronic renal disease in a cat
Hydronephrosis
Normal kidney in a cat
Normal kidney in a dog
Renal calculi
Renal infarction (1)
Renal infarction (2)
Renal lymphoma

Stomach, small and large intestines
Colonic carcinoma
Functional ileus
Gastric oedema
Gastric lymphoma
Hypereosinophilic syndrome
Inflammatory polyp
Jejunal foreign body
Jejunal lymphoma
Normal duodenal contractions
Normal duodenal papilla
Normal feline pylorus
Pseudolayering

Pancreas
Acute pancreatitis in a dog
Chronic pancreatitis in a cat
Insulinoma
Normal pancreas (cat)
Normal pancreas (dog)

Adrenal glands
Left adrenal gland tumour
Metastatic nodule
Normal left adrenal gland in a dog
Normal right adrenal gland in a cat
Normal right adrenal gland in a dog
Phaeochromocytoma

Bladder and urethra
Cystic calculi
Ectopic ureter
Ureteric jet

Prostate gland
Benign prostatic hyperplasia (1)
Benign prostatic hyperplasia (2)
Benign prostatic hyperplasia (3)
Normal prostate gland (1)
Normal prostate gland (2)
Prostatic abscess
Prostatic carcinoma (1)
Prostatic carcinoma (2)
Prostatic cysts (1)
Prostatic cysts (2)

Uterus
4-week pregnancy in a cat
4-week pregnancy in a Jack Russell Terrier
Normal uterus in a dog

Thyroid and parathyroid glands
Normal thyroid gland (1)
Normal thyroid gland (2)

Superficial soft tissues
Abdominal wall injury (1)
Abdominal wall injury (2)
Abscess
Foreign body (1)
Foreign body (2)
Lactating mammary gland
Lipoma
Mammary cysts
Nerve sheath tumour in the brachial plexus
Soft tissue neoplasm (1)
Soft tissue neoplasm (2)

Contributors

Matt Baron DVM DipACVR
VCA Veterinary Referral Associates, 500 Perry Parkway, Gaithersburg, MD 20877, USA

Frances Barr MA VetMB PhD DVR DipECVDI MRCVS
Department of Clinical Veterinary Science, University of Bristol, Langford House, Langford,
Bristol BS40 5DU, UK

Esther Barrett MA VetMB DVDI DipECVDI MRCVS
Wales & West Imaging, Jubilee Villas, Tutshill, Chepstow, Gwent NP16 7DE, UK

Livia Benigni DVM CertVDI DipECVDI FHEA MRCVS
The Royal Veterinary College, University of London, Hawkshead Lane, North Mymms, Hatfield,
Hertfordshire AL9 7TA, UK

Susanne A.E.B. Boroffka Dr.med.vet. PhD DipECVDI
Diagnostic Imaging Section, Clinic for Companion Animals, University of Utrecht, Postbus 80.154,
3508 TD, Utrecht, The Netherlands

Kate Bradley MA VetMB PhD DVR DipECVDI MRCVS
Department of Clinical Veterinary Science, University of Bristol, Langford House, Langford,
Bristol BS40 5DU, UK

Lorrie Gaschen PhD Dr.habil DVM Dr.med.vet. DipECVDI
School of Veterinary Medicine, Louisiana State University, Skip Bertman Drive, Baton Rouge,
Louisiana, LA 70803, USA

Daniela Gorgas Dr.med.vet. DipECVDI
Division of Clinical Radiology, Department of Clinical Veterinary Medicine, University of Bern,
Länggassstrasse 128, 3012 Bern, Switzerland

John P. Graham MVB MSc DVR DipACVR DipECVDI MRCVS
Affiliated Veterinary Specialists, 9905 South US Highway 17-92, Maitland, FL 32751, USA

Gawain Hammond MA VetMB MVM CertVDI DipECVDI FHEA MRCVS
School of Veterinary Medicine, University of Glasgow, Bearsden Road, Glasgow G61 1QH, UK

Silke Hecht Dr.med.vet. DipACVR DipECVDI
Department of Small Animal Clinical Sciences, University of Tennessee College of Veterinary
Medicine, C247 Veterinary Teaching Hospital, 2407 River Drive, Knoxville, TN 37996, USA

Jennifer Kinns BSs VetMB DipECVDI DipACVR MRCVS
Dunbartonshire, Scotland, UK

Robert M. Kirberger BVSc MMedVet(Rad) DipECVDI
Diagnostic Imaging Section, Department of Companion Animal Clinical Studies, Faculty of
Veterinary Science, University of Pretoria, Private Bag X04, Onderstepoort 0110, South Africa

Patrick R. Kircher Dr.med.vet. PhD DipECVDI
Section of Diagnostic Imaging, Vetsuisse Faculty, University of Zürich, Winterthurerstrasse 260, 8057 Zürich, Switzerland

Martin Kramer PhD Dr.med.vet DipECVDI
Department of Veterinary Clinical Sciences, Clinic for Small Animals, Justus-Liebig-University Giessen, Frankfurter Strasse, 108, 35392 Giessen, Germany

Paul Mahoney BVSc DVR DipECVDI CertVC FHEA MRCVS
Willows Veterinary Centre and Referral Service, Highlands Road, Solihull, West Midlands B90 4NH, UK

Stefanie Ohlerth Dr.med.vet. Dr.habil. DipECVDI
Section of Diagnostic Imaging, Vetsuisse Faculty, University of Zürich, Winterthurerstrasse 260, 8057 Zürich, Switzerland

Romain Pariaut DVM DipACVIM (Cardiology) DipECVIM-CA (Cardiology)
School of Veterinary Medicine, Louisiana State University, Skip Bertman Drive, Baton Rouge, Louisiana, LA 70803, USA

Nathalie Rademacher Dr.med.vet. DipECVDI DipACVR
School of Veterinary Medicine, Louisiana State University, Skip Bertman Drive, Baton Rouge, Louisiana, LA 70803, USA

Daniel Rodriguez MVZ Esp DipACVR
School of Veterinary Medicine, Louisiana State University, Skip Bertman Drive, Baton Rouge, Louisiana, LA 70803, USA

Federica Rossi DVM SRV DipECVDI
Clinica Veterinaria dell'Orologio, Sasso Marconi, Bologna, Italy

Gabriela Seiler Dr.med.vet DipECVDI DipACVR Cert Clin Res
College of Veterinary Medicine, North Carolina State University, 4700 Hillsborough Street, Raleigh, NC 27606, USA

Nerissa Stander BVSc MMedVet(Diag Im)
Diagnostic Imaging Section, Department of Companion Animal Clinical Studies, Faculty of Veterinary Science, University of Pretoria, Private Bag X04, Onderstepoort 0110, South Africa

Olivier Taeymans DVM PhD DipECVDI
Department of Clinical Sciences, Cummings School of Veterinary Medicine, Tufts University, 200 Westboro Road, North Grafton, MA 01536, USA

Foreword

The field of small animal ultrasonography has expanded widely over the past 20 years, creating a huge craving for compiled and updated information on the numerous applications of ultrasonography in veterinary medicine. Despite the advancement and development of cross-sectional imaging modalities such as CT and MRI, ultrasonography remains a very useful, cost-effective and widely available diagnostic method for our patients.

The *BSAVA Manual of Canine and Feline Ultrasonography* provides an excellent resource to the novice or more experienced reader. The Manual, which is made of about 230 pages and richly illustrated, has a user-friendly format. It is well organized and addresses first the physics and artefacts, followed by the main clinical applications using a systematic organ approach. In addition, a companion DVD is a pertinent complementary resource to the book, offering numerous video clips in support of information provided in each chapter.

The renowned editors have selected an international group of experienced authors to compile the Manual.

This Manual greatly complements the existing BSAVA imaging collection, which includes titles dedicated to abdominal, musculoskeletal and thoracic imaging, and should proudly take its place on the bookshelf of every small animal hospital.

Dominique Penninck DVM PhD DipACVR DipECVDI
Professor, Diagnostic Imaging Section,
Tufts Cummings School of Veterinary Medicine

Preface

Ultrasonography in veterinary medicine has become as invaluable a tool today to the general practitioner as it is in referral and academic institutes. Previous BSAVA Manuals on musculoskeletal, abdominal and thoracic imaging have included sections on ultrasonography; however, this is the first BSAVA Manual dedicated solely to the subject. It is a comprehensive resource aimed at both the beginner and the more experienced ultrasonographer. This has allowed us to explore the subject in more depth and provide information on both basic and advanced topics. The importance of radiography is emphasized throughout the Manual, and indications for the use of radiography, ultrasonography, CT and MRI are included to demonstrate the value of the individual modalities for each organ system or disease. However, CT and MRI are still not always readily available or affordable, and this Manual demonstrates where ultrasonography can be of value when cross-sectional imaging cannot be performed.

Ultrasonography is now used routinely for investigation of the thorax, superficial tissues and the musculoskeletal system, as well as for the abdomen. This Manual is ideal for the practitioner who is seeking a text that concentrates exclusively on small animal ultrasonography, with reference to diseases specific to both the dog and cat, and who is looking to expand their experience beyond that of the routine abdominal ultrasound examination.

The Manual begins with chapters on the physical principles of ultrasound, choosing equipment and the basic concepts of scanning. Subsequent chapters explore each organ system, including the superficial soft tissues, heart, eye and the musculoskeletal system. Every chapter includes practical approaches on how to perform the examination or explore the region of interest, with a description of normal anatomy, and is followed by a comprehensive description of abnormalities based on the most current medical literature. The Manual is packed with images of both normal and abnormal structures to accompany the text. However, the moving image is a vital part of interpreting ultrasound studies, thus there is reference to relevant video clips throughout the chapters, which are included on a DVD-ROM provided with each Manual.

Ultrasound-guided tissue sampling procedures such as fine-needle aspiration and Tru-cut biopsy have become an important part of the ultrasound examination. Differentiating inflammatory from neoplastic disease in many organ systems is not possible with ultrasonography, and this aspect is discussed throughout the Manual. For this reason, we have included a separate chapter that outlines the equipment required and the technique for obtaining tissue samples, so that we can improve the specificity of the ultrasound examination when abnormalities are detected.

The contributors to this Manual were chosen for their nationally and internationally recognized reputations and expertise in the field of ultrasonography. Their dedication to the advancement of veterinary ultrasonography through their clinical experience and research studies has made this Manual a must-have, current standard for anyone already performing ultrasound examinations or thinking of taking their first steps with the modality. We have greatly enjoyed the efforts of all the contributors for making this Manual what is sure to be another pearl of the BSAVA Manuals, and it was a pleasure to work with Nicola Lloyd and Marion Jowett at BSAVA.

Frances Barr
Lorrie Gaschen
December 2010

Physical principles

Daniela Gorgas

Production of ultrasound waves

Diagnostic ultrasonography is a cross-sectional imaging technique based on the physical principles of sound waves. Unlike electromagnetic waves, which can be transmitted within a vacuum, sound waves need a medium (liquid, solid or gas) for propagation. The particles of the medium are oscillated by a sound wave due to alternating pressure deviations from the equilibrium pressure, causing local regions of compression and rarefaction.

Characteristics of the ultrasound beam

Sound waves are characterized by wavelength (λ), frequency (f) and amplitude (A) (Figure 1.1a). Frequency refers to the number of waves that pass a given point in one second. It is usually described in units of cycles per second or Hertz (Hz). The frequency of sound detectable by human hearing is 16,000–20,000 Hz; sound of lower frequencies is called infrasound and that of higher frequencies is called ultrasound. The wavelength (λ) is the distance between corresponding points of two consecutive waves and can be calculated according to the following formula (if the speed of sound is known):

$$\lambda = c/f$$

Where: λ = wavelength; c = velocity; f = frequency.

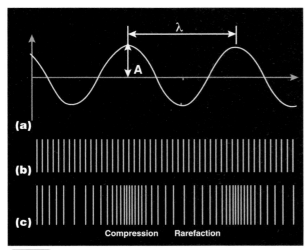

1.1 **(a)** Sound waves are characterized by wavelength (λ), frequency and amplitude (A). **(b)** Particles of matter at rest. **(c)** Sound waves cause compression and rarefaction of the particles of matter.

Ultrasound waves travel through the body. The body is comparable to a semi-fluid medium, and the speed of sound within the body is assumed to be 1540 m/s. However, the speed of sound within the body varies; stronger binding forces within a specific medium, such as bone, increase the speed of sound. The speed of sound within the body can not be changed and is considered a constant; frequency and wavelength are inversely proportional. Thus, a higher frequency sound wave always has a shorter wavelength and *vice versa*.

Propagation of sound waves

Within gases, liquids or semi-solids (such as the body), sound and ultrasound are transmitted as longitudinal waves, also called compression waves. Particles in the medium are periodically displaced by a sound wave due to alternating pressure deviations from the equilibrium pressure, and therefore oscillate. The region of increased pressure in relation to the equilibrium is called **compression**; the region of decreased pressure in relation to the equilibrium is called **rarefaction** (Figure 1.1bc). The energy carried by the sound wave converts back and forth between the potential energy of the compression and the kinetic energy of the oscillations of the medium. A single vibrating point sends out waves in all directions from the point of origin as concentric circles. The direction of propagation of the wave is the same as the direction of initiation, which is the direction of expansion of the piezoelectric crystal.

How are ultrasound waves produced?

The formation of ultrasound waves is based on the so-called piezoelectric effect, which was detected in 1880 by Pierre and Jacques Curie. The name's origin is the Greek word 'piezein' which means to press or squeeze, because the effect describes the ability of a crystal to convert pressure – a mechanical energy – into an electric energy. The opposite is used for the production of an ultrasound wave: an electric voltage is applied to a crystal, which is converted into mechanical energy, causing oscillation of the crystal. The oscillation is transmitted as an ultrasound wave into the body.

A modern ultrasound wave transducer contains multiple crystals, which work as piezoelements. Today, synthetic piezoelectric ceramics are employed, most often lead–zirconate–titanate (PZT).

Detection of returning echoes

The transducer acts not only as a transmitter of sound waves but, as described above, the piezo-elements are also able to act as a receiver. The reflecting echoes carry energy and transmit their energy to the transducer, causing a mechanical compression of the piezoelectric crystal. The compression forces the dipoles within the crystal to change their orientation, resulting in an electric voltage at the surface of the crystal which is amplified and converted for display.

The transducer is not able to send and receive echoes at the same time and alternates between a sending and receiving mode. Receiving or listening to echoes takes about 99% of the time, whilst sending the echoes takes about 1% of the time. The echoes are sent out as pulses and each pulse consists of several (normally two or three) waves. The length of the pulse is defined by the number of waves and their wavelength (**spatial pulse length**). The pulse rate or **pulse repetition frequency (PRF)** refers to the number of separate little packets of sound waves that are sent out each second.

Interaction of ultrasound waves with tissues

As sound waves propagate through a medium, different interactions occur (Figure 1.2), including:

- Reflection
- Refraction
- Diffraction
- Attenuation.

Reflection

The sound wave reflected back towards the source (probe) is called an echo, which is used to generate the ultrasound image. The reflection of echoes occurs mainly at tissue interfaces, which cause reflection of ultrasound waves due to differences in the acoustic impedance. The **acoustic impedance (Z)** is an indicator of the resistance or flexibility of a medium, which is determined by its density (ρ) and the speed of sound (c) within the medium according to the following formula:

$$Z = \rho c$$

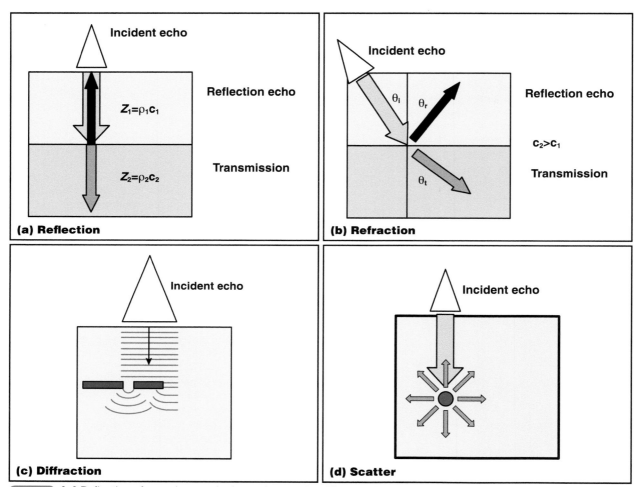

(a) Reflection

$Z_1 = \rho_1 c_1$

$Z_2 = \rho_2 c_2$

Incident echo

Reflection echo

Transmission

(b) Refraction

Incident echo

θ_i θ_r

Reflection echo

$c_2 > c_1$

Transmission

θ_t

(c) Diffraction

Incident echo

(d) Scatter

Incident echo

1.2 **(a)** Reflection of sound waves is dependent on the difference in impedance of two media. If the incident echo hits the reflecting surface at a 90 degree angle, the reflecting echo goes back to the transducer. **(b)** If the incident echo does not hit the reflecting surface at a 90 degree angle, the angle of incidence is the same as the angle of reflection ($\theta_i = \theta_r$). At boundaries between two media with different acoustic velocities, refraction occurs at an angle θ_t. **(c)** Diffraction is a change of direction of waves caused by an obstacle or a hole. **(d)** Scatter causes the beam to diffuse in many directions with only parts of the incident echo returning to the transducer.

The proportion of sound waves that is transmitted or reflected at an interface is dependent on the difference in impedance of both media (Figure 1.3). The greater the difference in impedance of two adjacent media, the greater the proportion of reflection. For a typical muscle–fat interface, approximately 1% of the ultrasound wave intensity is reflected and thus almost 99% of the intensity is transmitted to greater depths in the tissues. At a muscle–air interface, nearly 100% of incident intensity is reflected, preventing the anatomy beyond an air-filled cavity from being visualized. This also explains the need for acoustic coupling gel to fill the air space between the transducer and the skin.

Tissue	Density (ρ) (g/cm^2)	Velocity (c) (m/s)	Acoustic impedance (Z) (10^6 kg/m^{2}s)
Fat	0.97	1470	1.42
Muscle	1.04	1568	1.63
Liver	1.05	1570	1.65
Spleen	1.06	1565	1.66
Kidneys	1.03	1560	1.61
Water	0.998	1492	1.49
Compact bone	1.7	3600	6.12
Air	0.0013	331	0.004

1.3 Acoustic impedance, density and velocity of sound waves within various tissues of the body.

The incident angle of the sound wave when it interacts with an object also plays a role in whether the beam is reflected back to the transducer. As with the reflection of light, the angle of incidence and angle of reflection of the sound wave are equal. As the angle of incidence increases, reflected sound waves are less likely to reach the transducer (see Figure 1.2).

Refraction
Sound waves travel at various speeds through the different body tissues. When a sound wave passes from one medium to another at different acoustic velocities, its frequency remains the same but its wavelength changes. This causes the course of the ultrasound beam to deviate, a phenomenon called refraction. The angle of refraction (θ_t) is determined by the change in speed of the sound wave and is related to the angle of incidence (θ_i) by **Snell's law**:

$$\sin \theta_t / \sin \theta_i = c_2/c_1$$

If the speed of sound in the second medium (c_2) is greater than that in the first medium (c_1), the refraction angle (θ_t) is greater than the angle of incidence (θ_i) (see Figure 1.2b). If the speed of sound in the second medium is less than that in the first medium, the refraction angle is less than the angle of incidence.

No refraction occurs when the acoustic velocity is the same in the two media, or when the wave is perpendicular to the interface between the two media. The ultrasound machine assumes a straight line of propagation of the wave and places the returning echoes in a straight line beyond the transducer. When refraction occurs, artefacts in the image such as edge shadowing or speed displacement (see below) are seen.

Diffraction
Diffraction involves a change in the direction of waves as they pass through an opening or around a barrier in their path. Due to diffraction sound waves can be detected around a corner (see Figure 1.2c). There is an increase in the amount of diffraction with longer wavelengths and a decrease in the amount of diffraction with shorter wavelengths. As the wavelength becomes smaller than the obstacle, the wave is no longer able to diffract around the obstacle, and instead reflects off the obstacle.

Attenuation
Attenuation is a composite effect of loss of energy by **scatter** and **absorption**. The **absorption** of sound waves is a conversion of the sound wave energy into heat, and depends on the frequency of the sound wave and the temperature of the medium. The higher the frequency, the greater the absorption of the ultrasound beam. The absorption of ultrasound waves due to loss of acoustic energy also increases with the distance travelled through the medium. In soft tissues there is an almost linear relationship between the frequency and attenuation (dB/cm); a rule of thumb is a loss of 0.5 dB per cm per MHz.

Scatter of sound waves is due to either reflection or refraction by small particles within the medium, and causes the beam to diffuse in many directions (see Figure 1.2d). Acoustic scattering usually originates from objects within a tissue that are about the size of the wavelength. The internal structure of the parenchymal organs causes a certain pattern of scatter, which is characteristic for each organ. This pattern is responsible for the echotexture of each organ, with a speckling of echoes which range from fine to coarse.

Ultrasound image

Display mode
As the pulse passes through the patient, sound waves are reflected back to the transducer from each tissue interface. Assuming an average speed of sound of 1540 m/s in soft tissues, time can be converted into distance. The depth recorded on the display is proportional to the time it takes for the echo to return from the reflector (Figure 1.4).

A-mode
The earliest image representation in diagnostic ultrasonography was with amplitude modulation or

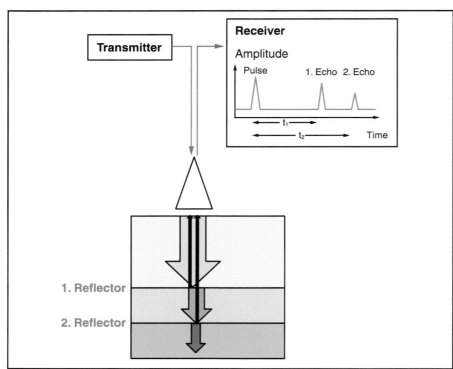

1.4 The transducer sends a pulse and records the time taken for the echo to return. The depth of the reflector recorded on the display is proportional to the distance of the reflector from the transducer. Due to attenuation, returning echoes are weaker with increased depth.

A-mode. It is a one-dimensional (1D) representation of the reflected sound wave as a peak on a display (Figure 1.5). The x axis represents the penetration depth and the y axis represents the amplitude (intensity) of the echo. The greater the reflection at the tissue interface, the larger the signal amplitude. Historically used for cerebral midline shift detection or exact distance measurements in ophthalmology, A-mode imaging is of no diagnostic importance today.

B-mode
B-mode displays a static image of a section of tissue. The peaks of A-mode are converted into dots, and brightness replaces the amplitude (brightness modulation). The intensity of the returning echo is converted into greyscale information: the greater the amplitude, the brighter the dot on the image. Every reflected sound wave is displayed as a dot as a function of location and intensity. In modern ultrasonography, the B-mode image is constantly updated, resulting in 'real-time' imaging.

M-mode
M-mode displays moving structures over time (motion mode). The echo data from a single ultrasound wave passing through moving anatomy are acquired and displayed as a function of time on the horizontal axis. The motion pattern allows functional evaluation of moving structures such as the heart.

Resolution
B-mode images are the result of a cross-section through a three-dimensional (3D) body. **Spatial resolution** describes the ability of a modality to discern objects in close contact. Resolution along the direction of the ultrasound beam is called **axial resolution**. It is determined by the ability of the transducer to detect two reflecting echoes separately without an overlap in the returning echoes; therefore, both echoes have to be separated by half the spatial pulse length (Figure 1.6). The shorter the transmitted pulse and likewise its returning echo pulse, the better the axial resolution. The pulse length is determined by

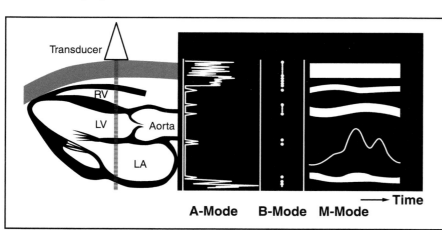

1.5 Different image display modes (A, B, M) using the heart as an example. LA = left atrium; LV = left ventricle; RV = right ventricle.

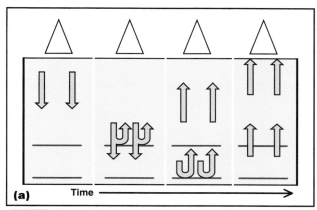 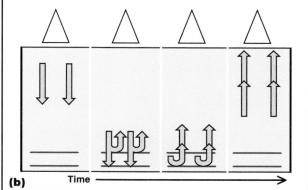

1.6 **(a)** Reflectors are detected separately if they are separated by a distance of >0.5 spatial pulse lengths. **(b)** Overlap of the returning echoes occurs if the distance between the two reflectors is <0.5 spatial pulse lengths; the two reflectors cannot be distinguished from one another in the resulting image. Reduction of spatial pulse length results in better axial resolution because reflectors that are closer to each other can be distinguished.

the number of cycles emitted multiplied by the wavelength. Typically, in diagnostic ultrasonography the pulse consists of three cycles. The higher the frequency, the shorter the wavelength and the spatial pulse length.

Lateral resolution is the ability to separate two adjacent objects perpendicular to the beam direction (Figure 1.7). Lateral resolution is determined by the beam width, which must be narrower than the space separating the objects. As beam diameter varies with distance in the near- and far-field, lateral resolution is depth-dependent. The best lateral resolution occurs at the interface between near- and far-field, where the beam diameter is approximately equal to half the transducer diameter. Greater lateral resolution can be reached by focusing the beam (see below).

Focusing the beam

Beam properties
Ultrasound waves interfere with each other, either in a constructive way (reinforcement) or by cancelling each other out, depending on the phase when they meet. Piezoelectric crystals do not behave as a single point source; an infinite number of vibrating points produce multiple concentric rings of waves. Wave interactions cause multiple constructive and destructive interference patterns, resulting in a wave front parallel to the transducer surface. As the beam courses away from the transducer, a slightly converging beam profile forms in the near-field. Beyond that, in the far-field, the beam diverges (Figure 1.8).

Near-field: The length of the near-field or Fresnel zone is determined by the diameter of the transducer and the wavelength of the ultrasound wave:

$$x'=r^2/\lambda$$

Where: x' = length of Fresnel zone (cm); r = radius of transducer (cm); λ = wavelength (cm). The Fresnel zone is longest with a large transducer and high transmitter frequency.

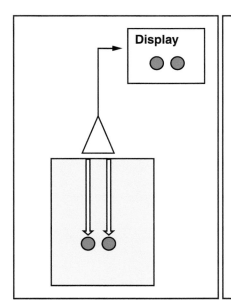 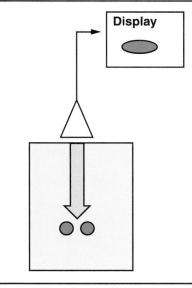

1.7 Lateral resolution is the ability of the transducer to separate two reflectors perpendicular to the beam direction and is dependent on beam width.

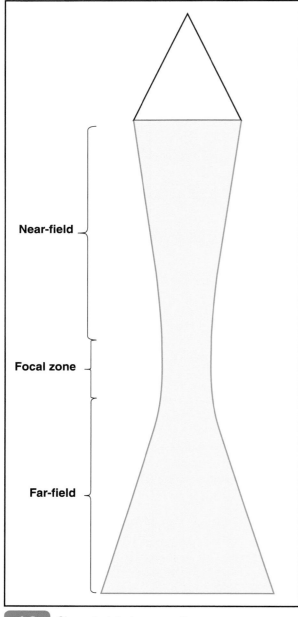

1.8 Characteristic beam profile.

Focal zone: The point of narrowest beam width is called the focal point, and the region over which the width of the beam is less than two times the width of the focal point is called the focal zone. Lateral resolution is best in this region.

Far-field: The amount of dispersion in the far-field or Fraunhofer zone is determined by the angle θ:

$$\sin θ = 1.22 \, λ/D$$

Where: θ = dispersion angle of far zone; λ = wavelength (mm); D = diameter of transducer (mm). An increase in frequency (resulting in a shorter wavelength) with a constant transducer diameter leads to a smaller dispersion angle. Lower frequency transducers cause a higher angle of dispersion.

Beam steering
Focused transducers restrict beam width and improve lateral resolution at a specific depth. Single-element transducers are focused by using a curved piezoelectric element or a curved acoustic lens. Focusing moves the transition point between the near-field and far-field from its determined position.

Effect of frequency
Higher frequency beams have two advantages over low frequency beams: depth resolution is superior; and the near-field is longer. However, tissue absorption rises with increasing frequency; therefore, a lower frequency beam is required to penetrate thick tissues.

- High frequency beam: increased attenuation, decreased penetration with increased resolution
- Low frequency beam: less attenuation, better penetration with decreased resolution.

Artefacts
An artefact on B-mode greyscale ultrasound images is any alteration in the image which does not represent an actual structure. Artefacts may be produced by technical imaging errors or echo distortions caused by ultrasound wave/matter interactions. In this section artefacts caused by physical interactions between the ultrasound beam and matter are discussed. Understanding and identifying artefacts is necessary to avoid interpretation errors. One main reason for artefact formation is the manner in which the ultrasound machine registers data from echoes, assuming that:

- Sound waves travel at a constant speed
- Sound waves travel in straight lines (transmitted and reflected echo)
- Attenuation of sound waves in tissue is constant.

Reverberation
Reverberation artefacts are produced by a pulse bouncing back and forth between two interfaces. They may be produced by sound waves reflecting between the transducer and tissue interfaces, or internally between two reflecting interfaces.

Transducer–interface reverberation echoes: These are produced each time the sound wave pulse returns to the transducer. Only the initial recorded echoes are real; other reverberation echoes that appear deeper in the tissue are multiples of the original transducer–interface echo. The time lapse that occurs between the second, third and fourth returning echoes places them at a greater depth in the tissue on the recorded image. Reverberation echoes will be smaller because of higher attenuation.

Transducer–interface reverberations (also called repetition artefacts) are more likely to occur from highly reflective interfaces such as gas and bone, particularly if the reflecting interface is near the transducer.

Internal structure–structure reverberation echoes: These occur when the sound wave pulse bounces back and forth between two tissue interfaces. This delays the sound wave pulse from returning to the transducer, and the reverberation echoes are recorded deeper than the original reflecting interface (Figure 1.9). Due to its typical appearance, the artefact is also called a comet tail artefact.

Mirror image
A strongly reflective, obliquely oriented surface may reflect the sound beam distally instead of returning it to the transducer (angle of incidence is equal to the angle of reflection). Objects within the direction of the beam reflect the sound beam back to the reflective surface and from there back to the transducer (Figure 1.10). Because it takes the sound waves longer to return, the object will be shown deeper to the oblique reflector surface on the image. A mirror image artefact is recognized as the object and its mirror image are equidistant from the mirror. The shape of the artefact is distorted when the mirror is curved. A typical example is the diaphragm: this is an obliquely oriented surface with high acoustic impedance (air-filled lung behind the diaphragm), and as a result on ultra-

sound images the liver and gallbladder are often misregistered as being cranial to the diaphragm. It is important to recognize this artefact to avoid the false conclusion of diaphragmatic rupture. This artefact will not occur in the presence of pleural effusion, because of lack of a highly reflective surface.

Attenuation

Shadowing: This is created by complete reflection or attenuation of the sound beam (Figure 1.11). The zone deep to the reflecting or attenuating structure is anechoic; however, some reverberation echoes may appear in the shadowed area. Shadowing may be produced by bone, gas, or calculi and can impede adequate imaging of deeper structures. The artefact is very useful to identify calculi within the urinary bladder, and to recognize that a hyperechoic structure is solid in nature.

Refractive and reflective acoustic shadowing zones may occur distal to the margins of rounded structures containing material of lower acoustic velocity, such as fluid-filled cavities. The sound waves penetrating the edge of such a structure may be slightly refracted or reflected, producing a linear anechoic

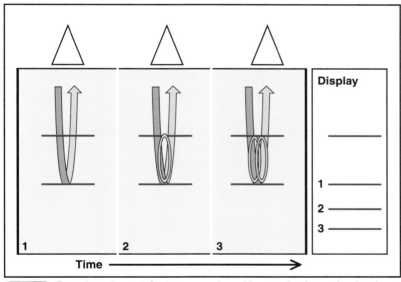
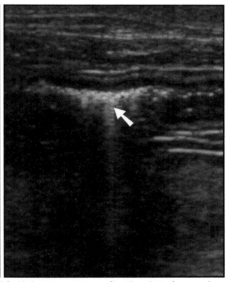

1.9 Reverberation artefacts are produced by a pulse bouncing back and forth between two reflecting interfaces. An example of this artefact (arrowed) is gas bubbles in an intestinal loop.

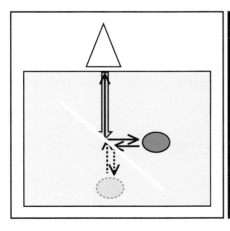
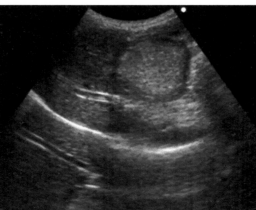

1.10 Mirror image artefacts are produced by a strong reflective, obliquely oriented surface which reflects the sound beam into an organ instead of returning it to the transducer. An example of this artefact is the appearance of a vessel and liver parenchyma distal to the diaphragm.

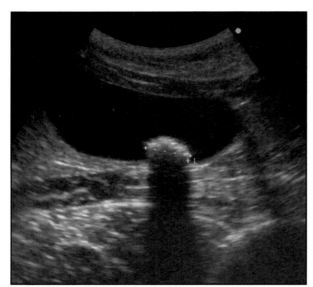

1.11 Complete reflection of the sound beam due to highly reflective surfaces (such as a urolith) within the urinary bladder creates acoustic shadowing, which appears as an anechoic zone deep to the structure preventing that region from being examined.

zone deep to the cystic structure. This is called **edge shadowing**. Such zones are evidence of a rounded structure such as a cystic cavity or even the kidney, and should not be mistaken for shadows produced by calculi, gas or bone (Figure 1.12).

Enhancement or through transmission: This is caused by a relative lack of sound wave attenuation. When sound waves pass through a fluid-filled structure, there is less tissue reflectance and attenuation (see Figure 1.12). A bright or echogenic area is produced immediately deep to the cystic structure because more sound waves are present in this area compared with tissues at the same depth not beneath the cyst. The bright or echogenic area may be confused with increased tissue echoes if it is not associated with an overlying fluid-filled cystic structure. Acoustic enhancement can be helpful in differ-

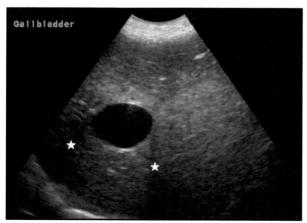

1.12 The gallbladder causes a relative lack of sound wave attenuation and distal enhancement. The hypoechoic lines tangential to the gallbladder wall are caused by edge shadowing (white stars).

entiating fluid-filled structures from solid structures of low echogenicity.

Sound wave speed
The ultrasound machine assumes a constant speed of sound of 1540 m/s within the body and calculates the distance of the reflector according to this. The speed of sound is in fact different in every tissue (see Figure 1.3). For instance, sound is slower in fat, resulting in the machine calculating the position of reflectors deeper than they actually are. The same happens to reflectors beyond tissues within which sound travels faster: they are represented closer to the transducer than they are in reality.

Secondary lobes
Secondary lobes are unwanted ultrasound beams originating from the transducer in a direction different from that of the primary beam. **Side lobes** and **grating lobes** are types of secondary lobes. These lobes have a different origin but both produce image artefacts due to error in positioning of the returning echo. Altering the plane of the image will usually abolish artefactual echoes, whilst real structures will remain.

Side lobes: These are present in all transducers and arise from the expansion of the piezoelectric elements perpendicular to the main beam. Returning echoes from the side lobes are positioned in the image as if they occurred along the main beam. This occurs in imaging of the gallbladder or urinary bladder, where side lobes produce artefactual 'pseudosludge' in an otherwise echo-free organ.

Grating lobes: These are specific to linear arrays and are associated with the regular spacing of the individual crystals in the transducer. More precisely, they are due to constructive interferences of the ultrasound beam between adjacent elements of the array, and may be reduced by using transducers with very closely spaced array elements. The misdirected energy can cause ghost images of highly reflective off-axis objects.

Slice thickness/beam width
When part of the ultrasound beam includes a cystic structure and the other part includes surrounding tissues, the echoes from the tissue are displayed within the cystic structure, mimicking the presence of sediment (Figure 1.13). This does not happen when the entire width of the beam includes a cystic structure. Therefore, slice thickness artefacts are reduced if the beam width is narrow, such as in the focal zone of the beam. Slice thickness is widest close to the transducer and beyond the focal zone.

Ambiguity
Ambiguity artefacts are created when a high pulse repetition frequency (PRF) limits the amount of time spent listening for echoes during the pulse repetition period (PRP). As the PRF increases, the PRP decreases. If an echo originating from a greater depth returns after the next pulse is already initiated, it will be displayed close to the transducer.

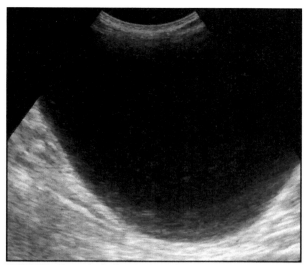

1.13 Pseudosludge in the urinary bladder. This artefact is due to the thickness of the ultrasound beam causing the false impression of sludge in the urinary bladder.

Doppler ultrasonography

Doppler ultrasonography is used to detect and evaluate blood flow, and offers information on its presence, direction, speed and character. The first description of the physical principles used in Doppler ultrasonography is attributed to Johann Christian Doppler, an Austrian mathematician and scientist who lived in the first half of the 19th century.

Doppler effect

The Doppler effect describes a change in the wavelength (or frequency) of energy transmitted as waves (e.g. sound or light) as a result of motion of either the source or the receiver of the waves. For example, the Doppler effect can be heard when an ambulance approaches, passes and retreats from an observer. A pedestrian ahead of the siren (in driving direction) perceives a higher frequency than the frequency sent out by the siren. As the ambulance passes and drives away from the pedestrian, the perceived frequency decreases.

In diagnostic ultrasonography the Doppler effect depends entirely on measurement of the relative change in the returned ultrasound wave frequency when compared with the transmitted frequency: the Doppler shift. It results from moving reflectors sending back to the stationary transducer ultrasound waves of a different frequency to those emitted (Figure 1.14).

Blood cells act as moving reflectors in the body. When the ultrasound wave is reflected back at a higher frequency, a positive Doppler shift results; when the returned frequency is lower, the Doppler shift is negative. If flow is perpendicular to the beam, no frequency change occurs and no Doppler shift is detected. The Doppler equation is expressed as follows:

$$f_d = 2f_i \, v \cos \theta / c$$

Where, the Doppler shift (f_d) of ultrasound waves depends on both the transmitted frequency (f_i) of the waves and the velocity (v) of the moving blood, but the speed of sound within blood is constant (c). Since the Doppler shift happens twice, first when the sound wave hits the reflector and second when the sound wave is reflected back from the still moving reflector, there is a factor of 2 included in the formula. The Doppler shift is highly dependent upon the angle (θ) between the beam transmitted and the moving red blood cells; this is expressed with the cosine in the formula. An angle of 0 degrees would not influence the formula (cosine 0° = 1), and an angle of 90 degrees would lead to no Doppler shift (cosine 90° = 0). All angles between 1 degree and 90 degrees would slightly reduce the amount of Doppler shift (Figure 1.15). Blood velocity can be calculated by rearranging the Doppler equation as follows:

$$v = f_d c / 2f_i \cos \theta$$

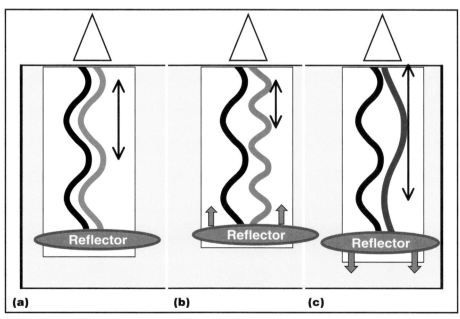

1.14 **(a)** A non-moving reflector reflects the echo (grey wave) at the same frequency and wavelength as the transmitted echo (black wave). **(b)** If the reflector moves towards the transducer, the ultrasound wave is reflected with a higher frequency and shorter wavelength (red wave). **(c)** A lower frequency and longer wavelength (blue wave) results if the reflector moves away from the transducer.

(a) (b) (c)

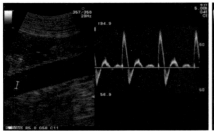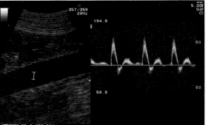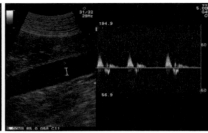

1.15 B-mode ultrasonograms of the abdominal aorta of a dog and the corresponding pulsed wave Doppler images showing the wave form spectrum and velocity of the aortic blood flow in m/s. As the angle between the transmitted beam (dotted green line and gate) and the moving red blood cells increases, the calculated velocity decreases according to the Doppler formula. Flow direction cannot be detected if the angle is 90 degrees.

Doppler shift

The Doppler signal depends on:

- Blood velocity – as velocity increases the Doppler shift increases
- Frequency of the transmitted ultrasound beam – the higher the ultrasound wave frequency the greater the Doppler shift. As in B-mode, lower ultrasound wave frequencies have better penetration. The choice of frequency is a compromise between better sensitivity to flow and better penetration
- The angle between the ultrasound beam and the moving reflectors – Doppler shift increases as the ultrasound beam aligns itself with the flow direction. This concept is paramount in optimal use of Doppler ultrasonography.

Types of Doppler system

There are two main types of Doppler system in common use today: continuous wave and pulsed wave. They differ in transducer design and operating features, signal processing procedures and in the type of information provided. Each has important advantages and disadvantages and the current practice of Doppler echocardiography requires some capability for both forms.

Continuous wave Doppler

Continuous wave (CW) Doppler is the older and electronically simpler of the two systems. CW Doppler involves continuous transmission of ultrasound waves coupled with simultaneous reception. A double crystal transducer accomplishes this dual function with one crystal devoted to each function.

Reflectors anywhere within the beam contribute to the Doppler signal until the ultrasound beam becomes sufficiently attenuated due to depth. CW Doppler ultrasonography gives information about velocity and flow direction, but is unable to determine the specific location of the reflector within the beam and cannot be used to produce colour flow images. The main advantage of CW Doppler is its ability to measure high blood velocities accurately. The main disadvantage of CW Doppler is its lack of selectivity or depth discrimination.

Pulsed wave Doppler

Pulsed wave (PW) Doppler systems use a transducer that alternates between transmission and reception of ultrasound pulses (as in real-time imaging). Doppler shift data are only selected from a small segment along the ultrasound beam, referred to as the 'sample volume', which can be positioned by the operator at any point along the axis of the PW Doppler ultrasound beam. Echoes return to the transducer during a specific time interval, so that reflector depth and frequency shift can be determined. All other returning information is essentially 'ignored'.

One main advantage of PW Doppler is the accurate determination of the depth from which the returning echoes originate. An additional advantage is that some imaging may be carried out simultaneously, with the sample volume shown superimposed on the two-dimensional (2D) image for guidance (Duplex ultrasonography). The main disadvantage of PW Doppler is its inability to accurately measure high blood flow velocities, such as those encountered in valvular stenosis. This limitation is technically known as 'aliasing' (see below) and results in an inability of PW Doppler to unambiguously record velocities >1.5 m/s.

It can usually be said that when an operator wants to know where a specific area of abnormal flow is located that PW Doppler is indicated. When accurate measurement of elevated flow velocity is required, then CW Doppler should be used.

Display modes

Various display modes are available in Doppler ultrasonography (Figure 1.16):

- Spectral Doppler
- Colour Doppler
- Power Doppler.

Spectral Doppler

Spectral Doppler is a form of ultrasound image display in which the spectrum of flow velocities is represented graphically on the y-axis, and time on the x axis; flow towards the transducer is displayed on top of the baseline and flow away from the transducer is displayed below the baseline (see Figure 1.15). Both PW and CW Doppler are displayed in this way. The spectral outputs from PW and CW Doppler have a different appearance:

	Spectral Doppler	Colour Doppler	Power Doppler
Properties	Examines the flow waveform within a specific part of the vessel	Provides a map of flow superimposed over an organ or structure	Colour brightness is related to the number of moving cells, not the velocity or frequency
Advantages	Provides directional information about flow	Provides directional information about flow	Sensitive: can detect low flow, smaller vessels, better penetration
	Provides velocity information and allows calculation of indices	Provides velocity information and shows vascular distribution	Not angle dependent
	Assesses the quality of blood flow	Detects turbulent flow, lack of flow	Free from aliasing
Disadvantages	Location only delivered in combination with additional images such as real-time B-mode	Limited flow information (only shows mean velocity)	No directional information
	Highly angle dependent – flow perpendicular to the transducer is very difficult to detect	Highly angle dependent – flow perpendicular to the transducer is very difficult to detect	No velocity information
		Low dynamics (frame rate can be low when scanning deep)	No flow character information
		Poor temporal resolution	Very poor temporal resolution
			Susceptible to noise and motion

1.16 Advantages and disadvantages of the various Doppler display modes.

- When there is no turbulence, PW Doppler will generally show a laminar (narrow band) spectral output
- CW Doppler rarely displays such a neat narrow band of flow velocities, even with laminar flow, because of the larger spectrum of velocities encountered.

Since CW Doppler imaging provides a limited amount of information over a large region, and spectral Doppler provides more detailed information about a small region, the two modes are complementary and, in practice, are used as such. Concurrent imaging with spectral Doppler and B-mode ultrasonography can also be used. Duplex Doppler employs a static or frozen B-mode image whilst the spectral Doppler waveform is observed. Triplex Doppler utilizes a real-time B-mode image with concurrent real-time spectral Doppler.

Colour Doppler

Colour Doppler or colour flow ultrasonography is a form of PW Doppler in which the energy of the returning echoes is assigned a colour. A colour Doppler instrument measures Doppler shifts in a few thousand sample volumes in the image plane. For each sample volume, the average Doppler shift is encoded as a colour and usually displayed as a map on top of the B-mode image; by convention, echoes representing flow towards the transducer are seen as shades of red, and those representing flow away from the transducer are seen as shades of blue (Figure 1.17).

Colour Doppler images are updated several times per second, thus allowing the flowing blood to be easily visualized. However, colour Doppler is very demanding on the electronics of the instruments, and

is therefore relatively expensive. Colour flow imaging can be used to identify the presence and direction of flow, determine the vascularity of normal organs and abnormal structures, to detect gross circulation anomalies, and to provide beam/vessel angle correction for velocity measurements. When B-mode, colour flow and PW Doppler are used simultaneously, their respective performances are decreased: frame rate is decreased, the colour flow box is reduced in size and the available PRF is reduced, leading to increased susceptibility to aliasing and a slower moving image.

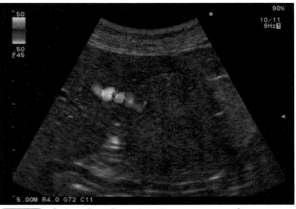

1.17 Colour flow Doppler ultrasonogram of an arteriovenous fistula within the liver of a dog. The mean Doppler shift is encoded to a colour and displayed on top of the B-mode image. The colour map is visible in the upper left corner, and shows the range of velocity which is encoded (–50 to +50 cm/s): flow toward the transducer is displayed in red and flow away from the transducer is displayed in blue. The course of the fistula is like a corkscrew and therefore both flow directions are present within one vessel.

Power Doppler

Power Doppler is based on the principles of PW Doppler and is also known as energy Doppler, amplitude Doppler and Doppler angiography. Instead of relying on Doppler frequency shift, the colour flow signal is derived from the total Doppler signal strength (amplitude) and ignores direction (frequency shift). The signal strength is determined by the concentration of moving reflectors being detected. Power Doppler does not display flow direction or different velocities. This method is free of aliasing and angle dependence, and is more sensitive to slow flow and/or flow in small vessels. The drawback is that due to a slower frame rate and PRF, it is highly susceptible to motion artefacts.

Artefacts

Aliasing

Aliasing is one of the most significant artefacts in Doppler examinations (Figure 1.18). The sampled nature of PW Doppler is at the origin of aliasing. When pulses are transmitted at a given PRF, sampling is performed at a rate equal to the PRF. When a signal is sampled at less than twice its frequency, the resulting signal is ambiguous and the digitized signal has a lower frequency than in reality.

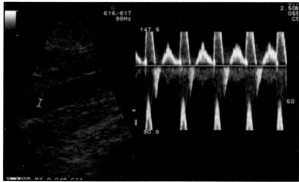

1.18 PW Doppler spectral tracing of the abdominal aorta of a dog showing aliasing. Aliasing occurs when the blood flow velocity exceeds the rate at which the PW system can record it properly. The aliased portion is cut off the top of the velocity spectrum and wraps around to point up from below the baseline.

The **Nyquist limit** is a descriptive term which specifies the maximum velocity that can be recorded without aliasing. It specifies that measurements of frequency shift will be appropriately displayed only if the PRF is at least twice the maximum velocity (or Doppler shift frequency). A similar effect is seen in movies where wagon wheels can appear to be going backwards due to the low frame rate of the film, causing misinterpretation of the movement of the wheel spokes.

Aliasing can be alleviated by increasing the PRF, decreasing the Doppler frequency shift using a lower insonating frequency, or by increasing the Doppler angle. However, as the PRF is increased, the sensitivity to low Doppler shifts, corresponding to low veloci-ties, is decreased. The time interval between sampling pulses is shorter with a higher PRF and might be insufficient for a pulse to travel from the transducer to the reflector and back. If a second pulse is sent before the first is received, the receiver cannot discriminate between the reflected signal from both pulses, and ambiguity in the range of the sample volume ensues. In colour Doppler this can cause a phantom image of a vascular structure seen midway between the transducer and the real structure. As the depth of the vessel of interest increases, return time of the pulse is increased, reducing the PRF for unambiguous imaging. The result is that the maximum Doppler shift decreases with depth.

Velocity scale error

The velocity scale controls the range of frequencies displayed and is critical in colour and spectral Doppler imaging. If the scale is too high, the dynamic range is too large and low velocity signals are missed. An error on the part of the ultrasonographer to lower the velocity scale can lead to a false diagnosis of lack of blood flow in a vessel. If the velocity scale is too low, the dynamic range is too small to display the high velocity signals accurately, and wrap around of the signal occurs, simulating aliasing.

Blooming

Blooming is more commonly known as 'colour bleed' because the colour spreads out from the vessel and into adjacent areas. The explanation for this artefact lies in the fact that the colour Doppler image consists of two images, namely the colour Doppler and the greyscale image. Thus, depending on how the parameters are set, the colour portion of the image can extend beyond the true greyscale vessel margin. This extension usually occurs deep to the vessels and, most commonly, is caused by excessively high gain settings.

Directional ambiguity

Directional ambiguity or indeterminate flow direction results when the interrogating beam intercepts a vessel at a 90 degree angle. The waveform of the spectral Doppler is displayed with nearly equal amplitude above and below the baseline in a mirror image pattern.

Pseudoflow

Pseudoflow is the motion of fluid imitating flow, and can sometimes be seen in colour or power Doppler. Pseudoflow occurs in ascites, urine within the urinary bladder, and jets created by urine entering the bladder at the ureterovesicular junction. However, the spectral Doppler tracing does not exhibit a normal arterial or venous waveform.

Flash

A flash artefact is a sudden burst of random colour that fills the frame, obscuring the greyscale image. This artefact may be caused by object motion or transducer motion. Flash artefacts may occur anywhere but are most commonly seen as a result of cardiac pulsation and in hypoechoic areas, such as cysts or fluid collections. Power Doppler is more susceptible to flash artefacts than colour flow Doppler.

Twinkling

The twinkling artefact is a colour Doppler signal that imitates motion or flow behind a strongly reflecting stationary interface. It can be seen behind any irregular or rough reflecting surface, but is commonly caused by urinary bladder calculi (Figure 1.19). Twinkling appears as a quickly fluctuating mixture of Doppler signals, with an associated characteristic spectrum of noise. With power Doppler, the signal location is the same, but the colour is uniform. A narrow band signal error generated by highly echogenic interfaces seems to be the primary cause of the artefact. Rough surfaces increase the delay in measuring the signal and amplify the errors, increasing the spectral bandwidth of the noise above the level of the wall filter.

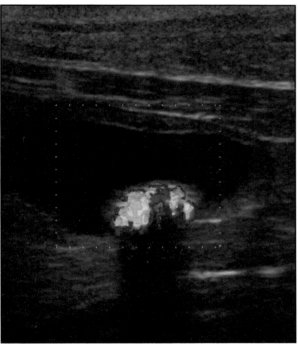

1.19 Colour flow image of the urinary bladder of a dog with a urolith showing twinkling. The rough reflecting irregular surface of the urolith imitates motion and causes a quickly fluctuating mixture of Doppler signals.

Harmonic ultrasonography

The ability of Doppler ultrasonography to detect blood flow in small parenchymal vessels is limited. To improve the detection of tissue perfusion and characterization of vascular patterns in organs and lesions, contrast media are used. An ultrasonography contrast medium needs different properties to those contrast media used in radiography, computed tomography (CT) and magnetic resonance imaging (MRI). To improve ultrasonic visibility, the contrast agent has to be a better reflector than the surrounding tissue.

The first ultrasonographic contrast medium was detected incidentally during echocardiography, where little gas bubbles were situated at the tip of an intra-cardiac catheter. The different acoustic impedance of gases makes microbubbles agitated in a saline solution an ideal contrast medium, and this is in fact still used to detect right-to-left cardiac shunts. However, the large size of the air bubbles (>50 µm) and their short half-life hamper their use in other parts of the body. Thus, other contrast media have been developed. Microbubble persistence and stability have been increased by encapsulating the gases in a shell, and this means that the diameter of the microbubbles can be decreased to 2–3 µm. Although highly reflective, these contrast agents also are highly attenuating, causing severe loss of signal strength as the sound waves travel through the body. The use of ultrasonographic contrast media in conventional ultrasonography is therefore relatively unsuccessful.

However, in the process of optimizing the imaging qualities of these stable microbubbles, it was discovered that they responded in a non-linear manner to incident sound waves. At low wave amplitude, the bubbles oscillate in sine wave fashion, generating echoes with the same frequency as the incident echo. At higher acoustic pressures, the waveform of the returning echo is distorted and no longer sinusoidal, containing the incident frequencies as well as their higher multiples. These frequencies are called **harmonic frequencies**, like the overtones of a musical note. In harmonic imaging the second (or higher) harmonic echo signals are also acquired and displayed. For example, in a 5 MHz transducer the transmitted frequency is 5 MHz, which is called the fundamental frequency or first harmonic frequency; the second harmonic frequency is 10 MHz; the third harmonic frequency is 15 MHz, and so on.

Contrast media are very efficient generators of harmonics, so the blood signal is greatly increased compared with that of the extravascular tissues. With contrast harmonic ultrasonography, fewer attenuation effects are observed from the contrast-enhanced region, and deeper structures can be seen more clearly than with contrast-enhanced fundamental ultrasonography.

Although harmonic imaging was originally developed for use in contrast ultrasonography, it was recognized that ultrasound images obtained in the 'second harmonic' mode had enhanced resolution and reduced acoustic noise. These naturally occurring harmonics are commonly called **native harmonic** or **tissue harmonic** imaging. Tissue harmonic imaging operates by transmitting a fundamental beam that has a low frequency. This fundamental pulse, as it propagates through the body tissues in a non-linear fashion, results in a gradual deformation of the wave shape and thus generates higher frequency harmonic sound waves. Echoes from the fundamental frequency are rejected and not used for image formation. The image is created only by the higher frequency harmonic sound waves.

Several techniques are currently used to detect harmonics and eliminate the unwanted fundamental echoes. Filtration techniques remove the echoes from the fundamental frequency and allow the harmonic frequencies to pass, so that the harmonic image can be formed. Other techniques cancel the fundamental echoes; for example, using a single line pulse inversion (PI) or a so-called side-by-side phase cancellation. Sophisticated transmit beam formation and signal detection is required to produce good quality harmonic images, which is not available in all ultrasound equipment. In addition, the transducers need special features and the range of harmonic frequencies capable of being detected and displayed depends mainly on the bandwidth of the transducer. The same is true for contrast harmonic imaging.

Recent publications indicate the use of contrast medium for the differentiation of benign from malignant lesions in the liver, spleen and lymph nodes. Potential other indications are perfusion studies of organs such as the kidney and heart, and superficial tumour perfusion. In addition, trauma patients with suspected haemorrhage might benefit from contrast harmonic ultrasound examinations. At this time the benefits have not been fully demonstrated and the availability of the equipment and the relatively high costs for the contrast medium hamper the routine use of this technique in veterinary practice.

References and further reading

Barthez PY, Léveillé R and Scrivani PV (1997) Side lobes and grating lobes artifacts in ultrasound imaging. *Veterinary Radiology* **38,** 387–393

Bushberg JT, Seibert JA, Leidholdt EM and Boone JM (2002) Ultrasound. In: *The Essential Physics of Medical Imaging, 2nd edn*, ed. JT Bushberg *et al.*, pp. 469–553. Lippincott Williams and Wilkins, Sacramento

Curry TS, Dowdey JE and Murry RC (1990) Ultrasound. In: *Christensen's Physics of Diagnostic Radiology, 4th edn*, ed. TS Curry *et al.*, pp. 323–371. Lea and Febiger, Philadelphia

Louvet A (2006) Twinkling artifact in small animal color Doppler sonography. *Veterinary Radiology* **47,** 384–390

Louvet A and Bourgeois JM (2008) Lung ring-down artifact as a sign of pulmonary alveolar–interstitial disease. *Veterinary Radiology* **49,** 374–377

Nyland TG, Mattoon JS, Herrgesell EJ *et al.* (2002) Physical principles, instrumentation and safety of diagnostic ultrasound. In: *Small Animal Diagnostic Ultrasound, 2nd edn*, ed. TG Nyland and JS Mattoon, pp. 1–18. WB Saunders, Philadelphia

Ohlerth S and O'Brien RT (2007) Contrast ultrasound: general principles and veterinary clinical applications. *The Veterinary Journal* **174,** 501–512

Park RD, Nyland TG, Lattimer JC *et al.* (1981) B-mode gray-scale ultrasound: imaging artifacts and interpretation principles. *Veterinary Radiology* **22,** 204–210

Penninck DG (2002) Artifacts. In: *Small Animal Diagnostic Ultrasound, 2nd edn*, ed. TG Nyland and JS Mattoon, pp. 19–29. WB Saunders, Philadelphia

Rubens DJ, Bhatt S, Nedelka S *et al.* (2006) Doppler artifacts and pitfalls. *Ultrasound Clinics* **1,** 79–109

Ziegler L and O'Brien RT (2002) Harmonic ultrasound: a review. *Veterinary Radiology* **43,** 501–509

2

Equipment

Patrick R. Kircher

Introduction

The technology of diagnostic ultrasonography is developing rapidly. Advances in new technologies, new transducer types, and new system designs are delivered every year by the diagnostic ultrasonography companies. Even for experts in ultrasonography it is difficult to follow this progress. 'The technology bought today is already outdated yesterday'; this is probably not entirely correct but shows one of the problems, especially when investment in equipment is planned. The multitude of vendors, ultrasound systems and different transducer types complicate the choice of the perfect product. Furthermore, the majority of the machines available on the market have not been designed for veterinary use, but built for the human medical market and adjusted to the needs of the veterinary ultrasonographer.

Knowledge of the different types of transducer and their respective advantages, together with an understanding of the tools available to improve the image during an ultrasonographic examination are essential. When sitting in front of an ultrasound unit it becomes apparent how many ways there are to manipulate image quality. For the novice it seems like sitting on the flight deck of an aeroplane, where lots of knobs and lamps are visible (Figure 2.1). Gain, power, focal zones, depth selection and frequency selection are the settings most frequently manipulated during an examination, but many other secondary adjustments exist,

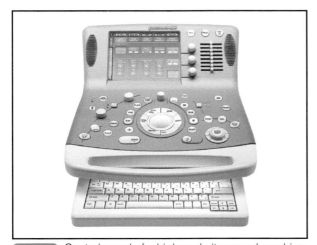

2.1 Control panel of a high-end ultrasound machine. The ergonomic and intuitive set-up of this unit make it easy to use.

such as line density, dynamic range and filters. Most of these are optimized in the factory and adjusted by the vendor's application specialist when the machine is purchased, and stored as 'presets'. For each transducer, several presets may be needed, taking into account the different areas of the body to be examined and the varying sizes of the prospective patients.

Transducers

Ultrasonic transducers (or probes) are manufactured for a variety of applications (e.g. the region of interest). Careful attention must be paid to selecting the most appropriate transducer for the application, taking into account transducer design and technology, and the available frequency range.

Types

There are two types of ultrasound transducer (Figure 2.2):

- Array transducers (linear or curved/convex), where the crystal elements are arranged in a line along the surface of the transducer
- Phased array transducers, containing only a small number of crystals that are fixed in position and activated sequentially to create a fan-type image.

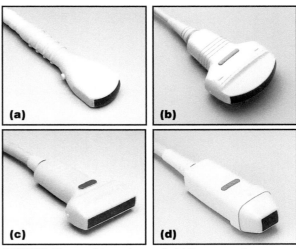

2.2 Types of transducer. **(a)** Microcurved array. **(b)** Curved array. **(c)** Linear array. **(d)** Phased array. Note the different sizes of the footprints of the transducers.

Array
Array transducers have the advantage of allowing a wide superficial field of view. Very superficial tissues are particularly well seen with linear arrays. They have the disadvantage of requiring a relatively large contact area between the skin and the transducer. In areas such as the thorax or the most cranial part of the abdomen, where an intercostal approach is required, the use of linear or large curved array transducers is limited (Figure 2.3a). To overcome this, small curved array transducers have been developed. These types are called microcurved or microconvex transducers (Figure 2.3b). Linear and curved array transducers are used for examination of the musculoskeletal system, abdominal organs, eyes, body wall and non-cardiac thoracic structures.

Phased array
Phased array (sector) transducers have the advantages of working with small footprints and creating pie-shaped images, which allow deep structures to be seen well. These transducers have poor near-field image resolution and are not a good choice for imaging superficial structures. Phased array transducers are used for echocardiography and for very deeply located abdominal or thoracic structures in large dogs.

Frequency
The ultrasound wave frequency produced by the transducer is characteristic of the crystals within it. Usually transducers have one characteristic frequency, determined by the size of the crystals. However, the frequency can be electronically altered within a certain range. For example, an 8 MHz probe can produce a range of frequencies from 5 to 10 MHz (Figure 2.4). These are commonly called 'multi-frequency transducers'. Low frequencies (2–3.5 MHz) have good tissue penetration and are therefore used to depict the deeper abdominal and thoracic

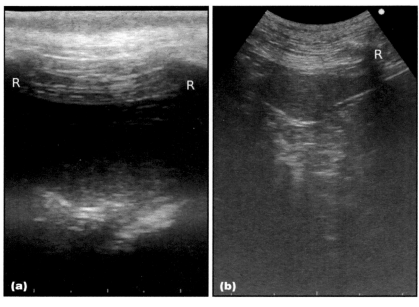

2.3 Ultrasonograms of the head of the spleen using a transcostal window. **(a)** With the linear array transducer the ribs (R) hamper the image, and the contact between the skin and transducer in this case was insufficient. **(b)** With the microcurved array transducer the window is more appropriate due to the small footprint of the transducer fitting in between a rib pair (R).

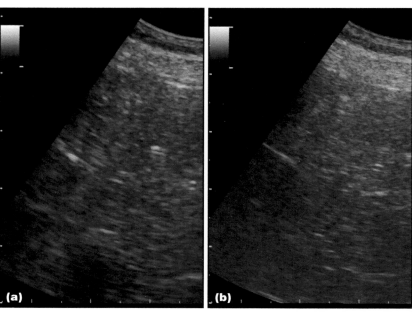

2.4 Ultrasonograms of the liver. **(a)** Transducer frequency is set relatively low at 5 MHz. **(b)** Transducer frequency is set at 10 MHz. Note the improvement in axial resolution: the image appears less grainy and the detail of the fine echotexture of the liver is clearer.

structures in large animals or giant-breed dogs. High frequencies (7.5–12 MHz or above) produce optimal image resolution but are limited in tissue penetration. They are selected for superficial structures where image detail is needed.

Stand-off pads

Stand-off pads are used to overcome limited resolution and image quality in the near-field. The near-field image using high frequency linear transducers is often very good without a stand-off pad. However, for very superficial structures (such as the body wall, skin surface, etc.) a stand-off pad moves the area of interest further from the probe and therefore out of the near-field and into the focal zone. For lower frequency linear probes and other probe types where the focal zone is even further distal, a stand-off pad will ultimately be required to improve the image quality of the superficial tissues. Stand-off pads are made of echolucent, gel-like material (Figure 2.5) and serve as an acoustic window between the transducer and the body surface. The stand-off pad increases the distance between the transducer and the body surface, placing the area of interest at a more optimal distance from the transducer for improved image quality. They are most commonly used for superficial imaging in musculoskeletal examinations (e.g. superficial tendons) and also for investigation of subcutaneous pathology.

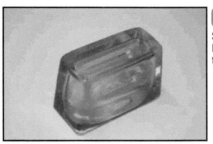

2.5
Stand-off pad for linear array transducers.

Image processing during examination

Power

The power control allows adjustment of the total ultrasound wave output from the transducer (Figure 2.6; see also **Changing acoustic power** clip on DVD). The higher the power is set, the higher the amplitude (dB) of the sound waves. This allows better tissue penetration and therefore higher echo intensities. Increasing the power has the effect of increasing the overall brightness of the image. The drawback is that the examined tissues have a higher mechanical exposure, measured by the mechanical index (MI). In addition, potential artefacts such as oversampling (see Gain) are possible. Usually the power control is not altered during an examination, but is rather given in the presets programmed for the different transducers and regions of interest. In general, although ultrasonography is considered biologically safe in the light of current knowledge, it is considered good practice to keep the power as low as possible without losing the details of structures being examined.

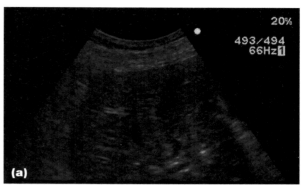

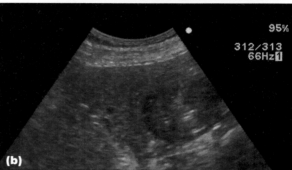

2.6 **(a)** Low acoustic power is selected. Note: the power is displayed as 20% of the maximum available (top right). The image appears dark, representing an insufficient amount of returning echoes. **(b)** The power is set to 95% of the maximum available (using the same gain settings), resulting in a better image. See also **Changing acoustic power** clip on DVD.

Gain

In contrast to power, the gain control is frequently adjusted during an examination. The gain controls do not affect sound wave output, but alter the electronic amplification of the returning echoes (Figure 2.7; see also **Changing gain** clip on DVD). Thus, increasing the overall gain has a similar effect on the image as increasing the power, and results in increased image brightness.

In general, echoes from deeper regions are weaker than those from superficial tissues near to the transducer. This is a result of the gradual attenuation of the beam over distance. Assuming that this attenuation is the same in all soft tissue types (an average over the different potential tissues is taken) the computer can calculate the gain to apply to echoes from each depth. In this way a homogeneous image intensity is created. As the depth is encoded by the time taken to receive the echo, this compensation is called time–gain compensation (TGC). As the assumed average does not apply to all tissues and regions imaged, the TGC can be influenced manually by the ultrasonographer via the TGC controls. This is essential when sound wave attenuation is less than expected (e.g. in the urinary and gallbladder regions) but also when attenuation is greater than expected (e.g. hyperattenuating liver tissue in cases of storage diseases). Newer equipment may provide automatic TGC functions. (See **Applying the 'image optimizer'** and **Time–gain compensation controls** clips on DVD.)

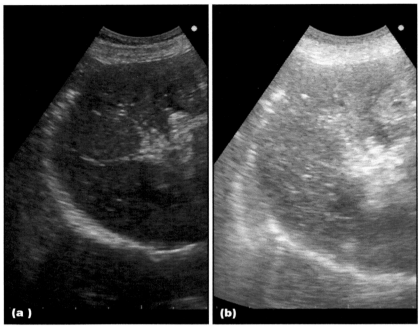

2.7 **(a)** The gain is set for optimal image quality. **(b)** Increasing the gain results in an overall increase in image brightness, and oversampling, creating a worsened signal-to-noise ratio. See also **Changing gain, Applying the 'image optimizer'** and **Time–gain compensation controls** clips on DVD.

Depth selection

Depth selection controls allow the depth of the image to be adjusted according to the area of interest (Figure 2.8). This effectively 'zooms in' on superficial tissues as the chosen depth is reduced. Reducing the selected depth also has a small effect on improving frame rate.

Positioning of the focal zones

The focal zone represents the zone of optimal image resolution (see Chapter 1). Irrespective of the design of the transducer, focusing of the sound beam is essential; an unfocused sound beam diverges rapidly, with consequent loss of image resolution. The focal zone of the transducer is that part of the sound beam where focusing, and therefore image quality, is optimal. Complex diffraction patterns can occur in the near-field (Fresnel zone). Beyond the focal zone is the far-field (Fraunhofer zone), where the beam diverges rapidly and image resolution decreases.

In modern equipment the focal zone can be selected along the axis of the sound beam electronically. The position of the focal zone is most often shown on the screen by a triangular marker on the side of the image. It is also possible to work with multiple focal zones within the displayed image. This optimizes a wider range of the image but results in a significant decrease in frame rate, as the different focal zones are a summation of single frames with differently positioned focuses (see **Changing the number of focal zones** clip on DVD). The aim is to keep the region of interest within the focal zone. If the tissues are deep to the focal zone, gentle pressure on the abdominal wall may decrease the distance

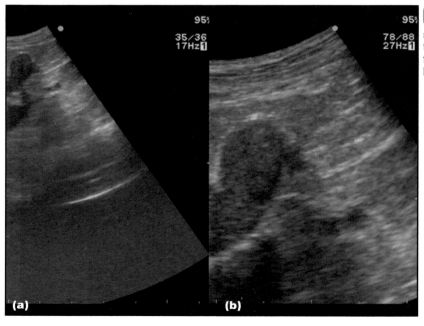

2.8 The difference between **(a)** and **(b)** is the depth selection. In (b) the region of interest in the near-field is enlarged. Note that the frame rate (upper right, Hz) is increased by selecting a lower depth.

between the transducer and the structure of interest. If the tissues are too superficial, use of an echolucent stand-off to increase the distance between the transducer and structure of interest may be helpful.

Sector angle and image width

The sector or beam angle describes the size of the field of view in sector and curved transducers. In linear transducers it is referred to as image width. In phased array transducers, the angle of the beam is altered, resulting in a narrower or wider pie-sector.

Reduction of the sector angle or image width can result in a decrease in the axial lines acquired, allowing an increase in frame rate, which may be advantageous in depicting moving objects. Depending on the settings of the unit, it can alternatively result in a higher line density, which improves lateral resolution and therefore image quality. With wider angles or image width, the field of view is larger. As more axial lines have to be computed to be displayed, the frame rate is reduced (see below). A wide angle is helpful for providing a good overview (Figure 2.9).

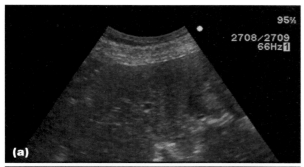

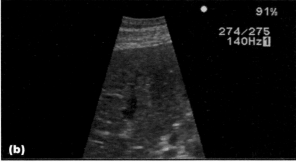

2.9 Changes in sector angle. **(a)** Maximum field of view for this transducer. **(b)** More narrow field of view. Note the increase in frame rate (upper right, Hz) in (b) compared with (a).

Frame rate

The frame rate describes the number of 'single' images built up and displayed per second. The frame rate therefore depends on the speed of the ultrasound unit in building up a single frame. Each frame consists of a certain number of axial lines; the number of lines is therefore one of the factors influencing the time taken to create a frame. There are two options which may be taken to reduce this time:

- The first is to narrow the sector angle or image width (see above), which reduces the number of axial lines computed for each image, but also reduces the size of the field of view

- The second is to reduce the line density (i.e. the number of lines per millimetre) in the spatial plane. This has the adverse effect of reducing the spatial resolution, leading to an inferior image quality.

There is therefore a trade-off between frame rate and either sector angle/image width or spatial resolution.

It may be necessary to increase the frame rate in animals or organs where excessive motion is occurring (e.g. in a rapidly breathing animal). The lower the frame rate, the less sharp motion is depicted on the image. Therefore, selecting a slower frame rate will improve image resolution, and selecting a faster frame rate will provide a more accurate evaluation of movement. In some units, the frame rate can be chosen and when increased, the machine reduces either line density or the image width. Other settings may also influence the frame rate, including the selection of multiple focal zones. In other machines, direct adjustment of the frame rate is not an option.

Image documentation and storage

As the images produced during the ultrasound examination are an important part of the patient record, image storage and retrieval is a crucial issue. Modern ultrasound machines contain hard disks on which a certain number of studies can be stored as raw data. The disk space is limited and usually, when full, older studies have to be deleted manually or the system reverts to the first in, first out mode and deletes the oldest study automatically. In some machines hard drive images are lost when a software update is performed during a service. Therefore, an external storage system is recommended. Some machines have the ability to export images in a .jpeg, .bmp or .tiff format to a local area network (LAN) on 'memory sticks' or CD/DVDs. With this form of storage the maintenance of the archive and retrieval of the images is difficult for many reasons, not least because files are only stored with file names.

An easier approach is to work with dedicated storage software. Almost all vendors provide storage of images and video clips in the DICOM format. DICOM (**D**igital **I**maging and **Co**mmunication in **M**edicine) is a standard for handling, storing, printing and transmitting medical imaging data. It has been developed by the American College of Radiology (ACR) and the National Electrical Manufacturers Association (NEMA). The current DICOM 3 standard is also known as NEMA Standard PS3 or ISO Standard 12052. All the manufacturers using this standard must provide a DICOM conformance statement for the US system model. The DICOM file provides the image format information, the image information, patient information, calibration information and additional data storage fields and is communicated through the TCP/IP protocol. It enables the integration of imaging equipment from various manufacturers into a network and Picture Archiving and Communication System (PACS).

The PACS is basically the archive system/server, where the images are stored and provided for all users in the network. With a PACS, studies can be queried by name, patient number, study ID and many other possibilities. Another advantage of storing the images in the DICOM format is the possibility to post-process the images and also to perform off-site measurements, as the calibration information of the studies is stored within the DICOM file. Video clips are usually stored as multi-frame files and can then be exported from the PACS as media (such as .avi or .mpeg) files.

Equipment and transducer care

As ultrasound units are expensive, their care is important. Most vendors provide manuals describing how to maintain their systems. In institutions where several people use the equipment, each individual should be thoroughly trained on how to care for the machine.

This starts with cleaning the air filters, which is often forgotten. As veterinary surgeons work with animals, much more dust, dirt and hair pollute the filters than in human medicine. The ultrasound units usually have a considerable ventilation system to cool the internal elements, so keeping the filters clean is important and has to be undertaken more often than the 'once a year' service by the vendor. The machines at the author's clinic are cleaned every 2 weeks by taking the filter pads out of the slots and vacuuming them. It is recognized very quickly how often this has to be done to prevent the ultrasound unit from overheating.

Care also has to be taken with the control panel, which is usually not waterproof and ultrasound gel on the fingers quickly leads to sticky buttons and the malfunction of the potentially available trackballs. For some units transparent protective covers for the panels exist and may be helpful. An important rule must be not to place any liquid containers on the unit. This may sound obvious, but it can prevent severe damage to the system.

The care of transducers is a frequently discussed topic. First of all, the surface material of the ultrasound transducer is delicate. Contact with needles, sharp objects and scraping cloths must be avoided. Specially dedicated microcidal wipes can be bought, but are expensive. Safe cleaning agents are usually described by the vendors. There is always a debate about the use of alcohol for cleaning transducers and/or the skin surface, or to promote good contact, e.g. during ultrasound-guided cystocentesis or fine-needle aspiration. The use of alcohol in such situations is widespread, but there is the potential danger of damaging the surface of the probe. Certain vendors allow isopropyl alcohol to be used with selected probes, at a maximum concentration of 70%. The probes should then be rinsed with water after use. Some vendors provide lists of usable disinfectants and alcohol for the probes. In general it is wise to discuss the matter with the vendors.

Choosing an ultrasound machine

Before starting the discussion about what to look for, one thing has to be kept in mind: the ideal system does not exist. Each system has its advantages and disadvantages, and personal preference plays an important role in choosing an ultrasound machine. However, it is good to seek the advice of an experienced person and to compare different systems before taking a decision.

As ultrasound machines are usually expensive, finances play a role in the process of evaluation. However, the first consideration must be the potential use of the machine, now and over the next few years. The more experience one gets with using ultrasound machines, the greater the range of potential applications. The more basic the system chosen, the faster the limits of the equipment are reached and frustration is created. For example, the question may be asked whether Doppler ultrasonography is really necessary. The answer to this is 'yes'. Blood vessels are important landmarks for finding smaller organs, such as adrenal glands. Furthermore, the differentiation between vessels and other tubular structures, such as ureters or bile ducts, is sometimes important. Thus, even beginners will quickly reach the stage where they find Doppler ultrasonography useful.

The size of the patient determines the frequency range and design of the transducers chosen. Hospital patient population may also play an important role. Where cats are the patients, a high frequency linear and microcurved transducer may serve best. If cardiac ultrasonography is planned, a phased array transducer is needed. If dogs are also within the patient population, lower frequency transducers have to be added.

Another question to consider is the mobility of the unit. Is it planned to have it stationary in a dedicated room or does it have to be mobile? Today's portable systems are of very high quality and also used by mobile ultrasonography specialists. Last, but not least, the service of the vendor has to be taken into account. Pricing and contents of the service contracts and warranties have to be evaluated carefully, together with the quality of the after-sales service.

Video extras

- Applying the 'image optimizer'
- Changing acoustic power
- Changing gain
- Changing the number of focal zones
- Time–gain compensation controls

Access via QR code or bsavalibrary.com/ultrasound_2

3

Principles of the ultrasound examination

Stefanie Ohlerth

Preparation of the patient

If possible, food should be withheld from animals for approximately 12 hours prior to the examination but access to water can be allowed. An empty stomach improves imaging of the cranial abdomen, in particular the liver, the porta hepatis, the stomach itself, and the pancreas. It can sometimes be useful to allow the animal a drink of water before undertaking ultrasound examination of the cranial abdomen. The water can highlight the stomach wall, intraluminal foreign material or mural masses of the stomach.

In addition, evacuation of the colon should be encouraged prior to conducting the examination. This helps to reduce artefacts produced by gas and ingesta from the gastrointestinal tract. Ideally, the urinary bladder should be moderately full for examination of the urogenital tract.

Abdominal ultrasonography may be easily performed in conscious animals. However, in uncooperative dogs and cats, animals with a painful abdomen, or in cases where an interventional procedure is planned, sedation, analgesia, or general anaesthesia is indicated. Medications that cause marked vasodilation, panting, aerophagia or gastric atony should not be used.

Preparation of the scanning site

For an abdominal ultrasound examination, animals are clipped from the xiphoid along the costal arch to the areas of the right and left kidney, respectively, and to the cranial aspect of the pubic bone (Figure 3.1). Clipping of the scanning site is necessary to remove hair, which otherwise traps small air bubbles and degrades the quality of the images acquired. In small dogs and cats, all dorsal abdominal structures may be imaged from a ventral acoustic window. It is important to extend the clipped area dorsally and cranially over the ribcage in larger and deep-chested dogs so that an acoustic window as close as possible to the organ may be chosen.

To improve rapid acoustic coupling, the skin may be prepared first by rubbing it gently with alcohol. Then, acoustic gel is applied to the skin and massaged in lightly. In general, an animal is gently restrained by one or two assistants and scanned in dorsal or right lateral recumbency (with its head to the left and feet facing the ultrasonographer). In dorsal

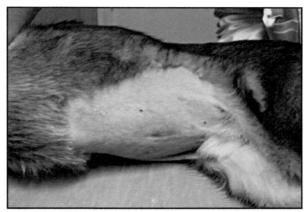

3.1 Clipped field for a complete abdominal ultrasonographic examination. The dog is in right lateral recumbency with the head to the left and legs facing the ultrasonographer.

recumbency, dogs and cats may feel more comfortable if they are positioned in a wide U-shaped foam plastic trough (Figure 3.2a) or on a cushion (Figure 3.2b). To scan the right cranial abdomen, in particular in deep-chested dogs, animals may be positioned in left lateral recumbency.

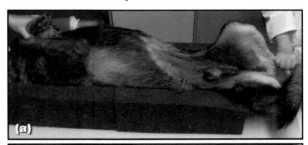

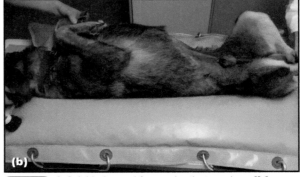

3.2 **(a)** A U-shaped foam plastic trough or **(b)** a cushion helps greatly with the positioning and restraint of the patient.

For examination of the thorax or musculoskeletal system, alternative positioning and patient preparation may be required. For example, in animals with pleural effusion, the ultrasound examination may be performed in sternal recumbency, especially if the patient is dyspnoeic. Clipping a large region for thoracic ultrasonography is generally not preferred and instead alcohol is used to scan for the appropriate acoustic window. These points are discussed in more detail in the Chapters specifically dealing with those body regions.

Selection of acoustic window

The acoustic window is the region of the body surface from which the tissue or organ of interest can be imaged. Selection of an appropriate acoustic window is important, and there are some basic principles to take into account.

- An acoustic window should be as close as possible to the organ of interest. This allows the selected region to be examined using the highest possible frequency, giving the best possible resolution.

- The size of the transducer should match with the coupling area. A microconvex probe is best suited for intercostal or parasternal approaches due to its smaller footprint. Linear array transducers, with their large footprint, are better suited to larger surface areas such as the mid-abdomen.
- Air interfaces degrade image quality and can be avoided by scanning from a dependent window. For example, the antrum, pylorus and duodenum are scanned best with the patient in right lateral or dorsal recumbency, because in this position the structures mainly contain liquid ingesta and only a little amount of gas. Similarly, to avoid gas artefacts from the lung, the cranial mediastinum is best imaged from the dependent intercostal site or via a thoracic inlet approach.
- The pubic bone may produce an acoustic shadow that prohibits visualization of the prostate gland or the urethra. In this instance a perianal approach may be chosen instead.
- Whilst the liver can be examined in most dogs using a substernal window, intercostal windows may be necessary to visualize the liver in deep-chested breeds.

Figure 3.3 is an overview of the common acoustic windows for major structures and regions.

Organ or region	Acoustic window
Cranial mediastinum	1st–4th intercostal space Parasternal approach for sternal lymph nodes Thoracic inlet
Liver	Caudal to xiphoid process, with cranial angulation of the ultrasound beam Left and right mid-abdominal to dorsal intercostal window
Spleen	Splenic head: • Left dorsal intercostal window • Left cranial ventral abdomen with sagittal beam angulation Splenic body and tail: • Along left costal arch • Left cranial ventral abdomen with sagittal beam angulation
Stomach	Caudal to xiphoid process, with cranial angulation of the ultrasound beam Fundus and body: along the left costal arch Antrum and pylorus: ventral to the right of midline or right intercostal window
Duodenum and pancreas	Ascending duodenum and body of the pancreas: • Right cranial mid-abdominal to dorsal window with sagittal and craniodorsal beam angulation • Right dorsal intercostal window Descending duodenum and right pancreatic limb: • Right mid-abdominal to dorsal window with sagittal beam angulation Left pancreatic limb: • Left mid-abdominal/sagittal window
Left kidney and left adrenal gland	Left cranial mid-abdominal to dorsal/sagittal window Left dorsal intercostal window (rarely)
Right kidney and right adrenal gland	Right cranial mid-abdominal to dorsal/sagittal window with craniodorsal beam angulation Right dorsal intercostal window
Ileum	Right mid-abdominal to dorsal window with sagittal beam angulation (just medial and parallel to the descending duodenum)
Colon	Ascending colon: • Right mid-abdominal to dorsal window with sagittal beam angulation (just medial and parallel to the descending duodenum) Transverse colon: • Ventral abdomen, caudal to the xiphoid process (just caudal to the stomach) Descending colon: • Left mid-abdominal to caudal window with sagittal beam angulation

3.3 Common acoustic windows for major structures and regions. For further information, the reader is referred to the Chapters on the various organs. (continues) ▶

Organ or region	Acoustic window
Urinary bladder	Caudal ventral or lateral abdomen, cranial to pubic bone
Prostate gland and urethra	Caudal abdomen, cranial to pubic bone with caudodorsal beam angulation Perianal approach
Uterus	Body: caudal abdomen, cranial to pubic bone (just dorsal to urinary bladder) Uterine horns: left and right mid-abdominal window with sagittal beam
Ovaries	Left and right mid-abdominal window (just caudal to the kidneys) with sagittal and dorsolateral beam angulation

3.3 (continued) Common acoustic windows for major structures and regions. For further information, the reader is referred to the Chapters on the various organs.

Principles of image interpretation

Orientation

Diagnostic ultrasonography is a cross-sectional imaging technology. The orientation of the image on the monitor should be consistent with the orientation of the transducer (i.e. the position of the marker on the probe should correspond with the position of the marker on the screen). Regardless of the orientation of the probe, the top of the image always represents the skin surface. With an animal in dorsal recumbency and an abdominal image in the transverse plane, the image on the monitor has the patient's left side on the right-hand side of the image and its right side on the left-hand side of the image. In this instance, if the probe marker faces the right side of the patient, the marker on the image will also be on the right (shown on the left-hand side on the monitor image). In a longitudinal plane, cranial or proximal should be to the left and caudal or distal to the right on the monitor image.

Echogenicity and echotexture

Tissues with a relatively homogeneous architecture such as the liver, spleen, pancreas, prostate gland or thyroid gland, typically present as a mixture of bright, grey and dark dots (speckles) like a salt and pepper mixture. However, the speckles do not represent true reflecting anatomical structures, but rather originate from complex interactions of reflection, absorption and scattering. Nevertheless, the resulting speckle pattern with a definite brightness (echogenicity) and dot size (echotexture) is often characteristic for a certain organ or pathological condition.

The echotexture of a tissue refers to a small or large dot size (fineness or coarseness) and dot spacing. Furthermore, the texture may be uniform (homogeneous) or non-uniform (heterogeneous). The echogenicity of normal parenchymal organs and tissues is depicted as various shades of grey and is usually described in relation to the echogenicity of neighbouring tissues. The normal liver, for example, is defined as hypoechoic in comparison with the hyperechoic spleen (Figure 3.4).

Fluid or blood that does not contain cells, debris or protein, appears black (i.e. anechoic), because only a few or no echoes are returned. The more cells, debris or protein that are contained in the fluid, the more echogenic it becomes. Regions producing few echoes are termed hypoechoic, whereas tissues that produce strong or numerous echoes are defined as hyperechoic. Similarly to echotexture, the echogenicity of a tissue may be further described as uniform (homogeneous) or non-uniform (heterogeneous).

In the normal patient, echogenicity increases from the more or less anechoic urine, bile and blood, through hypoechoic structures such as lymph nodes, the pancreas, liver, renal medulla and muscle to the relatively more hyperechoic tissues such as the spleen, the renal cortex and the prostate gland. Structural fat, organ capsules, vessel walls and other connective tissues appear even more hyperechoic, and bone, mineralization and gas are the most hyperechoic structures.

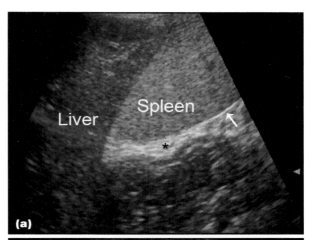

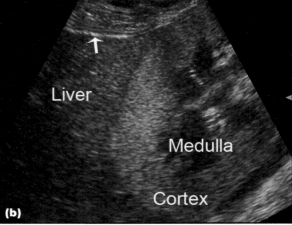

3.4 Longitudinal ultrasonograms of the normal liver, spleen and right kidney in a dog. **(a)** The liver is hypoechoic in comparison with the spleen. The structural fat (*) is hyperechoic in comparison with the liver. **(b)** The medulla of the right kidney is hypoechoic compared with the renal cortex, which in turn is hyperechoic compared with the liver. The capsule of the liver and spleen are partially seen as thin hyperechoic lines (arrowed).

4

Interventional procedures

Robert M. Kirberger and Nerissa Stander

Introduction

Interventional ultrasonographic procedures have been in common use in humans since the early 1980s and provide samples safely and with a high diagnostic yield. In veterinary practices with diagnostic ultrasound equipment, percutaneous fine-needle aspiration (FNA) and core tissue biopsy (CTB) should be routine procedures in order to make a diagnosis. The need for sedation when performing FNA is patient- and ultrasonographer-dependent. Puncture of superficial structures, such as the spleen, may not require sedation in cooperative animals. Sampling of deeper structures or sampling in uncooperative or panting animals requires sedation. If the samples are non-diagnostic, a CTB can be performed under deep sedation with or without local anaesthesia, or short-acting general anaesthesia.

Indications

Free abdominal or thoracic fluid, intraparenchymal fluid accumulation (e.g. cyst or abscess), urine and pericardial fluid can readily be aspirated. Extension tubes and three-way stopcocks may be used if complete drainage of substantial volumes of fluid is required. Diffusely affected organs, nodules and masses in any part of the body can undergo FNA or, if large enough, CTB provided the region of interest is not obscured by overlying gas. This includes evaluating bone lesions, particularly neoplasia that has penetrated the cortex, as well as superficially located lung pathology. Samples may be used for culture, biochemical tests, cytology and histopathology. Other less commonly used interventional procedures are discussed at the end of the Chapter. Being able to visualize the pathology and then guide a needle into it results in a much greater success rate than blind sampling, particularly if an organ is focally affected.

Equipment

Transducers

Linear and convex array transducers are preferred as superficial lesions are seen more easily due to the wide footprint. Freehand guiding of FNA or CTB is easier with linear array transducers in the authors' experience. Image quality should always be optimized before beginning the sampling procedure and the transducers operated at the highest possible frequency to enhance needle visibility.

Aspiration needles

A 22-gauge, 1.5 inch needle is most commonly used. Thinner needles may be used if the region involved is highly vascular or an abscess is suspected, and leakage of residual contents after aspiration needs to be minimized. Thicker needles are used where larger volumes of fluid have to be removed or viscous fluid is expected. Generally, the thinnest needle possible should be chosen. Spinal needles are available in lengths up to 3.5 inches and are thus used for deeper structures. The stylet helps to avoid aspiration of unwanted material along the needle tract and should only be removed once the area to be aspirated is reached. More sophisticated and expensive needles are also available. These may have a stylet, depth markings and a small butterfly spring system to act as an adjustable needle stop to set the depth required (Figure 4.1). These needles may have a normal bevelled edge (e.g. Chiba biopsy needle) or a crown-shaped tip (e.g. Franseen biopsy needle) for FNA of harder tissues such as bone (Figure 4.2). Other needles (e.g. Westcott) may have an additional slot similar to a Tru-Cut needle for collection of larger samples.

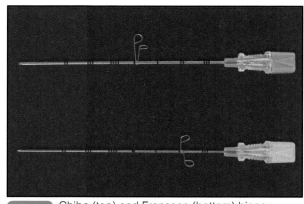

4.1 Chiba (top) and Franseen (bottom) biopsy needles. Note the centimetre markings and adjustable needle stop to set the depth.

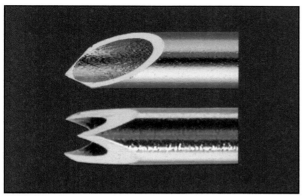

4.2 Close-up of Chiba (top) and Franseen (bottom) biopsy needles. Note the crown-shaped tip of the latter for bone sampling.

Core tissue biopsy instruments

CTB instruments are generally of the Tru-Cut type. Manually operated biopsy needles are rarely used nowadays and have been replaced by semi- or fully automated spring-loaded instruments. These have the advantages that they provide superior specimens and require only one operator who holds the transducer in one hand and the biopsy gun in the other. The trocar part of the needle has a sample notch, which can be up to 20 mm in length (Figure 4.3), and on some systems the size of the sample may be reduced by 50% for smaller nodules. The thickness of the needle usually varies between 14- and 18-gauge.

Disposable automated devices (Figure 4.4) are made of plastic but can usually be gas sterilized to use two or three times if required.

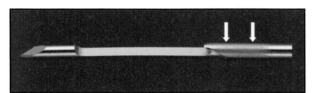

4.3 Close-up of a Tru-Cut type biopsy needle showing the sample notch and echo-enhancing coating (arrowed).

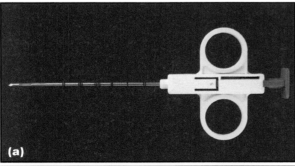

(a)

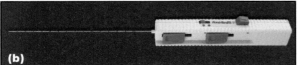

(b)

4.4 **(a)** Disposable semi-automatic biopsy device. The sample notch is adjustable to 9.5 or 19 mm. **(b)** Disposable automatic biopsy device. Note the safety button on top to avoid inadvertent firing.

Non-disposable devices (Figure 4.5) are made of metal and can be conventionally sterilized. The initial expense is quite high. However, although the disposable needles are cheaper and can be sterilized to use two or three times, this results in blunting of the needle and possible remnant infection.

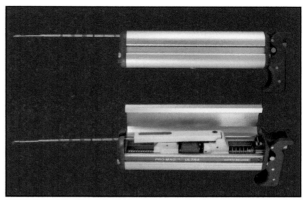

4.5 Sterilizable fully automated biopsy gun with disposable needle placement shown in the opened instrument.

Needle guidance systems

Specific adaptors are available for transducers to guide the needle to the affected area. These can accommodate a variety of needle sizes. The monitor will usually have centimetre markings along two white lines between which the needle can be seen as it enters the organ of interest (Figure 4.6). This greatly facilitates needle placement, but there can be less flexibility in the angle of introduction of the needle and its subsequent path.

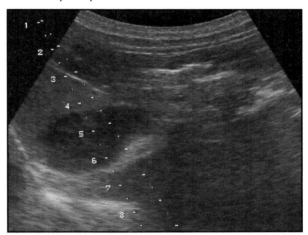

4.6 Ultrasonogram of the liver with diverging stippled guidelines, indicating the direction that needle angulation will take when using a transducer needle guide adaptor for cholecystocentesis. Numbered graduations on the side of the guidelines indicate a centimetre scale, which can be used to determine the correct depth of needle insertion.

Transrectal/vaginal/oesophageal/ gastrointestinal biopsy instruments

Special intraluminal transducers are available and may also have biopsy capabilities. Due to their cost these instruments are usually available only at selected specialized imaging institutions.

Sampling techniques

Patient preparation

For FNA the clipped skin needs to be suitably sterilized. Sedation or local anaesthesia are usually not required unless the patient is uncooperative. CTB must be performed in a sterile environment. Coagulation parameters should be checked and any coagulopathies should be treated before CTB is undertaken. The transducer is usually covered by a sterile glove or transducer sleeve. It is advisable to make a small skin incision adjacent to the transducer to avoid blunting the needle. Pressure can be applied to the overlying tissues, especially in the abdomen to displace interfering gas-filled structures and to bring the lesion closer to the skin surface.

If colour flow Doppler is available this should be used to check the vascularity of the lesion and to avoid major vessels, particularly arteries which are usually not visible ultrasonographically. If large volumes of ascites are present it may be better to reduce this before sampling as the organ of interest may tend to bounce around in the fluid. Potential post-biopsy haemorrhage is also difficult to detect in ascites cases if colour flow Doppler ultrasonography is not available.

Indirect sampling

An indirect sampling technique is usually used in circumstances where there are large amounts of free fluid or a large mass lesion. The area of interest is located ultrasonographically and the required needle depth determined. The point of needle entry can be marked by applying pressure to the sampling point for 30 seconds with the hub of a hypodermic needle. The transducer is then removed and the needle placed blindly in the affected region to obtain the sample. However, it may be easier to perform direct freehand sampling.

Direct freehand sampling

The plane of needle insertion must be in the midline plane of the transducer. Needles may be scarified or have an echo-enhancing coating (see Figure 4.3) to improve visibility. It should be ensured that the bevel of the needle faces the transducer as any gas trapped in the bevel will aid visibility. Needle visibility can be further maximized by positioning the focal zone at the region of interest, and moving the needle or stylet in and out or gently rocking the transducer to and fro to find the needle (Figure 4.7). The needle should pass obliquely across the ultrasound beam to enhance visibility. The needle is guided to the region of interest and the sample is taken. Freehand sampling does require some practice to place the needle accurately in the affected area, and using gelatine or agar tissue phantoms are useful ways to learn the technique (Finn-Bodner and Hathcock, 1993).

Direct sampling using a needle guidance system

Using guidance adaptors is an easy method of obtaining samples, but their use in collecting specimens from poorly positioned nodules may be limited, whereas the freehand technique allows more flexibility.

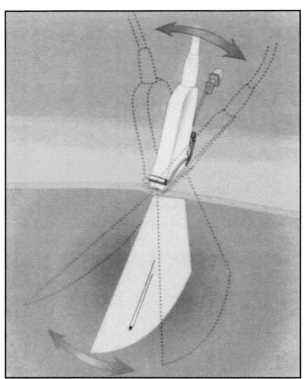

4.7 Technique of rocking the transducer to fan the ultrasound beam so that the beam is aligned with the needle. Note the needle guide adaptor attached to the transducer. (Reproduced from Dodd *et al.*, 1996 with permission from *Radiographics*).

Fine-needle aspiration

FNA is a cheap, easy technique with minimal risk of complications. The sampling methodology varies between operators and organs being aspirated. The stab technique involves getting the needle tip to the region of interest and stabbing the needle back and forth a few times and then withdrawing the needle. This is particularly useful in vascular lesions or the spleen, to avoid aspirating a very bloody sample. The suction technique involves 3–4 gentle suctions when the needle tip is in the area of interest, but may result in more blood contamination of the sample. Suction should not be applied whilst removing the needle to avoid tissues along the needle tract being aspirated.

Core tissue biopsy

Due to its more invasive nature CTB is usually only performed if FNA is non-diagnostic. It should be ensured that the length of needle advancement is known when the gun is fired to avoid penetrating the far side of the organ under investigation and possibly damaging other vital organs (Figure 4.8). It should also be ensured that there is some normal tissue superficial to the biopsy site, which can act as a seal for any potential haemorrhage. Particularly when performing CTB of the liver, the biopsy site should not traverse two liver lobes (i.e. the edges of adjacent lobes should be identified before sampling). Haemorrhage should be checked for at about 1 minute and 30 minutes after the procedure. Examining the biopsy site immediately after the procedure with colour flow Doppler ultrasonography

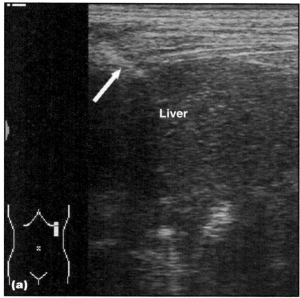

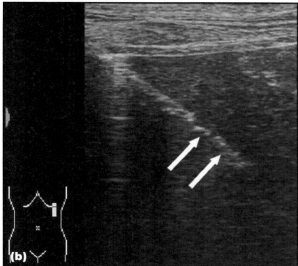

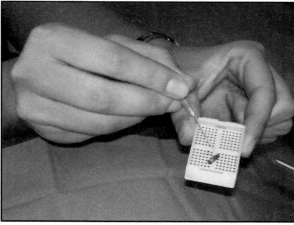

4.9 CTB sample being placed in a biopsy cassette prior to placement in formalin.

4.8 Sagittal ultrasonograms of the left liver lobe demonstrating the CTB technique. **(a)** The linear hyperechoic biopsy needle can be seen at the periphery of the liver prior to firing of the biopsy gun. **(b)** Firing the biopsy gun causes the needle to advance further into the hepatic parenchyma as the sample is collected. White arrows indicate the needle tip.

may show some haemorrhage, hence the 1 minute wait at which stage bleeding has usually stopped. As tissue samples may be fairly small they should be placed in a biopsy cassette (Figure 4.9) before putting the sample in formalin. At least two or three samples should be taken from different regions of the lesion to obtain representative samples. Where possible, some normal tissue at the periphery should be included and necrotic centres avoided.

Specimen quality and accuracy

Published data vary on the diagnostic accuracy of the various techniques. FNA may provide a cytological diagnosis in up to 84% of cases and CTB can provide up to 97% diagnostic quality samples. In the liver FNA is much less accurate than CTB, but still may be a useful first diagnostic approach. The correlation between cytological diagnoses and final histopathological diagnoses may also vary between organs. Lung FNA has been shown to be diagnostic in 82% of cases (DeBerry *et al.*, 2002). Splenic FNA samples were diagnostic in 61% of cases, whilst in the liver, feline samples were 51% and canine samples 30% diagnostic with respect to the final histopathological diagnosis (Wang *et al.*, 2004; Ballegeer *et al.*, 2007). Impression smears from the biopsy sample, whilst preserving the sample for histopathology, can give an immediate cytological sample, which is usually more diagnostic than FNA cytology (Bonfanti *et al.*, 2006).

Potential complications

Generally the advantages of obtaining a diagnostic sample far outweigh the risk of any possible complication, with one study reporting only three major post-biopsy complications from 233 cases (Léveillé *et al.*, 1993).

- Haemorrhage is rare and will usually stop within a few minutes unless a coagulopathy is present. The kidney has greater bleeding potential than other organs.
- Peritonitis is rare if infected lesions are sampled with thin needles, but appropriate antibiotics should be used.
- Penetrating hollow organs should be avoided, particularly with CTB.
- Tumour seeding along the needle tract is rare, but has been reported in bladder and prostate gland transitional cell carcinomas (Nyland *et al.*, 2002). It is also advisable to avoid passing the needle through two body cavities, but benefits may outweigh potential complications (for example, aspirating an accessory lung lobe lesion transhepatically).
- Adrenal gland biopsy of a potential phaeochromocytoma should be avoided as a hypertensive or paradoxical hypotensive crisis may be precipitated.
- Use of an automated biopsy gun to collect hepatic samples in cats has been associated with 19% of cats developing severe shock compared with 0% when a semi-automated biopsy gun was

used. This is believed to be due to the pressure wave created by the automatic device resulting in intense vagotonia (Proot and Rothuizen, 2006). However, this complication has not been encountered by the authors or editors.

- Post-biopsy arteriovenous fistulas are a rare complication and occur more commonly in the kidney.

Other interventional procedures

A number of other ultrasound-guided procedures are possible and are briefly mentioned here. Readers should refer to the relevant organ Chapters or references.

Intraoperative procedures

Sterile transducers may be used in the operating theatre to guide the surgeon to lesions not visible superficially, such as brain neoplasia or intrahepatic shunts close to the diaphragm. In addition, in cases with a spinal tumour or disc herniation ultrasonography can also be used to provide the surgeon with information on lesion borders and exact location.

Ultrasound-guided tissue ablation

Hepatic and renal cysts and abscesses have been successfully treated by means of alcoholization. The cavitary lesion is drained, filled with 95% ethanol for 3 minutes, and then drained again. Percutaneous ultrasound-guided chemical ablation of pathological parathyroid and thyroid nodules with ethanol have also been described.

Seldinger drainage techniques

Large intra-abdominal abscesses can be drained using this technique, but its use is limited to specialized institutions. Briefly, the technique involves passing a trocar into the affected region under ultrasound guidance, a round-tipped guide wire is then passed through the trocar into the abscess and the needle is withdrawn. A blunt cannula or drainage tube is then passed over the guide wire into the lesion, followed by removal of the guide wire and drainage. The technique is also commonly used in angiography.

Ultrasound-guided lymphography

Chylothorax secondary to thoracic duct rupture can be diagnosed by means of contrast-enhanced computed tomography (CT) following ultrasound-guided injection of contrast medium into the popliteal or mesenteric lymph nodes.

Percutaneous cholecystography and pyelography

Ureteral obstruction can be confirmed by means of percutaneous antegrade pyelography by passing a spinal needle into the distended renal pelvis, aspirating 50% of the hydronephrotic fluid and injecting iodinated contrast medium. Similarly, ultrasound-guided cholecystography or cholecystocentesis can be performed using a 22-gauge needle. Passing the needle through the liver apparently minimizes the rare risk of complications.

Ultrasound-guided urinary catheter suction samples

In dogs with suspected bladder or prostatic transitional cell carcinoma, a urinary catheter with side holes can be passed and placed adjacent to the mass using ultrasound guidance. Suction can then be applied to obtain cytological samples. This avoids potential seeding of tumour cells along an aspirating needle tract.

References and further reading

Ballegeer EA, Forrest LJ, Dickinson RM *et al.* (2007) Correlation of ultrasonographic appearance of lesions and cytologic and histologic diagnoses from aspirates from dogs and cats: 32 cases (2002–2005). *Journal of the American Veterinary Medical Association* **230**, 690–696

Bonfanti U, Bertazzolo W, Bottero E *et al.* (2006) Diagnostic value of cytologic examination of gastrointestinal tract tumours in dogs and cats: 83 cases (2001–2004). *Journal of the American Veterinary Medical Association* **229**, 1130–1133

Britt T, Clifford C, Barger A *et al.* (2006) Diagnosing appendicular osteosarcoma with ultrasound-guided fine-needle aspiration: 36 cases. *Journal of Small Animal Practice* **48**, 145–150

Chastain CB, Panciera D and Waters C (2001) Percutaneous ultrasonographically guided radiofrequency heat ablation of primary hyperparathyroidism in dogs. *Small Animal Clinical Endocrinology* **11**, 10

DeBerry JD, Norris CR, Samii VF *et al.* (2002) Correlation between fine-needle aspiration cytopathology and histopathology of the lung in dogs and cats. *Journal of the American Animal Hospital Association* **38**, 327–336

Dodd III GD, Esola CC, Memel DS *et al.* (1996) Sonography: the undiscovered jewel of interventional radiology. *Radiographics* **16**, 1271–1288

Finn-Bodner ST and Hathcock JT (1993) Image-guided percutaneous needle biopsy: ultrasound, computed tomography, and magnetic resonance imaging. *Seminars in Veterinary Medicine and Surgery (Small Animal)* **8**, 258–278

Higgs ZCJ, Macafee DAL, Braithwaite BD *et al.* (2005) The Seldinger technique: 50 years on. *The Lancet* **366**, 1407–1409

Johnson EG, Wisner ER, Kyles A *et al.* (2009) Computed tomographic lymphography of the thoracic duct by mesenteric lymph node injection. *Veterinary Surgery* **38**, 361–367

Léveillé R, Paugh Partington B, Biller DS *et al.* (1993) Complications after ultrasound-guided biopsy of abdominal structures in dogs and cats: 246 cases (1984–1991). *Journal of the American Veterinary Medical Association* **203**, 413–415

Long CD, Goldstein RE, Hornhof WJ *et al.* (1999) Percutaneous ultrasound-guided chemical parathyroid ablation for treatment of primary hyperparathyroidism in dogs. *Journal of the American Veterinary Medical Association* **215**, 217–221

Nyland TG, Wallack ST and Wisner ER (2002) Needle-tract implantation following US-guided fine-needle aspiration biopsy of transitional cell carcinoma of the bladder, urethra, and prostate. *Veterinary Radiology and Ultrasound* **43**, 50–53

Penninck DG and Finn-Bodner ST (1998) Updates in interventional ultrasonography. *Veterinary Clinics of North America: Small Animal Practice* **28**, 1017–1040

Proot SJ and Rothuizen J (2006) High complication rate of Tru-Cut biopsy gun device for liver biopsy in cats. *Journal of Veterinary Internal Medicine* **20**, 1327–1333

Rothuizen J and Twedt DC (2009) Liver biopsy techniques. *Veterinary Clinics of North America: Small Animal Practice* **39**, 469–480

Szatmári V, van Sluijs FJ, Rothuizen J *et al.* (2003) Intraoperative ultrasonography of the portal vein during attenuation of intrahepatic portocaval shunts in dogs. *Journal of the American Veterinary Medical Association* **8**, 1086–1092

Wang KY, Panciera DL, Al-Rukibat RK *et al.* (2004) Accuracy of ultrasound-guided fine-needle aspiration of the liver and cytologic findings in dogs and cats (1990–2000). *Journal of the American Veterinary Medical Association* **224**, 75–78

Zatelli A, D'Ippolito P, Bonfanti U *et al.* (2007) Ultrasound-assisted drainage and alcoholization of hepatic and renal cysts: 22 cases. *Journal of the American Animal Hospital Association* **43**, 112–116

5

Thorax

Gabriela Seiler

Indications

Non-cardiac thoracic ultrasonography complements radiography in the examination of patients with chest wall, pleural space, mediastinal and pulmonary disease (for information on cardiac ultrasonography, see Chapter 6). Since ultrasound waves are reflected at soft tissue–gas interfaces, indications for non-cardiac thoracic ultrasonography include evaluation of peripheral lesions that are not surrounded by air, or thoracic diseases that are associated with pleural effusion. Pleural effusion provides an ideal window for ultrasonographic evaluation of thoracic structures, and thoracocentesis should be postponed until after the examination unless the patient is in severe respiratory distress. Ultrasonography is often used to investigate the cause for the effusion (e.g. presence of a cranial mediastinal mass). Most thoracic lesions, if visible with ultrasonography, are also accessible for ultrasound-guided fluid or tissue sampling, which is essential for definitive diagnosis. Thoracic ultrasonography is often used to determine the origin of a thoracic mass if it is equivocal on radiography. Lesions such as pulmonary or mediastinal masses can be further characterized as cystic or solid, and vascularity can be determined using Doppler ultrasonography. Evaluation of thoracic wall masses is another indication for ultrasonography; presence of erosive rib lesions, fistulous tracts and foreign bodies, and extension of disease into the pleural cavity can be assessed.

Value of ultrasonography compared with radiography and computed tomography

Thoracic radiography and ultrasonography are complementary as the lesions surrounded by air are easily visualized on a radiograph, whereas soft tissue structures can be further characterized on an ultrasonogram. Ultrasonography is inherently limited to the non-aerated portion of the thorax; therefore, it should always be performed in conjunction with radiography for a full assessment of thoracic disease. Radiographs help determine whether a lesion is likely to be visible ultrasonographically and which acoustic window is the most appropriate.

One advantage of ultrasonography compared with radiography is the fact that the presence of pleural effusion allows better visibility of intrathoracic structures, whereas it can obscure lesions on radiographs. Observation in real time allows better differentiation of pulmonary and intrathoracic extension of thoracic wall lesions, as pulmonary lesions slide against the chest wall with respiratory movement, and blood flow can be assessed using Doppler ultrasonography. Cross-sectional imaging eliminates superimposition, and the internal architecture of thoracic structures can be assessed.

When compared with computed tomography (CT), the biggest advantage of ultrasonography is the ability to perform the examination in the conscious or lightly sedated patient. In patients with severe respiratory compromise, the general anaesthesia and prolonged recumbency necessary for CT scanning can be detrimental to their health. Similar to radiography, large volumes of pleural effusion also decrease the diagnostic quality of a CT study.

Imaging technique

Patient preparation

For optimal image quality, the area of interest should be prepared by clipping the hair coat, cleaning the skin with alcohol and applying ultrasound gel. However, it is often not reasonable to clip the entire thorax to identify the area of interest such as the location of a pulmonary mass. In these cases, wetting the hair coat generously with alcohol (without clipping) allows sufficient image quality to localize the lesion in most instances. Once the acoustic window is located that allows visualization of the lesion, the precise area can then be prepared as described above.

Positioning

Patients can be examined in either lateral or sternal recumbency. If tolerated by the patient, dorsal recumbency may be used as well. Small footprint transducers are ideal as they allow access to the thoracic cavity through several windows. Sector or microcurved transducers are recommended, at a frequency between 5 and 10 MHz, depending on the size of the patient. High frequency linear transducers are very useful for assessment of the superficial structures, especially in smaller patients.

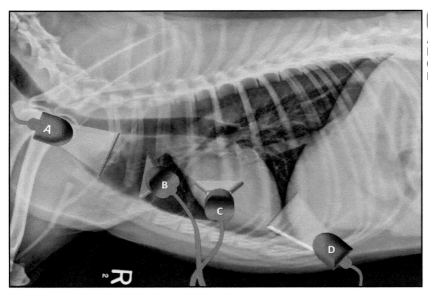

5.1 Transducer placement for different scan windows.
A = thoracic inlet window;
B = transverse intercostal window;
C = long-axis intercostal window;
D = substernal, transhepatic window.

Three different windows are commonly used for thoracic ultrasonography (Figure 5.1):

- Intercostal
- Thoracic inlet
- Substernal.

For an intercostal window, the transducer is placed between the ribs in both a longitudinal (across the ribs) and an oblique transverse (parallel to the ribs) direction. Moving the transducer in a ventral-to-dorsal direction along the intercostal space allows assessment of the chest wall, pleural space, lung surface and the ventral portion of the mediastinum. For assessment of the cranial aspect of the cranial mediastinum, the trachea and oesophagus as well as the large mediastinal vessels, the transducer is placed at the thoracic inlet and tilted caudally into the thorax. The scan window with this approach is limited, but there is less interference by air and no superimposed triceps musculature. For a substernal, transhepatic window the transducer is placed caudal to the sternal xiphoid and angled cranially. This approach allows assessment of the diaphragmatic surface and the caudoventral mediastinum.

Normal ultrasonographic appearance

The thoracic wall consists of skin and layers of subcutaneous fat and muscle, resulting in alternating layers of hyperechoic and hypoechoic bands (Figure 5.2). Normal ribs are seen as smooth hyperechoic surfaces, which are straight in a long-axis view and curved in a short-axis view. A clean shadow is cast deep to the rib. The pleural–lung interface is characterized by a smooth hyperechoic line. Distinct layers of parietal and visceral pleura are not seen in dogs and cats; however, the lung surface can be distinguished by observing the lung lobes slide along the parietal pleural surface during respiration (see **Normal lung** clip on DVD).

Assessment of the normal lung is limited to the surface, which should be smooth and hyperechoic with reverberation artefacts deep to the lung surface ('dirty shadowing') created by complete reflection of the sound waves at the soft tissue–air interface. Any superficial lung alteration such as atelectasis, consolidation or nodules may lead to an interruption of the smooth surface. The normal mediastinum, which is usually only visible if pleural effusion or pulmonary disease is present, consists of a small amount of echogenic, irregular fat surrounding the large vessels, extending to the thoracic inlet. Normal lymph nodes are not differentiated from the mediastinal fat.

In young animals, the thymus may still be visible as echogenic tissue with a coarse structure in the ventral mediastinum cranial to the heart; it is well vascularized when interrogated with colour Doppler ultrasonography. The intrathoracic trachea and oesophagus are rarely seen; even in the presence of

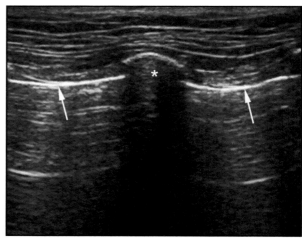

5.2 Long-axis view of the chest wall of a normal Cairn Terrier using a linear transducer. The lung surface is seen as a smooth, straight hyperechoic line (arrowed). The superficial soft tissues have a striated appearance consistent with layers of fat, muscle fibres and fascial planes. A rib (*) is seen in cross-section: it has a smooth, curved surface and creates a distal shadow.

pleural effusion, the remaining air in the dorsal lung obscures the dorsal mediastinal structures. Complete assessment of the diaphragm requires a combination of a substernal transhepatic and an intercostal approach. It is seen as a hyperechoic, smooth and continuous surface of the liver. Only in the presence of both peritoneal and pleural fluid is it visible separately as a thin, hyperechoic linear structure.

Thoracic wall lesions

The structure and content of a thoracic wall mass as well as the involvement of the ribs and invasion into the pleural space can be assessed with ultrasonography. Tumours of the thoracic wall originate in the soft tissues (sarcoma, infiltrative lipoma), the ribs or the sternum (chondrosarcoma, osteosarcoma). Inflammatory lesions such as abscesses and granulomas may be caused by superficial wounds or penetrating foreign bodies. Ultrasonography is usually successful at identifying fluid pockets and draining tracts. Small foreign bodies are difficult to identify, but if visible most foreign bodies present as a hyperechoic structure with distal shadowing. The subcutaneous tissues in the near-field should be scrutinized for the presence of a fistulous tract, seen as an irregular hypoechoic path leading towards the surface of the chest wall. Thoracic wall oedema or cellulitis presents as thickened subcutaneous tissues with a striated appearance caused by fluid in between the fascial planes and fat layers of the chest wall.

Thoracic wall masses can be differentiated from lung masses by observing the mass during respiration: lung masses slide along the thoracic wall with inspiration and expiration, whereas thoracic wall masses remain fixed in position relative to the ribs. Penetration of the thoracic cavity is recognized by an absence of the hyperechoic pleural surface and medial displacement of the lung lobes.

Rib lesions and fractures

Aggressive rib lesions typically present as an irregular bone surface; often the rib is expanded and surrounded by a hypoechoic mass (Figure 5.3). Discontinuity of the cortex or smooth thickening of the rib is seen with acute and chronic rib fractures and callus formation (Figure 5.4). Rib fractures are not usually associated with significant soft tissue thickening. Osteomyelitis or tumours such as osteosarcoma may involve the sternum and can be difficult to differentiate radiographically from commonly observed degenerative changes. Ultrasonography is useful to determine the presence of a soft tissue mass associated with an abnormal sternebra, and to obtain tissue samples if an aggressive lesion is suspected.

Pleural space disease

Pleural effusion is readily detected by thoracic ultrasonography and is visible as an anechoic or

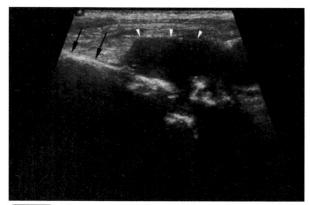

5.3 Ultrasonogram of an 8-year-old male neutered Golden Retriever with a thoracic wall mass. The transducer is aligned with the long axis of the 7th rib. Dorsal is to the left of the image. The proximal portion of the rib is normal with a smooth hyperechoic surface (black arrows); the distal portion of the rib is surrounded by a large hypoechoic mass (white arrowheads). The bone surface of the distal portion of the rib is interrupted and very irregular, consistent with lysis and periosteal reactions. Biopsy of the mass revealed a poorly differentiated sarcoma.

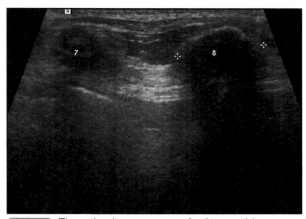

5.4 Thoracic ultrasonogram of a 6-year-old neutered Australian Shepherd bitch. The 7th and 8th ribs are seen in cross-section. The 8th rib is much larger in diameter than the 7th, but has a smooth surface and no associated soft tissue mass. This is consistent with callus formation following rib fracture. The dog had sustained thoracic trauma several months prior to this ultrasound examination.

hypoechoic layer between the chest wall and the lungs or mediastinum. The echogenicity of the effusion is related to its type:

- Exudate, haemorrhage and neoplastic effusions: very echogenic and consist of a large number of cells, fibrin or protein (Figure 5.5)
- Transudate, modified transudate and chylous effusions: anechoic (see **Pleural fluid** clip on DVD).

Chronic effusions are often characterized by loculation of fluid into pockets, a large amount of fibrin strands and increased rounding and irregularity of the lung lobes (Figure 5.6). Thickening and irregularity of the pleural surface can be seen with chronic

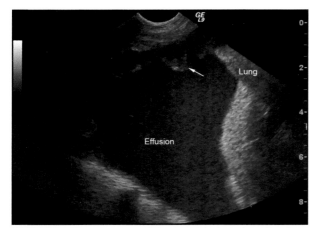

5.5 Ultrasonogram of the cranial pleural cavity of a 3-year-old male neutered mixed-breed dog with pyothorax. There is a large amount of very cellular pleural fluid present. The lung lobes are partially collapsed and there are multiple fibrin tags seen along the pleural surface (arrowed).

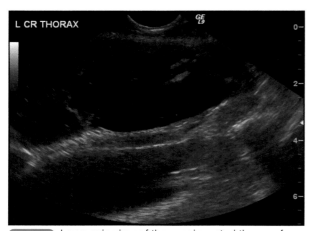

5.6 Long-axis view of the cranioventral thorax of a 6-year-old male neutered Borzoi with chronic idiopathic chylothorax. Note the round pockets of fluid separated by thick hyperechoic fibrin strands.

effusion, but may also be a sign of pleuritis or neoplastic pleural disease. Pleural masses are uncommon, and most often caused by metastatic disease such as carcinomatosis or by mesothelioma.

The presence of pneumothorax limits the value of thoracic ultrasonography, but it is very important that the ultrasonographer is able to recognize it, especially as a complication of thoracic interventional procedures such as biopsy or fine-needle aspiration (FNA). The air-filled lung and free gas within the pleural space both result in a hyperechoic surface beneath the chest wall with distal reverberations; however, no movement of the free pleural air relative to the chest wall is observed during respiration.

Mediastinal masses

Evaluation of a cranial mediastinal mass effect observed radiographically is a common indication for thoracic ultrasonography. Mediastinal masses are usually readily identified as hypoechoic nodules

in the otherwise hyperechoic mediastinal fat (Figure 5.7). Differential diagnoses include lymphoma, thymoma, histiocytic sarcoma, ectopic thyroid or parathyroid tissue, other tumours such as metastatic melanoma and lymphomatoid granulomatosis, as well as mediastinal haematomas, abscesses and granulomas, which can appear identical to neoplastic lesions. Enlarged lymph nodes tend to be round or lobulated, whereas thymomas often have a more complex heterogenic and cystic structure (Figure 5.8). Enlarged sternal lymph nodes are hypoechoic round to oval structures immediately dorsal to the sternum, whereas cranial mediastinal lymph nodes are found in a more dorsal location and surrounded by mediastinal fat. In the presence of a mediastinal mass, visible mediastinal vessels should be assessed for thrombosis or vascular invasion to determine surgical resectability.

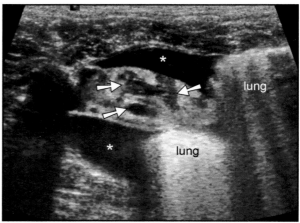

5.7 Long-axis view of the cranial thorax of a 10-year-old female neutered Domestic Shorthaired cat. Bilateral pleural effusion is present (*). The cranial mediastinum is thickened and contains multiple enlarged, hypoechoic lymph nodes (arrowed). The cranial lung lobes are partially collapsed and very rounded. The cat was diagnosed with idiopathic chylothorax. Histopathology showed reactive hyperplasia of the lymph nodes.

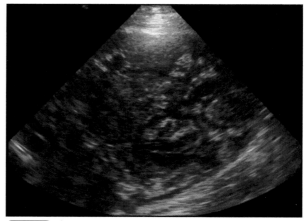

5.8 An 8-year-old neutered Labrador bitch was presented for regurgitation. Megaoesophagus and a cranial mediastinal mass were seen radiographically. On ultrasound examination of the cranial mediastinum, a large heterogenic mass with multiple cavitations was seen. Thymoma was diagnosed on cytology.

Cranial mediastinal cysts, more commonly seen in older cats than in dogs, can readily be differentiated from mediastinal masses by their thin wall, anechoic contents and distal acoustic enhancement (Figure 5.9). FNA typically yields clear, almost acellular fluid. Caudal mediastinal masses are rare (Figure 5.10). Caudodorsal mediastinal masses, often associated with the oesophagus, may be seen using a transhepatic approach. The transducer is placed in midline, pointing cranially, and then is slowly fanned to the left to identify the cardia and oesophageal hiatus. In deep-chested larger dogs it may not be visible. Paraoesophageal abscesses are uncommon, but may be recognized by a thick hyperechoic wall and hypoechoic to hyperechoic mobile contents. Cytology is needed to differentiate abscessation from necrotic neoplasia.

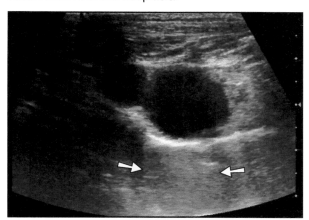

5.9 Ultrasonogram of the cranial mediastinum of an 18-year-old female spayed Domestic Shorthaired cat presented with lethargy and icterus. Liver neoplasia was subsequently diagnosed. On thoracic radiographs a cranial mediastinal mass was observed. Ultrasonographically there are two hypoechoic, thin-walled cystic structures seen cranial to the heart with distal acoustic enhancement (arrowed) of the larger structure. Cranial mediastinal cysts, unrelated to the liver disease, were diagnosed.

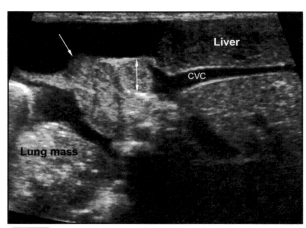

5.10 Long-axis view of the caudal mediastinum of a 16-year-old male neutered Persian cat with squamous cell carcinoma in the accessory lung lobe and metastasis into the caudal vena cava (CVC) diagnosed on necropsy. The accessory lung lobe mass is labelled. A second hypoechoic mass (arrowed) is seen in the caudal mediastinum, extending into the caudal vena cava (double-headed arrow). Pleural effusion is also present.

Diaphragmatic rupture and herniation

Ultrasonographic assessment of the diaphragm can be valuable if the diagnosis of diaphragmatic hernia is equivocal on radiographs due to the superimposition of pleural fluid. However, complete ultrasonographic assessment of the diaphragm is challenging, especially in larger breed dogs. Care should be taken to follow the outline of the diaphragm bilaterally, both from a substernal and an intercostal window.

In the presence of diaphragmatic rupture, the smooth outline is no longer continuous, the cranial hepatic margin is irregular and typically pleural effusion has accumulated in the caudal thoracic cavity. Abdominal organs identified within the thoracic cavity, either in direct contact with the pericardial sac or lateral to it, confirm the diagnosis (Figure 5.11). More difficult to diagnose are diaphragmatic tears with only mild cranial displacement of the liver or falciform fat, which cannot be differentiated from pericardial or mediastinal fat. In these cases, discontinuity of the diaphragmatic outline and absence or displacement of abdominal organs within the peritoneal cavity need to be taken into account.

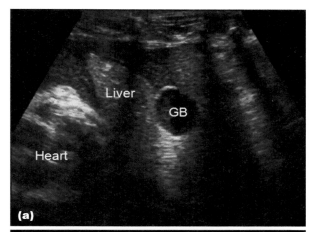

(a)

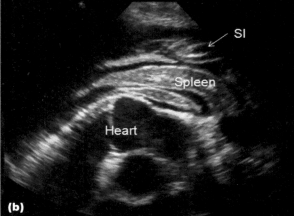

(b)

5.11 Ultrasonograms of the caudoventral thorax of (a) a cat and (b) a dog with traumatic diaphragmatic hernia. In the cat, the liver and gallbladder (GB) have herniated into the thoracic cavity; some of the liver lobes are adjacent to the heart and surrounded by echogenic pleural effusion (haemorrhage). In the dog, the spleen and some small intestinal (SI) loops are seen adjacent to the heart. Pleural effusion is also present.

Several artefacts present potential pitfalls and should be recognized. Sound waves reflected off the diaphragm and other reflective surfaces within the abdomen (such as the gallbladder wall) result in an image of liver parenchyma being displayed in the thoracic cavity. This 'mirror image' artefact can be recognized by the complete symmetry of the liver vasculature on each side of the diaphragm. Repositioning of the transducer using a different angle or window will often make the artefact disappear. This artefact is only visible if the diaphragm is intact and may in fact help rule out a diaphragmatic hernia. Refraction of the ultrasound beam on the diaphragmatic surface in the presence of peritoneal fluid may lead to a false appearance of a discontinuous diaphragm. Investigating the diaphragmatic surface from a different angle will also help in recognizing the artefact. Consolidated lung tissue can be confused with herniated liver, but following the vascular structures will aid differentiation.

Peritoneopericardial diaphragmatic hernia (PPDH) is readily identified with ultrasonography by the presence of abdominal contents in the pericardial sac. True diaphragmatic hernias can be recognized as such if an abnormal bulge containing liver or fat is protruding into the thorax but is still covered by a smooth hyperechoic border without any evidence of pleural effusion.

Lung lobe conditions

Ultrasonographic examination of the lungs is possible if alveolar air has been replaced by fluid or tissue, or if the lung lobes have collapsed. It is also often used to confirm suspicion of lung lobe torsion if radiographs are equivocal.

Consolidation

Mild or partial consolidation is often first seen as interruption of the smooth hyperechoic pulmonary surface with distal ring-down artefacts. These artefacts are characterized by vertical streaks, composed of densely spaced hyperechoic lines extending into the deep portions of the lung (Figure 5.12). With more severe consolidation, the periphery of the lung lobes increasingly loses aerated alveoli and becomes more hypoechoic. Residual air within the airspace results in hyperechoic speckles within the lung tissue, best seen during inspiration (Figure 5.13).

A consolidated lung lobe usually retains its size and shape. Differential diagnoses include pneumonia, pulmonary haemorrhage (contusions), oedema, fibrosis and lobar neoplasia. Linear hyperechoic structures creating reverberation artefacts represent gas-filled airways. Once all the air is replaced with fluid or cells, the lung tissue has an echotexure similar to that of the liver; this appearance is called 'hepatization'. Fluid-filled bronchi may be seen as hypoechoic tubular structures with hyperechoic walls ('fluid-bronchograms') and are differentiated from vessels by means of Doppler ultrasonography.

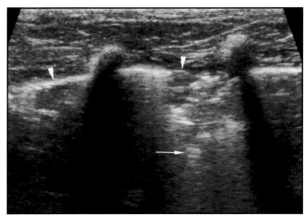

5.12 Long-axis view of the thorax of an 18-month-old Domestic Shorthaired cat presented for lethargy and coughing. Multiple areas of focal consolidation are seen in the periphery of the lung lobes (arrowheads). Some of the consolidations create ring-down artefacts (arrowed) seen as a narrow strip of densely spaced hyperechoic lines. *Mycoplasma* infection was the final diagnosis.

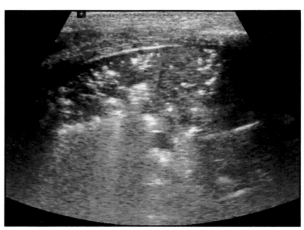

5.13 Ultrasonogram of the cranial lung lobe of an 11-week-old Dogue de Bordeaux bitch presented for dyspnoea and vomiting. The lung lobe is partially consolidated but hyperechoic foci consistent with residual air in the airways or alveolar space are seen throughout the lobe. Necrotizing pneumonia was the final diagnosis.

Atelectasis

Atelectatic lung lobes, commonly identified in the presence of pleural effusion, present as small triangular structures with a smooth surface and various amounts of residual gas in the airways (Figure 5.14). If observed during respiration, increased air content resulting in more reverberation artefacts can be appreciated during inspiration.

Pulmonary masses

Pulmonary masses are round to irregular but still convex structures within the lung and may distort the surface and architecture of the affected lobe (Figure 5.15). The pulmonary origin of a mass can usually be determined by observing movement with respiration and by the presence of gas foci within the mass (see **Pulmonary mass (1)** clip on DVD). Although the margins may be irregular, they are usually still

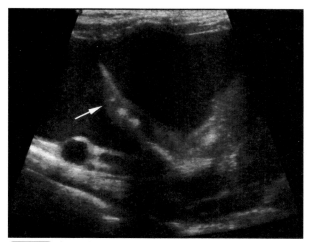

5.14 Lung lobe atelectasis in a dog with a large volume pleural effusion. The lung lobe is collapsed to a thin triangular structure (arrowed). The hyperechoic foci in the centre represent gas-filled bronchi.

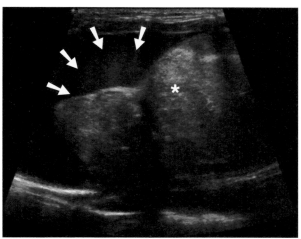

5.15 Long-axis view of the thorax of a 3-year-old male neutered Domestic Shorthaired cat with pulmonary adenocarcinoma. The affected lung lobe is distorted and contains a hypoechoic mass (*). The tip of the lung lobe is surrounded by cellular effusion due to carcinomatosis (arrowed).

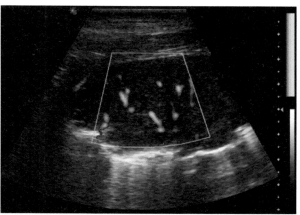

5.16 Power Doppler ultrasonogram of a pulmonary mass in a 9-year-old male neutered Poodle. The mass is hypoechoic, well delineated towards the aerated lung tissue (hyperechoic) and is well perfused. Pulmonary carcinoma was diagnosed with fine-needle aspirates.

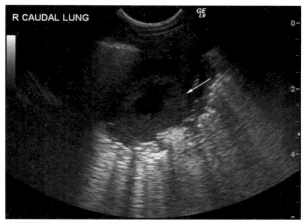

5.17 A 2-year-old Weimaraner was presented for lethargy, fever and coughing. Pleural effusion and a mass lesion in the right caudal lung lobe were seen radiographically. On ultrasound examination, a fluid-filled mass with a thick hyperechoic capsule (arrowed) was seen. The lung lobe was resected and a pulmonary abscess was diagnosed.

relatively distinct towards the normal lung tissue, whereas pulmonary consolidation resulting from non-neoplastic disease tends to have indistinct margins. Blood flow may be detected within the mass using Doppler ultrasonography (Figure 5.16).

Anechoic areas within the mass lesion are consistent with necrotic tissue or abscessation. Cavitated lung masses may contain cystic, fluid-filled or air-filled areas. Abscesses tend to have a thick wall structure and larger fluid-filled cavitations (Figure 5.17). Metastatic neoplasia or granulomatous lung disease results in well defined, round hypoechoic nodules throughout the lung lobes, but, normally, since the remainder of the lobe is still aerated, only the very superficial ones are visible (Figure 5.18; see also **Pulmonary mass (2)** clip on DVD). Cytology is needed for a definitive diagnosis in all cases.

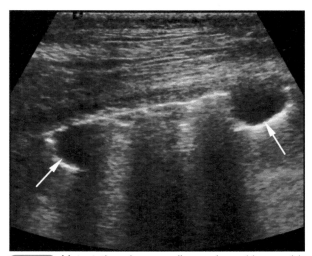

5.18 Metastatic pulmonary disease in an 11-year-old neutered Labrador Retriever bitch. Two hypoechoic nodules are seen on the surface of the lung (arrowed). Nodules deeper in the parenchyma are obscured by the air-filled lungs.

Torsion

Typically, torsed lung lobes are enlarged and hypo-echoic, and the tip of the lung lobe is somewhat blunted. An abnormal position, with the tip pointing dorsally for instance, may be recognized. Pockets of gas within the torsed lung lobe, seen radiographically as a vesicular gas pattern, can be recognized ultrasonographically as irregular hyperechoic regions within the lung lobe that create distal reverberation artefacts. The central bronchus may be fluid-filled, resulting in a 'fluid-bronchogram'; a linear hypoechoic tube with hyperechoic wall structure (Figure 5.19). Pleural effusion often surrounds the torsed lung lobe (see **Lung lobe torsion** clip on DVD). If the patient is calm and the respiratory rate low enough to avoid significant motion artefact, colour Doppler examination of the torsed lung lobe can be used to confirm absence of venous blood flow. If the torsion is relatively acute, arterial blood flow may still be present and should not be used to rule out lung lobe torsion. Adjacent lung lobes are usually at least partially atelectatic, especially in the presence of pleural effusion.

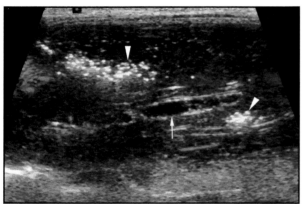

5.19 Ultrasonogram of a 9-year-old male neutered Pug with torsion of the left cranial lung lobe. The rotated lung lobe is very hypoechoic, enlarged and contains multiple hyperechoic speckles, consistent with trapped gas (arrowheads). The tubular hypoechoic structure with hyperechoic walls (arrowed) represents a fluid-filled bronchus. No blood flow could be detected in this lung lobe with Doppler ultrasonography and the diagnosis of lung lobe torsion was confirmed during surgery.

Particular considerations for sampling

The general principles of fluid collection are covered in Chapter 4. Ultrasound-guided thoracocentesis is very helpful in the presence of loculated effusion or if the fluid is associated with a large amount of fibrin strands that may obstruct the needle. For diagnostic thoracocentesis and drainage of transudate, 22-gauge needles are sufficient, but larger needles may be needed for therapeutic removal of large amounts of viscous fluid. If a large volume has to be drained, the needle should be attached to an extension set with a three-way stopcock. As with any type of thoracocentesis, the caudal margin of the ribs should be avoided during needle placement to avoid laceration and bleeding of the intercostal vessels.

FNA of thoracic masses or pulmonary consolidations should only be attempted by experienced ultrasonographers and in patients that are immobilized. If the targeted structure is very large, deep sedation may be sufficient; whereas for smaller targets, especially if located in the lungs, general anaesthesia is required in order to stop respiration for the duration of the sampling procedure (see **Fine-needle aspiration of a pulmonary mass** clip on DVD). For biopsy, general anaesthesia is recommended. Complications of FNA and biopsy of pulmonary lesions include haemorrhage and pneumothorax. Personnel should always be prepared to do an emergency thoracocentesis before starting the procedure, in case the lung tissue is lacerated and results in leakage of air into the pleural space.

References and further reading

d'Anjou MA, Tidwell AS and Hecht S (2005) Radiographic diagnosis of lung lobe torsion. *Veterinary Radiology and Ultrasound* **46**, 478–484

Hecht S (2008) Thorax. In: *Atlas of Small Animal Ultrasonography, 1st edn*, ed. D Penninck and MA d'Anjou, pp. 119–150. Blackwell Publications, Iowa

Konde LJ and Spaulding K (1991) Sonographic evaluation of the cranial mediastinum in small animals. *Veterinary Radiology and Ultrasound* **32**, 178–184

Lamb CR, Mason GD, and Wallace MK (1989) Ultrasonographic diagnosis of peritoneopericardial diaphragmatic hernia in a Persian cat. *Veterinary Record* **125**, 186

Larson MM (2009) Ultrasound of the thorax (non-cardiac). *Veterinary Clinics of North America: Small Animal Practice* **39**, 733–745

Louvet A and Bourgeois JM (2008) Lung ring-down artefact as a sign of pulmonary alveolar-interstitial disease. *Veterinary Radiology and Ultrasound* **49**, 374–377

Mattoon JS and Nyland TG (2002) Thorax. In: *Small Animal Diagnostic Ultrasound, 2nd edn*, ed. JS Mattoon and TG Nyland, pp 325–353. WB Saunders, Philadelphia

Mellanby RJ, Villiers E and Herrtage ME (2002) Canine pleural and mediastinal effusions: a retrospective study of 81 cases. *Journal of Small Animal Practice* **43**, 447–451

Reichle JK and Wisner ER (2000) Non-cardiac thoracic ultrasound in 75 feline and canine patients. *Veterinary Radiology and Ultrasound* **41**, 154–162

Schultz RM and Zwingenberger A (2008) Radiographic, computed tomographic and ultrasonographic findings with migrating intrathoracic grass awns in dogs and cats. *Veterinary Radiology and Ultrasound* **49**, 249–255

Seiler G, Dukes-McEwan J and Gaschen L (2008) Basics of thoracic ultrasonography. In: *BSAVA Manual of Canine and Feline Thoracic Imaging*, ed. T Schwarz and V Johnson, pp. 20–66. BSAVA Publications, Gloucester

Spattini G, Rossi F, Vignoli M et al. (2003) Use of ultrasound to diagnose diaphragmatic rupture in dogs and cats. *Veterinary Radiology and Ultrasound* **44**, 226–230

Tidwell AS (1998) Ultrasonography of the thorax (excluding the heart). *Veterinary Clinics of North America: Small Animal Practice* **28**, 993–1015

Wood EF, O'Brien RT and Young KM (1998) Ultrasound-guided fine needle aspiration of focal parenchymal lesions of the lung in dogs and cats. *Journal of Veterinary Internal Medicine* **12**, 338–342

Zekas LJ and Adams WM (2002) Cranial mediastinal cysts in nine cats. *Veterinary Radiology and Ultrasound* **43**, 413–418

Video extras

- **Fine-needle aspiration of a pulmonary mass**
- **Lung lobe torsion**
- **Normal lung**
- **Pleural fluid**
- **Pulmonary mass (1)**
- **Pulmonary mass (2)**

Access via QR code or bsavalibrary.com/ultrasound_5

6

Heart

Romain Pariaut

Introduction

Transthoracic cardiac ultrasonography, or echo-cardiography, provides high-quality images of the heart, great vessels and paracardiac structures. It has developed into an essential diagnostic tool for the evaluation of dogs and cats with cardiac disease.

Indications

The range of indications for echocardiography is large and includes:

- Auscultation abnormalities:
  o Heart murmurs
  o Muffled heart sounds
  o Arrhythmias.
- Physical examination abnormalities:
  o Ascites
  o Jugular vein distension and increased pulsation
  o Central cyanosis
  o Weak femoral pulse; pulse deficit.
- Electrocardiography abnormalities:
  o Variation in electrocardiogram (ECG) wave amplitude or duration; changes in the cardiac electrical axis
  o Arrhythmias.

- Radiography abnormalities:
  o Cardiac silhouette enlargement
  o Pulmonary vein enlargement
  o Pulmonary artery enlargement; tortuous pulmonary artery
  o Pleural effusion
  o Interstitial to alveolar lung pattern associated with pulmonary vein enlargement.
- Hypertension
- Dyspnoea with radiographic changes suggesting cardiac involvement
- Syncope
- Arterial thromboembolism
- Cardiac tamponade
- Use of a cardiotoxic agent (e.g. doxorubicin)
- Identification of phenotypically normal animals prior to use in a breeding programme.

Value of echocardiography compared with radiography

Thoracic radiography and echocardiography are complementary techniques in the evaluation of the patient with cardiac disease (Figure 6.1). Echocardiography provides more detailed information on the structure and function of the heart; however, there are limitations to the technique. Thoracic radiography allows detailed evaluation of the pulmonary

Echocardiography	Thoracic radiography
Mild or no sedation	Mild or no sedation
Detailed, dynamic image of the cardiac chambers and great vessels in real time	Image of the cardiac silhouette
Examination of the heart from multiple imaging planes	Examination of the cardiac silhouette limited to four views in two orthogonal planes (left lateral, right lateral, dorsoventral, ventrodorsal)
Information on cardiac function and intracardiac blood flow	No information on cardiac function or intracardiac blood flow
Evaluation of the heart possible in the presence of pleural effusion	Evaluation of the cardiac silhouette impaired by pleural effusion
Pneumothorax, dyspnoea and tachypnoea may hinder ultrasonographic examination	Dyspnoea and tachypnoea may result in movement blur on radiographs
Does not provide information on lung disease or presence of pulmonary oedema	Provides critical information on lung disease, most importantly pulmonary oedema and pulmonary vascular disease
Expensive and requires ultrasound system equipped with dedicated software and transducers	Available in most veterinary practices and inexpensive
Safe for the patient and operator	Exposes patient and personnel to ionizing radiation

6.1 Comparison of echocardiography and thoracic radiography.

vasculature and parenchyma, which is important for completing the assessment of cardiac function.

Imaging technique

Positioning

In order to decrease lung interference, an echocardiogram is usually performed with the patient in lateral recumbency on a 'cut out' table (Figure 6.2), which allows transducer manipulation from beneath the animal. One or two assistants can help restrain the patient in left or right lateral recumbency. Sedation is usually not needed. Dogs and cats can also be examined in a standing position.

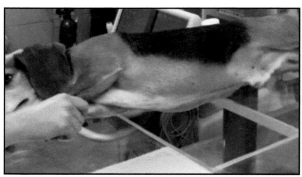

6.2 A dog restrained in right lateral recumbency on a 'cut out' table, which allows echocardiographic examination from underneath.

Transthoracic images of the heart can be obtained where lung tissue is not interposed between the heart and the chest wall. A parasternal window is present on the right side of the thorax, between the sternal border and costochondral junction, from the 3rd to the 6th intercostal space. On the left side of the thorax the windows are adjacent to the sternal border, between the 5th and 7th intercostal spaces (caudal or apical views), and between the sternum and the costochondral junction at the 3rd or 4th intercostal space (cranial views). A subcostal window is located just caudal to the xiphoid process.

Protocol

Both cardiac anatomy and function can be assessed using echocardiography. A comprehensive examination utilizes various imaging modalities (Figures 6.3 and 6.4), including:

- Two-dimensional (2D)
- M-mode
- Doppler.

Right parasternal acoustic window

The transducer is placed on the right ventral thorax. Long-axis and short-axis views can be recorded from this approach. An initial qualitative evaluation of cardiac chamber size and function is performed. In addition, the diameter of the left ventricle and the thickness of the interventricular septum and left ventricular free wall can be measured in diastole and systole, and the left atrial diameter to aortic diameter ratio can be calculated. From the right parasternal acoustic window, the direction of blood flow is, for the most part, oriented perpendicular to the ultrasound beam and therefore cannot be reliably assessed by Doppler techniques.

Long-axis views: Two standard views can be obtained from a right parasternal position: the right parasternal long-axis 4-chamber view and the right parasternal long-axis outflow view (Figure 6.5).

2D echocardiography
Obtain standard long-axis and short-axis views from right parasternal, left parasternal and subcostal acoustic windows Assessment of cardiac chamber, valve and great vessel anatomy Qualitative evaluation of cardiac chamber size and systolic function of the ventricles Measurement of the left atrium, left ventricle and aortic annulus Detection of pericardial effusion and/or cardiac masses
M-mode echocardiography
Obtain views at the left mid-ventricular, mitral valve and aortic valve level from a right parasternal acoustic window Quantification of left ventricular diameter and wall thickness at end-diastole and end-systole Quantitative assessment of left ventricular function (shortening fraction) Provides high temporal resolution, allowing detection of fine, rapid motion of the cardiac structures (valves and chordae)
Doppler echocardiography
Evaluation of laminar and turbulent blood flow across the valves Detection of blood flow across intracardiac and extracardiac shunts Quantitative assessment of blood flow velocity and volume Determination of pressure gradients across valves and obstructions • Pulsed wave Doppler is limited to low velocity, non-turbulent blood flow (e.g. normal flow within the left and right ventricular outflow tracts, mitral and tricuspid valve inflow in diastole, and pulmonary vein flow) • Colour flow Doppler is used to detect valve insufficiencies, stenosis and septal defects • Continuous wave Doppler is indicated to determine the severity of subvalvular, valvular and supravalvular stenosis, to detect and quantify valve regurgitation, and to detect intracardiac and extracardiac shunts

6.3 Applications of the different echocardiographic imaging modalities.

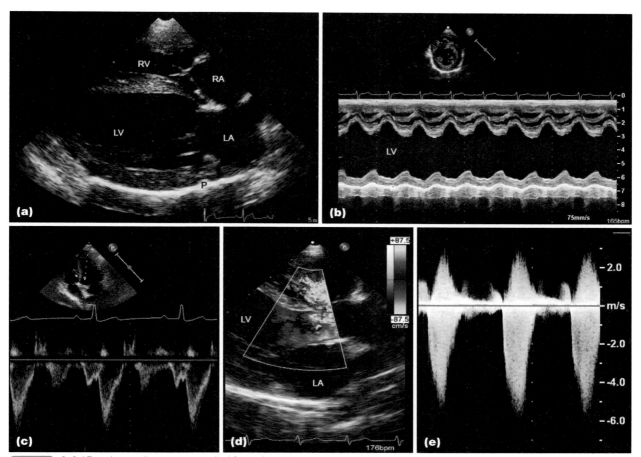

6.4 **(a)** 2D echocardiogram recorded from the right parasternal long-axis window, revealing the left and right cardiac chambers. Ultrasound waves reflected by structures closer to the transducer are displayed at the top of the image, which is shown in greyscale. Note the ECG tracing at the bottom of the image, which is used to identify the phases of the cardiac cycle. **(b)** M-mode echocardiogram recorded through the left ventricle at the level of the papillary muscles. Motion of the interventricular septum and left ventricular free wall is shown over many cardiac cycles. **(c)** PW Doppler echocardiogram of blood flow, obtained by placing the sample volume within the left ventricular outflow tract. Note that the envelope of the Doppler tracing is empty, indicating laminar blood flow during systole. The Doppler tracing is displayed below the baseline, indicating that blood flow is away from the transducer. **(d)** Colour flow Doppler echocardiogram recorded in a cat with a ventricular septal defect. Note the pyramid-shaped region of interest, in which colour Doppler is performed and superimposed on to the 2D image. Red indicates blood travelling towards the transducer; blue indicates blood travelling away from the transducer; and turbulent blood flow is displayed as a mosaic of colours. **(e)** CW Doppler echocardiogram recorded from a subcostal window in a dog with subaortic stenosis. Note that the Doppler flow profile is filled, indicating that many different blood flow velocities have been recorded along the ultrasound beam at the same time. LA = left atrium; LV = left ventricle; P = pericardium–lung interface; RA = right atrium; RV = right ventricle.

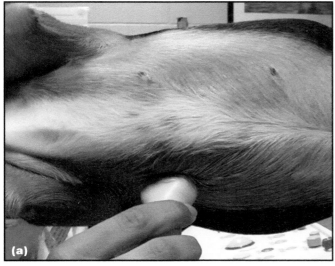

6.5 2D right parasternal long-axis views. **(a)** Transducer placement between the sternum and the costochondral junction at the level of the precordial impulse. The transducer is aligned with the long axis of the heart (from apex to base). In most dogs and cats, the long axis of the heart is along a line connecting the xiphoid process to the caudal border of the scapula at a 45-degree angle with the spine. On the monitor, the image should be oriented with the base of the heart to the right side of the screen, with the reference mark symbol on the top right side of the image and the reference index of the transducer pointing towards the heart base (i.e. oriented towards the patient's head in most cases). (continues) ▶

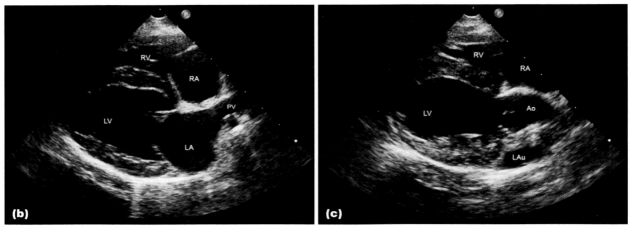

6.5 (continued) 2D right parasternal long-axis views. **(b)** The right parasternal long-axis 4-chamber view allows visualization of the right atrium (RA), right ventricle (RV), left atrium (LA) and left ventricle (LV). Note the pulmonary vein (PV) entering the left atrium. **(c)** The aortic root (Ao) and aortic valve are visualized from the right parasternal long-axis outflow view. Starting with the 4-chamber plane, the outflow view is obtained by tilting the transducer more vertically with a slight clockwise rotation when the animal is in right lateral recumbency. LAu = Left auricular appendage.

Short-axis views: Right parasternal short-axis views (Figure 6.6) are obtained with the animal and the probe in the same basic position as for the right parasternal long-axis view. Short-axis views are acquired by rotating the transducer 90 degrees towards the animal's sternum, so that the imaging plane is perpendicular to the long axis of the heart.

Left parasternal acoustic window
The animal is restrained in left lateral recumbency. Blood flow patterns are usually best assessed by Doppler ultrasonography from the left-sided window.

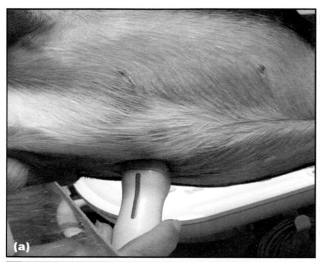

6.6 2D right parasternal short-axis views. **(a)** Transducer orientation with the ultrasound beam perpendicular to the long axis plane. The reference mark of the probe is oriented towards the animal's elbow. The transducer is positioned so that the pulmonary artery is visualized on the right side of the screen when the base of the heart is imaged. By sweeping the ultrasound beam between the apex and the base of the heart, the operator can examine various cardiac structures (displayed as successive 2D planes). **(b)** Left ventricular papillary muscle level. The right ventricle (RV; displayed at the top of the screen) has a crescent-shaped appearance and is positioned above the left ventricle (LV). The anterolateral (ventral) papillary muscle (PM) is visible on the right side of the screen; it may also be visualized on the right parasternal long-axis outflow view. The posteromedial (dorsal) papillary muscle is on the left side of the screen. **(c)** Mitral valve level. In this view the mitral valve looks like a 'fish mouth' in diastole. (continues) ▶

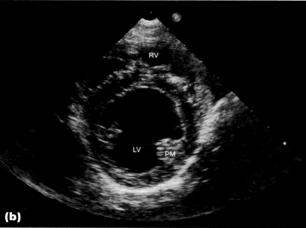

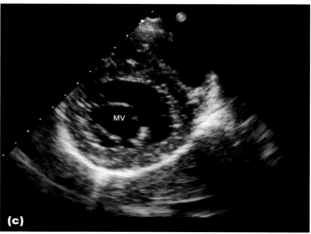

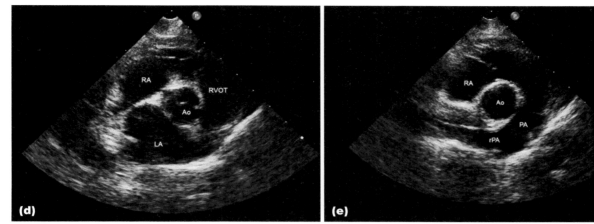

6.6 (continued) 2D right parasternal short-axis views. **(d)** Aorta level. The transducer is angled towards the base of the heart. In this view, the right atrium (RA), right ventricle and right ventricular outflow tract (RVOT) are visualized. The left atrium (LA) lies below the aorta (Ao). **(e)** Pulmonary artery level. With further tilting of the transducer, a view of the pulmonic valve and pulmonary artery (PA) with its bifurcation is obtained. rPA = right pulmonary artery.

Caudal (apical) views: Two standard views can be obtained from a left parasternal position: the left apical 4-chamber view and the left apical 5-chamber view (Figure 6.7).

Cranial views: From a left parasternal position, a long-axis view of the ascending aorta and a view of the pulmonary artery and its bifurcation can be obtained (Figure 6.8). The pulmonary artery view is very useful for visualization of patent ductus arteriosus (PDA) in dogs. From a cranial position, the transducer can be oriented caudally to obtain a view of the cranial and caudal venae cavae, the right atrium (see **Left cranial view of the right atrium** clip on DVD), the tricuspid valve and a portion of the right ventricular inflow.

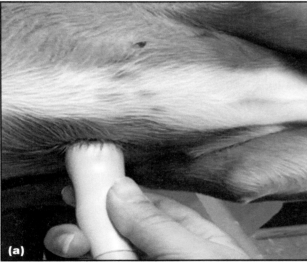

6.7 2D left caudal (apical) views. **(a)** The transducer is placed in the left intercostal space where the precordial impulse is palpated; usually the 6th intercostal space. This is also the region of the apex of the left ventricle. With the animal in left lateral recumbency, the transducer is placed on the left sternal border, held at a 30–40 degree angle to the animal's sagittal plane and oriented towards the left shoulder of the patient with the reference index facing the floor. With the transducer in this position, the heart is displayed upside down on the monitor, with the apex on top of the screen and the left cardiac chambers on the right side. **(b)** 4-chamber view. This view shows all four cardiac chambers, the interatrial septum, the interventricular septum and the atrioventricular valves. LA = left atrium; LV = left ventricle; RA = right atrium; RV = right ventricle. **(c)** 5-chamber view. This view allows visualization of the left ventricular outflow tract and the aorta (Ao).

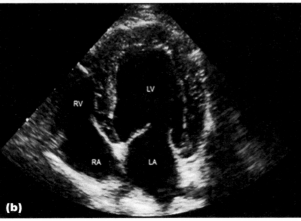

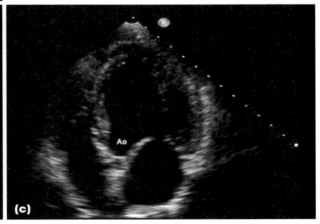

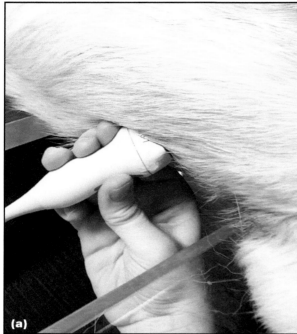

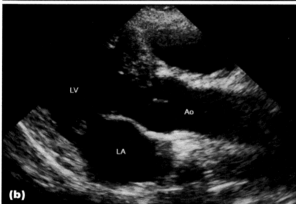

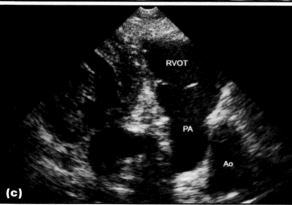

6.8 2D left cranial views. **(a)** The transducer is moved along the sternal border towards the left axillary region. The transducer is oriented towards the spine of the animal. **(b)** This view shows the long axis of the ascending aorta (Ao), the left ventricle (LV) and the left atrium (LA). The index mark of the transducer is directed towards the head of the animal and the transducer is kept in contact with the left sternal border. **(c)** This view allows visualization of the pulmonic valve and main pulmonary artery (PA). It requires the transducer to be held almost parallel to the animal's sagittal plane. Portions of the aortic root and descending aorta (Ao) are also visible. RVOT = right ventricular outflow tract.

Subcostal window

The only indication for using a subcostal approach is the measurement of blood flow velocity within the left ventricular outflow tract by continuous wave (CW) Doppler in dogs suspected to have subaortic stenosis. Peak aortic velocity is usually higher when recorded from the subcostal window compared with the left apical 5-chamber view. The heart is imaged by placing the transducer just caudal to the xiphoid process and orientating it cranially towards the head of the animal with the index mark within the mid-sagittal plane. The depth of the image is increased and a significant amount of manual pressure against the abdomen is usually necessary to display the heart in the far-field. The liver is seen in the near-field. When the transducer is adequately oriented, the left ventricular outflow tract and the long axis of the aortic root are visible.

Outcomes

At the end of an echocardiogram, the following questions should have been answered:

- What is the primary lesion?
- What is the likely aetiology of the primary lesion?
- Are there coexisting abnormalities?
- What is the size and function of all four cardiac chambers?
- What is the severity of the lesion (mild, moderate, severe)?

In addition, the initial echocardiographic assessment provides baseline information to determine the progression of the disease and monitor the response to treatment on follow-up examinations.

Equipment

Electrocardiogram

Ultrasound systems used for echocardiography should be equipped with ECG cables in order to display a continuous ECG tracing on the monitor during the examination. The electrodes should be connected to the limbs of the animal before the examination is started; lead II is usually recorded. Electrocardiographic waves help identify the diastolic (ventricular filling) and systolic (ventricular contraction) phases of the cardiac cycle.

Transducer selection

Transducers with a small contact surface are preferred to prevent shadowing artefacts from the ribs. Newer transducers use phased array technology. High frequency transducers provide better resolution in the near-field, whilst low frequency transducers facilitate the examination of deeper structures and usually provide the best colour Doppler signal. The optimal transducer frequency is therefore determined by the size of the animal: 8–10 MHz for cats and small-breed dogs; 5–8 MHz for medium-sized dogs; and 2–5 MHz for large-breed dogs.

Transducer manipulation

The ultrasound beam fans out of the transducer in a plane; its orientation is indicated by an index mark on the probe (Figure 6.9). The index mark is a plastic ridge on the transducer itself, so the operator holding the probe is aware of its position without having to look at the transducer. By convention, the location of the index mark on the transducer corresponds to the part of the image plane that appears on the right side of the screen.

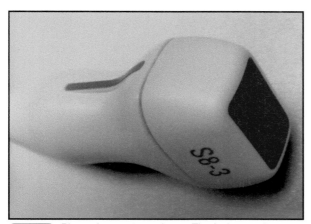

6.9 Phased-array transducer. The index mark on the transducer indicates the plane of the ultrasound beam.

Normal echocardiographic appearance

Initial screening
The examination starts from a right parasternal approach with qualitative assessment of the cardiac structures and function using real-time 2D echocardiography (Figure 6.10).

- The right atrium and left atrium are of similar size
- The diameter of the left atrium is 1–1.5 times the diameter of the aortic annulus
- The right ventricular internal diameter is approximately one-third of the left ventricular internal diameter in diastole
- The free wall of the right ventricle is equal to one-third or half the thickness of the left ventricular free wall
- The interventricular septum and the left ventricular free wall are similar in thickness
- The mitral valve leaflets should be thin, and should close on the plane of the mitral valve annulus in systole with no apparent bulging towards the left atrium
- The internal diameter of the left ventricle should decrease by 30–40% in systole compared with diastole
- For the experienced operator, a qualitative evaluation of ventricular contraction is usually sufficient to determine when cardiovascular dysfunction is present. This knowledge is only gained by frequent evaluation of normal animals

6.10 Qualitative evaluation of cardiac structure and function.

Left ventricle

Structure
The left ventricle is the largest cardiac chamber. It is conical in shape and forms the apex of the heart. The cavity of the left ventricle is divided into an inflow and an outflow region. The interventricular septum delimits the outflow tract medially, and the septal leaflet of the mitral valve forms an intermittent lateral boundary

at the base of the heart. There is no anatomical partition of the outflow tract in the apical and mid-ventricular regions. The outflow tract is best seen on the right parasternal long-axis outflow view and the left apical 5-chamber view. The interventricular septum separates the left ventricle from the right ventricle, and is best seen on the right parasternal long-axis view. It is thick and muscular for most of its length, but has a thin membranous part at the origin of the aorta.

Dimensions
Studies have shown that, in dogs, coefficients of variation of echocardiographic parameters vary between 3 and 26% and on average between 10 and 15% (Chetboul *et al.*, 2005). The level of expertise of the operator and external factors that can impair optimal image acquisition may further decrease the accuracy of these measurements. Therefore, measurements should be interpreted in conjunction with the qualitative assessment of cardiac structure and function, as well as the patient's history and physical examination.

Standard measurements include:

- Interventricular septum thickness
- Left ventricular internal diameter at end-diastole and end-systole
- Left ventricular free wall thickness at end-diastole and end-systole.

End-diastole occurs at the onset of the QRS complex on the ECG, which also corresponds to the frame following mitral valve closure or the frame in which the left ventricular internal diameter is at its maximum. End-systole occurs at the end of the T wave. In the absence of an ECG, systole coincides with the frame preceding mitral valve opening or the frame in which the left ventricular internal diameter is at its minimum. Measurements are made on the right parasternal short-axis view at the chordae tendinae level, either directly with callipers on a 2D still frame or on an M-mode image (Figure 6.11). Alternatively, the right parasternal long-axis view at the chordae tendinae level, just below the tip of the mitral valve, may be used (Figure 6.12). If an M-mode image is used to take measurements, the cursor should be placed perpendicular to the long axis of the left ventricle.

Allometric scaling on M-mode measurements in dogs
Mean left ventricle measurements (cm) in normal dogs can be predicted from bodyweight (BW, kg) (Cornell *et al.*, 2004)

Left ventricle internal diameter:
- Diastole = $1.53\ BW^{0.294}$
- Systole = $0.95\ BW^{0.315}$
Interventricular septum:
- Diastole = $0.41\ BW^{0.241}$
- Systole = $0.58\ BW^{0.240}$
Left ventricular free wall:
- Diastole = $0.42\ BW^{0.232}$
- Systole = $0.64\ BW^{0.222}$

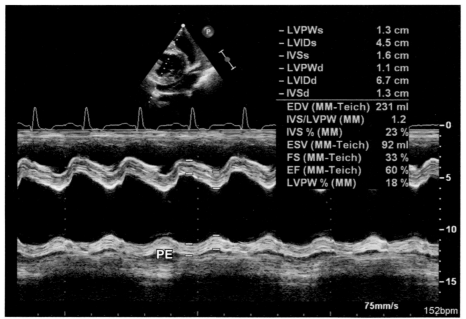

– LVPWs	1.3 cm
– LVIDs	4.5 cm
– IVSs	1.6 cm
– LVPWd	1.1 cm
– LVIDd	6.7 cm
– IVSd	1.3 cm
EDV (MM-Teich)	231 ml
IVS/LVPW (MM)	1.2
IVS % (MM)	23 %
ESV (MM-Teich)	92 ml
FS (MM-Teich)	33 %
EF (MM-Teich)	60 %
LVPW % (MM)	18 %

75mm/s   152bpm

6.11 M-mode echocardiogram of the left ventricle from a right parasternal short-axis view at the chordae tendinae level. The M-mode cursor is positioned perpendicular to the interventricular septum (IVS) and bisects the free (posterior) wall of the left ventricle between the papillary muscles. The left ventricular internal diameter at end-diastole (LVIDd) is measured at the onset of the QRS complex on the ECG. The left ventricular internal diameter at end-systole (LVIDs) is measured at the point of maximal posterior excursion of the interventricular septum. The shortening fraction (FS) is calculated from the LVIDd and LVIDs. The ejection fraction (EF) is automatically calculated using the Teichholz's formula (Teich), which is based on the cube formula with correction factors for the increasingly spherical shape of the ventricle with increasing dilatation. The interventricular septum wall thickness in diastole and systole, and the left ventricular posterior wall (LVPW) thickness in diastole and systole have also been measured. Note that the echolucent line at the epicardium–lung interface is consistent with a small amount of pericardial effusion (PE).

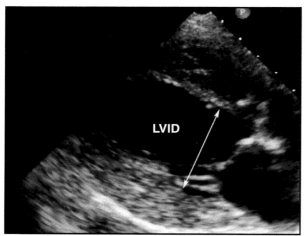

6.12 Right parasternal long-axis 4-chamber view showing measurement of the left ventricular internal diameter (LVID). The diameter is measured between the papillary muscles and the mitral valve, perpendicular to the long axis of the heart.

Function

Systolic function: Qualitative assessment of left ventricular function should be complemented with quantitative measurements (see Figure 6.11). In dogs and cats, left ventricular systolic function is usually determined by calculating the shortening fraction (FS) from linear measurements of the left ventricular internal diameter at end-diastole (LVIDd) and end-systole (LVIDs). Shortening fraction (expressed as a percentage) is calculated from the following formula:

$$FS = \frac{(LVIDd - LVIDs)}{LVIDd} \times 100$$

Example
An FS of 30% indicates that the left ventricular internal diameter is 30% smaller in systole than it is in diastole. In the author's echocardiography laboratory, normal dogs have an FS of 25–45%. However, it seems that the FS can be as low as 22–25% in normal large-breed dogs. The FS is around 40% in cats.

Changes in preload, afterload and left ventricular contractility affect the shortening fraction. Preload represents ventricular filling pressure during diastole. In normal animals, it corresponds to the end-diastolic volume. Afterload represents the resistance the left ventricle has to overcome during systole. In normal animals, an approximation of afterload is the arterial blood pressure. Contractility represents the inherent capacity of the left ventricle to contract independently from a change in end-diastolic volume or arterial blood pressure. The shortening and ejection fractions increase with increased preload, decreased afterload or increased contractility.

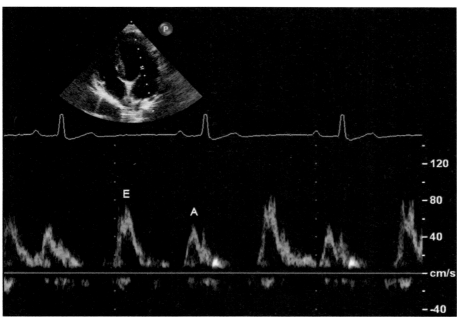

6.13 PW Doppler echocardiogram of the normal mitral valve inflow velocities. From the left apical 4-chamber view, the ultrasound beam is aligned parallel to the blood flow across the mitral valve. The sample volume is placed at the level of the tips of the mitral valve leaflets. Mitral valve inflow is recorded as a biphasic flow. The early rapid filling wave (E) is larger than the second wave resulting from atrial contraction (A).

Diastolic function: Diastole represents two-thirds of the cardiac cycle. Diastole refers to the filling phase of the ventricles. It starts with the closure of the aortic and pulmonic valves and the active relaxation of the ventricular myocardium. The filling phase starts with the opening of the atrioventricular valves when ventricular pressure decreases below atrial pressure. The filling phase is divided into an initial rapid phase and a slow phase. Diastole ends with atrial contraction, which contributes 10–20% of the left ventricular end-diastolic volume. Diastolic dysfunction is the cause of heart failure in cats with hypertrophic cardiomyopathy. It is present in addition to systolic dysfunction in dogs with dilated cardiomyopathy. Diastolic function can be assessed non-invasively by Doppler echocardiography. However, it is technically challenging to identify diastolic dysfunction. Doppler evaluation of mitral inflow is the most commonly used technique (Figure 6.13).

Right ventricle

Structure
The right ventricle has a complex geometry, described as crescent-shaped or pyramid-shaped. This, in addition to its smaller size and thinner walls, makes the echocardiographic assessment of the right ventricle difficult. The right ventricle chamber is divided into an inflow and an outflow region by a ridge of muscular tissue known as crista supraventricularis. Both regions cannot be fully examined on the same echocardiographic view. The inflow region is directly beneath the tricuspid valve. It is best assessed from the right parasternal long-axis 4-chamber view and the left apical 4-chamber view (see Figures 6.5b and 6.7b). The outflow region extends upward and to the left. It is best imaged from the right parasternal short-axis view at the level of the aorta and the left cranial short-axis views (see Figures 6.6d and 6.8c). Small papillary muscles originate from the apical portion of the interventricular septum.

Dimensions
In clinical practice, the assessment of the right ventricle is mostly qualitative (Figure 6.14). Measurements of the inflow portion of the right ventricle can also be obtained from the left apical 4-chamber view (Figure 6.15).

Severity of dilatation	Comments
Mild	Right ventricular width between 35 and 50% of the left ventricle
Moderate	Right ventricular width between 50 and 100% of the left ventricle
Severe	Right ventricle larger than the left ventricle

6.14 Qualitative assessment of right ventricle dilatation from the left apical and right parasternal 4-chamber views (Gordon *et al.*, 2009).

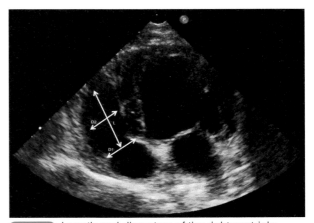

6.15 Length and diameters of the right ventricle inflow portion measured on an apical 4-chamber view. D1 represents the diameter of the right ventricle at the tricuspid valve annulus. D2 is the diameter of the right ventricle at the level of the left ventricular papillary muscles. L is the length of the right ventricular inflow portion from the tricuspid annulus to the apex.

Left atrium

Structure

The left atrium is positioned caudal to the aorta and above the left ventricle. It is divided into the body of the atrium and the auricular appendage. The auricular appendage is heavily trabeculated. It is best seen from a right parasternal short-axis view at the aortic valve level (see Figure 6.6d). Contraction of the left atrium delivers 15–30% of left ventricular filling. The left atrium receives blood from five to eight (usually seven) pulmonary veins, which enter the craniodorsal and caudodorsal parts of the chamber. They are usually not clearly visible on the echocardiogram, but pulmonary venous inflow can be identified and studied by pulsed wave (PW) Doppler ultrasonography. The interatrial septum separates the left atrium and the right atrium. The flap of the foramen ovale may be seen from a right parasternal long-axis 4-chamber view on the left atrial side in animals with a patent foramen ovale.

Dimensions

Linear measurements of the left atrium are used to calculate the left atrium to aortic ratio (LA/Ao). The LA/Ao ratio is independent of bodyweight (Figure 6.16). In normal dogs, the LA/Ao ratio is between 1.3 and 1.5. It is usually not greater than 1.6.

Right atrium

Structure

The right atrium is divided into a main chamber and the right auricular appendage. The right auricular appendage is difficult to image with transthoracic echocardiography. The right atrium receives blood from the caudal vena cava, the cranial vena cava and the coronary sinus. The cranial vena cava is difficult to assess on a 2D echocardiogram. Blood inflow can be identified by PW Doppler ultrasonography. The caudal vena cava can be imaged from a modified right parasternal short-axis view at the level of the aortic valve, and from an oblique view of the base of the heart with the transducer placed in a left cranial position (see **Left cranial view of the right atrium** clip on DVD). The coronary sinus is the dilated end of the great coronary vein (Figure 6.17).

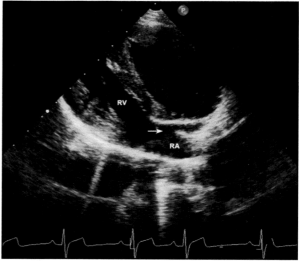

6.17 Modified left apical 4-chamber view obtained by tilting the transducer medially. The coronary sinus (arrowed) is seen as an echo-free linear structure opening in the right atrium (RA) at the level of the atrioventricular junction. A dilated coronary sinus is usually seen with cardiac conditions associated with elevated right atrial pressures. RV = right ventricle.

Dimensions

In clinical practice, qualitative assessment of the right atrium is made by comparing its size to the left atrium (Figure 6.18).

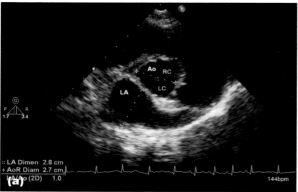

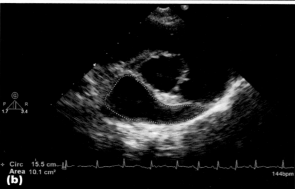

6.16 **(a)** Left atrial (LA) and aortic (Ao) diameters obtained from a right parasternal short-axis view at the level of the aortic valve. The measurement is made on the first frame following aortic valve closure. The aortic diameter is measured along the commissure between the left coronary and right coronary aortic valve cusps. The left atrial diameter is measured on the same frame on a line extending from and parallel to the commissure, between the non-coronary and left coronary aortic valve cusps to the blood–tissue interface of the left atrial wall. **(b)** Left atrial circumference and area can also be determined by tracing the contour of the atrium on a 2D frame. LC = left coronary cusp; RC = right coronary cusp.

Severity of enlargement	Comments
Mild	Area of the right atrium is between 100 and 150% of the left atrium
Moderate	Area of the right atrium is between 150 and 200% of the left atrium
Severe	Area of the right atrium is more than twice the size of the left atrium

6.18 Qualitative assessment of right atrial dilatation from the left apical and right parasternal 4-chamber views (Gordon *et al.*, 2009).

Cardiac valves

The echocardiographic appearance of the mitral valve, tricuspid valve, aorta and aortic valves, and pulmonary arteries and pulmonic valve are shown in Figures 6.19 to 6.22.

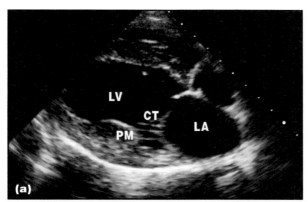

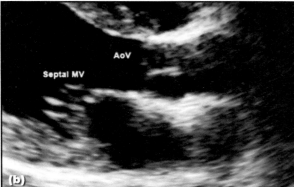

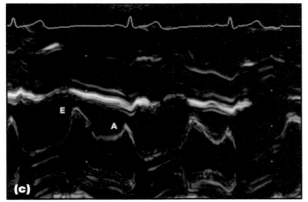

6.19 Mitral valve anatomy. **(a)** Right parasternal long-axis 4-chamber view recorded in early systole in a dog with normal mitral valve apparatus. The mitral valve apparatus comprises the parietal (posterior, caudal) and septal (anterior, cranial) leaflets, the annulus, the underlying left ventricular wall and the chordae tendinae (CT). Chordae tendinae are attached to the tip and mid portion of the leaflets and anchor them to the papillary muscles. **(b)** The septal leaflet of the mitral valve (MV) is continuous with the aortic valve (AoV) and together with the interventricular septum define the anatomical region of the left ventricular outflow tract. **(c)** M-mode recording of the mitral valve. The interrogation beam transects the tip of the leaflets. The septal leaflet motion follows a typical 'M' shape pattern in diastole. This corresponds to the valve opening during early diastole (E point), slowly returning to a closed position and re-opening during atrial contraction (A point). LA = left atrium; LV = left ventricle; PM = papillary muscles.

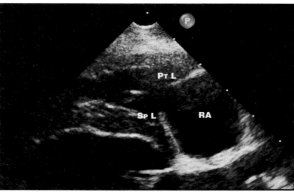

6.20 Tricuspid valve anatomy. Right parasternal long-axis view. The tricuspid valve apparatus consists of the parietal (PT L) and septal (SP L) leaflets, the tricuspid valve annulus, which is slightly more apical than the mitral valve annulus, and the chordae tendinae, which are much thinner in the right ventricle than in the left ventricle. Note that the tricuspid valve is made of only two leaflets in dogs and cats. RA = right atrium.

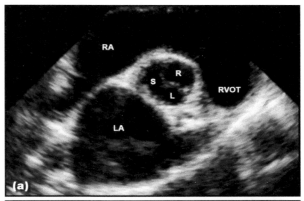

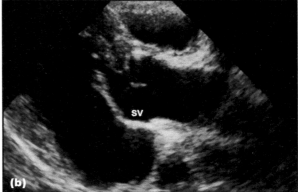

6.21 Aortic valve and aorta anatomy. **(a)** The three cusps are visualized from the right parasternal short-axis view at the level of the aortic valve. In this plane, the three lines of closure form a Y shape in diastole. Starting from the left coronary cusp (L), which faces the left auricular appendage, and rotating clockwise, there are the non-coronary cusp (S) and the right coronary cusp (R). The right cusp faces the right ventricular outflow tract (RVOT). The cusps are crescent-shaped. They open fully in systole and their commissures form a tight seal in diastole preventing backflow from the aorta into the left ventricle. **(b)** Three aortic sinuses or sinuses of Valsalva (SV) appear as dilatation of the aorta, just above the aortic valve. The left and right coronary arteries originate from the left and right sinuses, respectively. The ascending aorta is also visualized from this right parasternal long-axis outflow view. LA = left atrium; RA = right atrium.

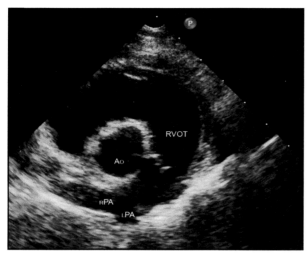

6.22 Pulmonic valve and pulmonary artery anatomy. The pulmonary trunk originates from the right ventricular outflow tract (RVOT). It wraps around the ascending aorta (Ao) with its medial surface in contact with the aortic wall. This is visualized best on a right parasternal short-axis view at the aortic valve level. The pulmonary trunk bifurcates into the right pulmonary artery (rPA), which leaves the main pulmonary artery at nearly a right angle, and the left pulmonary artery (LPA), which is shorter and more difficult to image on a transthoracic echocardiogram. The pulmonic valve is similar in structure to the aortic valve. The cusps of the valve are thinner than the aortic cusps, and are more difficult to image.

Congenital cardiac diseases

Patent ductus arteriosus

Patent ductus arteriosus (PDA) is a persistent communication between the cranial portion of the descending aorta and the main pulmonary artery at the level of its bifurcation.

Left-to-right shunting

PDA is the most common congenital cardiac defect in dogs. It is usually diagnosed during physical examination by the characteristic continuous machinery-type murmur, auscultated best in the left axillary region, and bounding femoral pulses. It is a hereditary disease with a higher prevalence in small-breed dogs (Toy and Miniature Poodles, Pomeranians, Maltese, Yorkshire Terriers). German Shepherd Dogs are also predisposed to this condition. PDA is rare in cats. PDA is usually present as an isolated defect; however, rarely, accompanying congenital cardiac defects are identified during the transthoracic echocardiographic examination.

In the fetus, the ductus arteriosus allows venous blood from the right ventricle to bypass the pulmonary circulation and the non-functional lungs. Blood flow from the right ventricle is directed into the descending aorta and is oxygenated in the placenta. Failure of the ductus to close shortly after birth results in left-to-right shunting, causing volume overload of the left ventricle and atrium. The degree of volume overload depends on the size of the PDA and the amount of blood re-circulating, as well as the age of the animal at diagnosis, because left ventricular

enlargement worsens with time. Pulmonary hypertension is another complication of large PDAs that have been left untreated, as the chronic increase in pulmonary blood flow causes vascular damage.

The presence of a PDA is usually confirmed by demonstrating continuous blood flow from the aorta into the main pulmonary artery on Doppler imaging (Figure 6.23; see also **Patent ductus arteriosus viewed from the left cranial window** clip on DVD). Direct visualization of the PDA can be obtained from a left parasternal cranial view (Figure 6.24). The ampulla diameter and minimal ductal diameter should be measured if transcatheter occlusion of the vessel is the selected treatment option. The minimal ductal diameter corresponds to the point of insertion of the PDA into the pulmonary artery. At the time of the procedure, better visualization of the PDA and more detailed measurements can be obtained by transoesophageal echocardiography (Figure 6.25; see also **Patent ductus arteriosus viewed from a transoesophageal approach** clip on DVD).

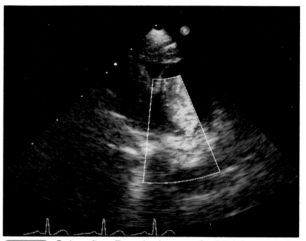

6.23 Colour flow Doppler image of a PDA from a left cranial view. Turbulent flow (displayed as a mosaic of colours) delineates the walls of the ductus. The colour jet narrows at the junction between the PDA and the main pulmonary artery. Laminar blood flow within the pulmonary artery is shown in blue.

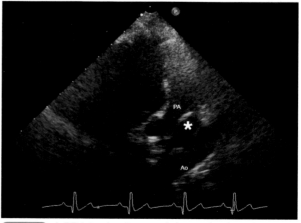

6.24 A PDA is clearly seen (*) opening into the pulmonary artery (PA) on this left parasternal cranial view. Note that part of the PDA seems to travel within the wall of the descending aorta (Ao).

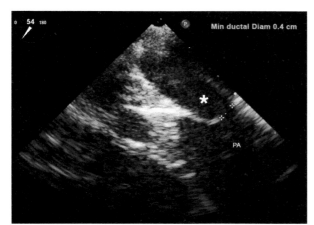

Min ductal Diam 0.4 cm

6.25 This view of a PDA (∗) was obtained by transoesophageal echocardiography with the transducer placed in a cranial position and oriented at 54 degrees. The minimal ductal diameter, which corresponds to the junction between the PDA and the pulmonary artery (PA), was measured prior to transcatheter occlusion of the PDA with a canine ductal occluder. Transoesophageal echocardiography can be used to assess placement of the occlusion device and the presence of residual blood flow (on colour Doppler imaging) prior to its release.

The magnitude of the left-to-right shunt and the clinical significance of the PDA are usually estimated indirectly by assessing the degree of left ventricle overload and severity of left atrial dilatation. In young dogs with moderate to severe shunting, left ventricular end-diastolic and end-systolic diameters are increased, and the shortening fraction is within normal limits (see **Patent ductus arteriosus** clip on DVD). The shortening fraction may decrease over time (Figure 6.26).

The presence of pulmonary hypertension may affect prognosis following occlusion of the PDA. Pulmonary artery pressure is estimated by measuring

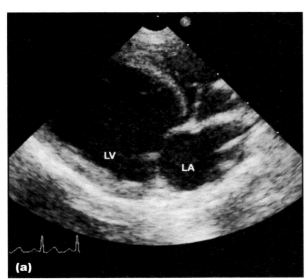

6.26 **(a)** Right parasternal long-axis 4-chamber view showing left ventricular (LV) and left atrial (LA) enlargement in a dog with a PDA. Note that left ventricular enlargement occurs sooner and is more pronounced than left atrial dilatation. However, with time, left atrial pressures increase, causing signs of left-sided congestive heart failure. (continues) ▶

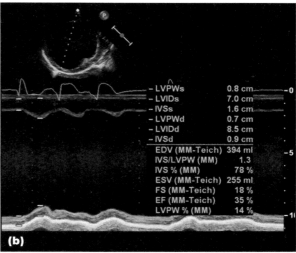

– LVPWs	0.8 cm
– LVIDs	7.0 cm
– IVSs	1.6 cm
– LVPWd	0.7 cm
– LVIDd	8.5 cm
– IVSd	0.9 cm
EDV (MM-Teich)	394 ml
IVS/LVPW (MM)	1.3
IVS % (MM)	78 %
ESV (MM-Teich)	255 ml
FS (MM-Teich)	18 %
EF (MM-Teich)	35 %
LVPW % (MM)	14 %

6.26 (continued) **(b)** M-mode image of the left ventricle of a 4-year-old, 15 kg dog with a PDA. There is severe left ventricular enlargement and a decreased shortening fraction. Note the irregular ECG rhythm caused by frequent ventricular premature beats. At this stage of the disease, it is still recommended to occlude or ligate the PDA. However, long-term prognosis is guarded.

the peak systolic pressure gradient across the PDA by CW Doppler (Figures 6.27 and 6.28). This can be undertaken from a right parasternal short-axis view at the level of the pulmonary artery, or more accurately from the left parasternal cranial view. CW Doppler (Figure 6.29) measures the peak velocity of blood as it reaches the main pulmonary artery. The pressure gradient is derived from the simplified Bernoulli equation:

Pressure gradient = 4 x peak velocity^2.

General information

- Pulsed wave and continuous wave Doppler echocardiography can be used to determine blood flow velocity
- Blood flow velocity across a stenotic area (e.g. stenotic valve, restrictive ventricular septal defect, mitral or tricuspid valve insufficiency) is proportional to the difference in pressure between the two cardiac chambers across the stenosis (e.g. left and right ventricles, left ventricle and left atrium)
- The simplified Bernoulli equation states that:

Pressure gradient = 4 x peak velocity^2

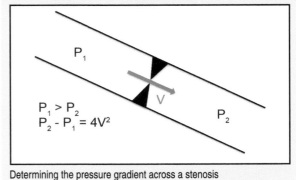

P_1

$P_1 > P_2$
$P_2 - P_1 = 4V^2$

P_2

V

Determining the pressure gradient across a stenosis

6.27 Use of Doppler echocardiography to measure pressure gradients. (continues) ▶

Application: determining the pulmonary artery pressure

- Systolic pulmonary artery pressure can be estimated if a jet of tricuspid valve regurgitation is present
- In systole, pulmonary artery pressure (PPA) is equal to right ventricular pressure
- It is important to confirm that there is no right ventricular outflow tract obstruction
- According to the simplified Bernoulli equation:

$$P_{RV} - P_{RA} = 4V_{TR}^2$$

Where:
P_{RA} = right atrial pressure
P_{RV} = systolic right ventricular pressure
V_{TR} = peak velocity of tricuspid valve regurgitation

$$P_{PA} = P_{RV}$$

Therefore: $P_{PA} = 4V_{TR}^2 + P_{RA}$

- V_{TR} is measured by continuous wave Doppler from an apical 4-chamber view
- P_{RA} can be measured invasively by placing a catheter in the right atrium. However, P_{RA} is usually estimated according to the size of the right atrium (Serres *et al.*, 2007):
  o Normal sized right atrium = 5 mmHg
  o Enlarged right atrium, no heart failure = 10 mmHg
  o Enlarged right atrium with right-sided heart failure = 15 mmHg
- Pulmonary hypertension is usually considered to be present when:
  o V_{TR} is >3 m/s, which corresponds to a P_{PA} of 35–40 mmHg. Tricuspid valve regurgitation is almost always present with pulmonary hypertension
  o Right ventricular free wall hypertrophy, interventricular septal flattening, right atrial dilatation and right ventricular dilatation are visualized by 2D echocardiography

6.27 (continued) Use of Doppler echocardiography to measure pressure gradients.

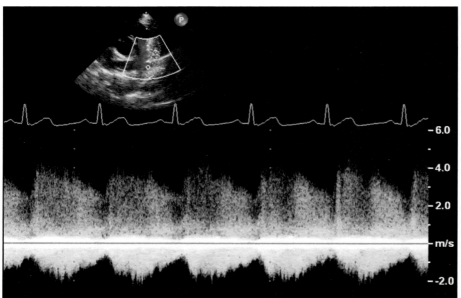

6.28 CW Doppler is used to measure the velocity of flow through a PDA from a left parasternal cranial view. The flow is continuous. The maximal flow velocity can be used to estimate the pressure gradient between the aorta and the pulmonary artery. In this case, a peak velocity of 4 m/s corresponds to a pressure gradient of 64 mmHg (using the simplified Bernoulli equation, see text for details), suggesting elevated pulmonary artery pressure. The normal pressure gradient is expected to be around 85 mmHg (peak systolic pressure in the aorta of 120 mmHg; peak systolic pressure in the pulmonary artery of 25 mmHg).

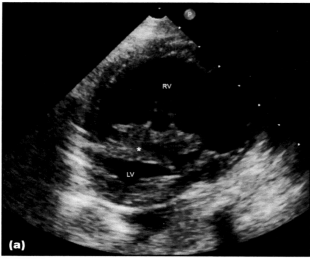

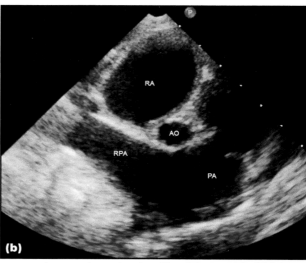

6.29 **(a)** Right parasternal short-axis view of a dog with severe pulmonary hypertension. The right ventricle (RV) is severely dilated and there is flattening of the interventricular septum (∗) throughout the cardiac cycle.
(b) Severe dilatation of the main pulmonary artery (PA) and right pulmonary artery (RPA) as visualized from a right parasternal view. AO = aorta; LV = left ventricle; RA = right atrium. (continues) ▶

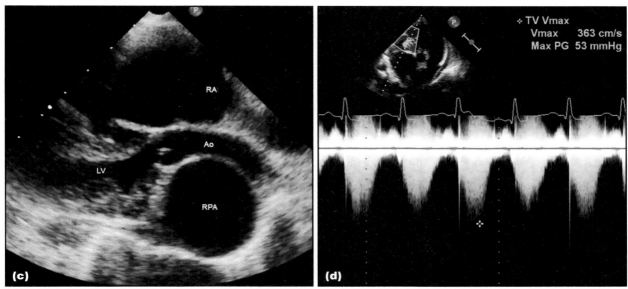

6.29 (continued) **(c)** A severely dilated right pulmonary artery (RPA) is visualized in cross-section from the right parasternal long-axis outflow view. Note that the right atrium (RA) is markedly dilated. **(d)** CW Doppler recording of a tricuspid valve regurgitant jet. The pressure gradient between the right ventricle and the aorta is estimated from the peak velocity of the tricuspid jet, measured at 53 mmHg. This indicates that pulmonary artery pressure is at least 53 mmHg. This is consistent with moderate pulmonary hypertension. Ao = aorta; LV = left ventricle.

Right-to-left shunting

A right-to-left shunting PDA is rarely diagnosed. Two conditions must be present for right-to-left shunting to occur. Firstly, a large PDA that does not taper on the pulmonary side, offering little or no resistance to blood flow, must be present. Secondly, the pulmonary artery pressure must approach systemic arterial pressure (Eisenmenger physiology). In many dogs, right-to-left shunting is most likely the consequence of the absence of a drop in pulmonary vascular resistance soon after birth. In these dogs, left-to-right shunting may never be present. In some dogs, pulmonary vascular obstructive disease develops as a consequence of a large pre-existing left-to-right shunt; a continuous murmur may be present initially and then disappears when the direction of flow reverses. Reversal of a left-to-right PDA is rare and almost always occurs in puppies.

Dogs with a right-to-left PDA are usually presented for signs associated with polycythaemia. Many dogs do not manifest clinical signs, but suspicion of a right-to-left PDA is raised by a high haematocrit in the absence of dehydration. The presence of differential cyanosis (i.e. cyanosis of the mucous membranes in the caudal region and normal mucous membrane colour cranially) is almost always diagnostic of a right-to-left PDA. Dogs with a right-to-left PDA do not have a murmur associated with blood flowing from the pulmonary artery to the descending aorta because the amount of blood shunting may be small. In addition, blood flow is laminar when the ductus does not taper and has a diameter similar to that of the aorta.

Echocardiographic signs of a right-to-left PDA include right ventricular hypertrophy associated with severe pulmonary hypertension. From a right parasternal short-axis view at the level of the papillary muscles, flattening of the septum is often noted in diastole. On a short-axis view at the level of the pulmonary artery, dilatation of the pulmonary artery is visible. Tricuspid valve regurgitation is usually present with severe pulmonary hypertension. CW Doppler interrogation of the jet of tricuspid valve insufficiency provides an estimate of the right ventricle to right atrium pressure gradient. The left atrium and left ventricle are small or normal size. Direct visualization of the PDA is possible, but usually difficult because of the absence of turbulent blood flow to detect its location by colour Doppler echocardiography. Agitated saline echocardiography is used to confirm the presence of an extracardiac right-to-left shunt (Figure 6.30; see also **Bubble study** clip on DVD). When a right-to-left PDA is present, microbubbles are visualized within the abdominal aorta following injection of agitated saline into a peripheral vein, despite the lack of intracardiac shunting.

- An indwelling peripheral venous catheter placed in the right cephalic vein or a saphenous vein facilitates the procedure
- 3–5 ml of 0.9% heparinized saline should be drawn up. It can be mixed with 0.5–1 ml of blood, which may increase the stability of the microbubbles
- Microbubbles are created by agitating the syringe vigorously, or by running the saline back and forth between two syringes connected to each other by a three-way stopcock
- The agitated saline is rapidly injected through the catheter. On a real-time right parasternal long-axis 4-chamber view of the heart, the contrast medium should only be visible in the right cardiac chambers. The size of the air-filled microbubbles prevents them from crossing the pulmonary capillary bed and reaching the left atrium. Contrast medium in the left cardiac chambers is consistent with a right-to-left intracardiac shunt

6.30 Preparation of agitated saline (see also **Bubble study** clip on DVD).

Abnormalities of cardiac septation

Atrial septal defects

An atrial septal defect (ASD) is a communication between the left and right atria, resulting from the incomplete closure of a portion of the interatrial septum. ASDs are rarely diagnosed in dogs and cats, although a recent study suggested the prevalence may be higher than previously thought. In the population studied, ASDs represented 37.7% of all congenital heart diseases diagnosed during a 4-year period (Chetboul *et al.*, 2006). In dogs, the prevalence is higher in Standard Poodles and Boxers.

Three types of ASD have been documented in dogs and cats (Figure 6.31):

- Ostium primum septal defects involve the lower portion of the atrial septum
- Ostium secundum septal defects are in the area of the fossa ovalis (i.e. the middle of the atrial septum). The vast majority of ASDs diagnosed in dogs and cats are of this type (Figure 6.32)
- Sinus venosus septal defects involve the upper portion of the atrial septum, near the junction of the septum with the cranial vena cava.

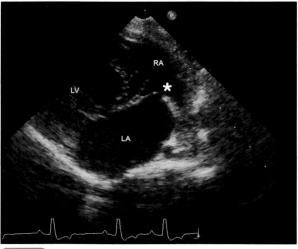

6.32 Echocardiogram showing an ASD (∗) in a dog with left atrial (LA) enlargement secondary to chronic degenerative mitral valve disease. The location of the defect is consistent with an ostium secundum defect. It is possible that marked stretching of the atrial septum may restore patency at the level of the foramen ovale, if the membrane of the foramen has not fused with the atrial septum soon after birth. LV = left ventricle; RA = right atrium.

The presence of an ASD usually results in a left-to-right shunt across the interatrial septum (Figure 6.33; see also **Atrial septal defect** clip on DVD). In normal conditions, left atrial pressure is higher than right atrial pressure. Moreover, the compliance of the left side of the heart is lower than the compliance of the right side of the heart, which facilitates shunting of blood into the right atrium and ventricle. However,

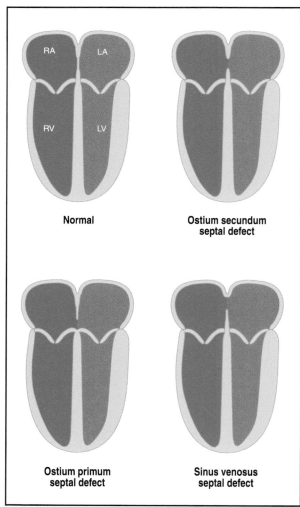

6.31 Different types of ASD. LA = left atrium; LV = left ventricle; RA = right atrium; RV = right ventricle.

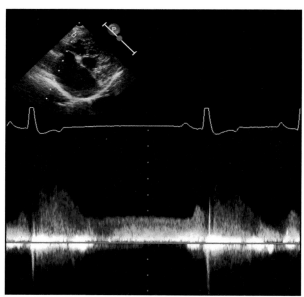

6.33 Left-to-right flow, demonstrated by Doppler imaging from a modified left apical view, in a dog with an ostium secundum ASD and a markedly enlarged left atrium secondary to mitral valve regurgitation. Note that left-to-right shunting increases following the P wave on ECG (i.e. atrial contraction). Shunting is also increased during ventricular systole. This is most likely due to elevated left atrial pressures caused by mitral valve regurgitation.

the direction of shunting can be reversed if pressure increases or compliance decreases in the right side of the heart. This may occur if tricuspid valve regurgitation or pulmonary hypertension develops.

Possible haemodynamic consequences of an ASD include volume overload of the right atrium and ventricle and pulmonary hypertension. Enlargement of the right atrium and ventricle depends on the volume of blood shunting from the left atrium to the right atrium. The size of the ASD and the differences in pressure and compliance between the left and right side of the heart determine the volume of shunt. Dogs with right-sided volume overload develop signs of right-sided heart failure, including ascites. Increased blood flow through the pulmonary circulation may promote pulmonary hypertension. This seems to be a rare occurrence in animals with ASDs.

Echocardiography is performed to assess the nature and haemodynamic consequences of the lesion. The right parasternal long-axis 4-chamber view provides the best visualization of the atrial septum. The left apical 4-chamber view may also provide a good image of the defect. However, the position of the septum parallel to the ultrasound beam may cause echo dropout in the region of the fossa ovalis and increase the number of false-positive results. Direct visualization of small ASDs can be challenging. Colour Doppler imaging of the atrial septum region from a right parasternal long-axis view may help identify blood flow across the septum.

The clinical significance of ASDs is based on qualitative assessment of the degree of enlargement of the right atrium and ventricle from a right parasternal long-axis 4-chamber view and a left apical 4-chamber view. Pulmonary hypertension is estimated by assessing the degree of right ventricular concentric hypertrophy, and measuring the pressure gradient across the tricuspid valve when tricuspid valve regurgitation is present. Clinically significant pulmonary hypertension is usually associated with detectable tricuspid valve regurgitation.

The direction of blood flow through an ASD is determined by injection of a small volume of agitated saline into a peripheral vein. Right-to-left shunting is identified by visualizing microbubbles crossing the interatrial septum. A small number of microbubbles can be seen crossing the interatrial septum in predominantly left-to-right ASDs because, for a short period of time during the cardiac cycle, atrial pressure or ventricular compliance may be lower in the left side than in the right side. Evidence of left-to-right shunting relies on the visualization of blood free from bubbles originating from the left atrium within the right atrium during the injection of agitated saline. This is called a negative contrast effect.

Ventricular septal defects

A ventricular septal defect (VSD) is an abnormal communication between the left and right ventricles at various levels within the interventricular septum. VSDs represent the most common congenital heart disease in the human paediatric population, but their prevalence is much lower in dogs and cats. English Springer Spaniels are predisposed to VSDs.

Anatomically, VSDs are classified as:

- Perimembranous or membranous
- Muscular.

Membranous or perimembranous defects are located in the membranous portion of the septum. Perimembranous VSDs have extensions into the trabecular, inlet or outlet region of the septum. On the left side they are located just below the aortic valve, and on the right side they are adjacent to the septal leaflet of the tricuspid valve. They represent the vast majority of the VSDs identified in dogs and cats.

Muscular VSDs are bordered entirely by myocardial tissue. They can be further classified as trabecular, inlet or outlet VSDs.

- The trabecular septum extends from the membranous septum to the cardiac apex.
- The inlet septum is posterior to the membranous septum and between the mitral and tricuspid valves.
- The outlet septum is anterior to the membranous septum and between the trabecular septum and the great arteries. VSDs in this portion of the septum are described as supracristal. They are situated just below the aortic valve on the left side and the pulmonic valve on the right side.

VSDs are also described as restrictive or non-restrictive. Restrictive VSDs are small in size and provide high resistance to blood flow. They do not interfere with the pressure gradient that normally exists between the left and right ventricles, but allow left-to-right shunting of blood during systole. A small amount of blood may flow in diastole. Restrictive VSDs may result in left-sided volume overload, as blood shunting across the VSD re-circulates to the left side of the heart, but this is not usually the case. The defect is typically located just below the aortic valve and may result in progressive aortic valve regurgitation caused by the prolapse of an aortic cusp through the defect. This is a more common complication.

Non-restrictive VSDs are large in size and do not offer resistance to blood flow. There is therefore equalization of pressures between the left and the right ventricles. Non-restrictive VSDs are associated with severe pulmonary hypertension, and may result in severe left ventricular volume overload if pulmonary vascular resistance is significantly lower than systemic resistance. More commonly, they result in right-to-left shunting across the defect because of progressive development of pulmonary vascular disease (Eisenmenger physiology). Spontaneous closure of VSDs is rare in dogs.

Echocardiography is performed to assess the location, size and haemodynamic consequences of the VSD. Most VSDs are first detected with colour flow Doppler, which displays the rapid and turbulent jet of blood across the VSD.

- Perimembranous VSDs can usually be identified on a right parasternal short-axis view. They are located just below the tricuspid valve at the 10 o'clock position (see **Ventricular septal defect (1)** clip on DVD).

- Outlet VSDs are located between the 12 and 2 o'clock position, usually just below the pulmonic valve. Due to the complex 3-dimensional (3D) shape of the interventricular septum, multiple echocardiographic views are necessary to fully assess the defect. Outlet and perimembranous VSDs can be seen on a right parasternal long-

axis outflow view (Figure 6.34a; see also **Ventricular septal defect (2)** clip on DVD) and a left apical 5-chamber view. The right parasternal short-axis view allows differentiation between perimembranous and outlet VSDs (Figure 6.34f).
- Inlet VSDs are visualized from a left apical 4-chamber view.

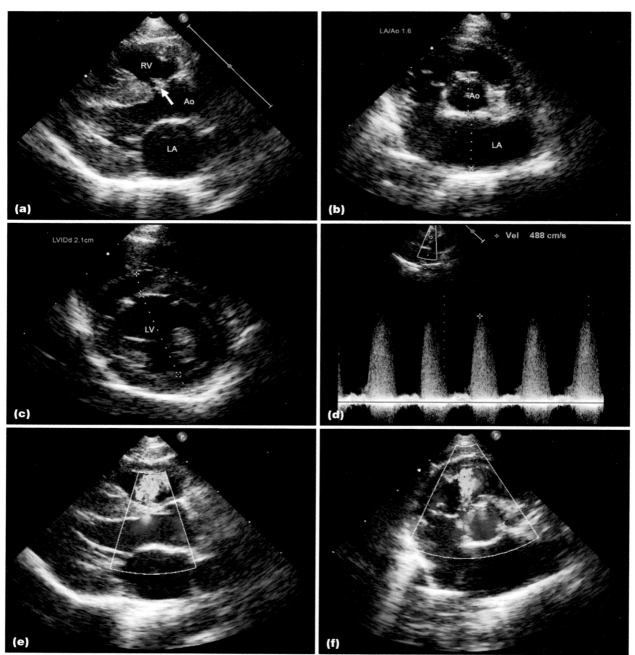

6.34 Restrictive perimembranous VSD in a cat. **(a)** The VSD (arrowed) is visualized just below the aortic valve (Ao) on a right parasternal long-axis outflow view. The left atrium (LA) appears to be mildly dilated. **(b)** The clinical significance of a VSD is determined by calculating the left atrial (LA) to aortic (Ao) diameter ratio from a right parasternal short-axis view. A LA/Ao ratio of 1.6 indicates mild atrial enlargement. **(c)** Linear measurements of the interventricular septum, left ventricular internal diameter in diastole (LVIDd) and left ventricular free wall can be obtained using this image. The LVIDd is 2.1 cm, which is consistent with moderate left ventricular (LV) dilatation (normal LVIDd in cats is approximately 1.3 cm). **(d)** Blood flow velocity (Vel) is measured across the defect using CW Doppler. The pressure gradient between the ventricles is determined using the simplified Bernoulli equation. In this case the pressure gradient was 95.3 mmHg. **(e)** Colour Doppler imaging confirms the presence of a VSD. The dimensions of the colour flow jet across the defect may provide an estimate of the size of the VSD. **(f)** The position of the VSD at 10 o'clock and the blood flow turbulence across the defect, as shown by Doppler imaging from a right parasternal short-axis view at the level of the left ventricular outflow tract, confirm that the VSD is perimembranous and restrictive. RV = right ventricle.

The size of the VSD can be compared with the diameter of the aortic annulus. Small VSDs are <25%, moderate VSDs are between 25 and 75% and large VSDs are >75% of the diameter of the aortic annulus.

Various parameters are assessed to determine the clinical significance of restrictive VSDs. The direction and velocity of blood flow across small defects is recorded using Doppler imaging. Colour Doppler echocardiography is used to scan the surface of the interventricular septum from different views, and can demonstrate a left-to-right turbulent, high velocity jet during systole (Figure 6.34e). The velocity of blood flow across a perimembranous defect can usually be measured accurately using CW Doppler from a right parasternal short-axis or right parasternal long-axis outflow view (Figure 6.34d). The beam should be oriented as parallel as possible to the blood flow. Blood flow velocity measurements, as recorded by CW Doppler, can be used to estimate the pressure gradient across the defect using the simplified Bernoulli equation. The normal pressure gradient between the ventricles is around 100 mmHg (which corresponds to blood flow velocity of approximately 5 m/s).

The size of the restrictive VSD relates to the risk of left ventricular volume overload and congestive heart failure. However, clinical significance is better determined by measuring the size of the left-sided cardiac chambers. Follow-up examinations are usually necessary to evaluate the long-term haemodynamic consequences of a VSD. Most small VSDs are not clinically significant (Figure 6.34bc). Finally, it is important to assess the structure and motion of the aortic valve for signs of cusp prolapse and aortic valve insufficiency. This is a complication that may lead to left ventricular volume overload secondary to aortic valve insufficiency.

Right-to-left VSDs are large and directly visualized on 2D transthoracic echocardiography. They are typically associated with severe pulmonary hypertension, and on occasion pulmonic stenosis, which results in marked concentric hypertrophy of the right ventricular free wall and hypertrophy of the right ventricular papillary muscles, flattening of the interventricular septum and dilatation of the pulmonary arteries. Right-to-left shunting is confirmed by injection of agitated saline into a peripheral vein. After injection, microbubbles can be identified within the left ventricle.

Aortic stenosis

Aortic stenosis is an obstruction of the left ventricular outflow tract that can occur at the subvalvular, valvular and supravalvular levels. Subvalvular stenosis is caused by a fibrous membrane or a fibromuscular narrowing of the left ventricular outflow tract just below the aortic annulus. The fibrous ring may extend to the septal leaflet of the mitral valve. Subaortic stenosis is usually an isolated congenital heart disease, and is one of the most common congenital defects in dogs. It is more common in large-breed dogs; Boxers, Golden Retrievers, Newfoundlands and Rottweilers are over-represented. The severity of the stenosis typically worsens from birth until 12 months of age.

Subaortic stenosis results in left ventricular concentric hypertrophy, secondary to pressure overload and decreased perfusion of the left ventricle when severe hypertrophy is present. As a result, ventricular arrhythmias are frequently detected. In some dogs, subaortic stenosis progresses to myocardial failure and secondary mitral valve insufficiency. Valvular stenosis results from abnormal valve development. The cusps are usually partially fused. In the case of a dysplastic valve, the cusps are thickened and poorly mobile. Valvular aortic stenosis is uncommon. Supravalvular stenosis is extremely rare.

Echocardiography is indicated to assess the nature and haemodynamic consequences of subaortic stenosis. Evidence of subaortic stenosis is first obtained by colour flow Doppler scanning of the left ventricular outflow tract region, which reveals turbulent blood flow. Mild aortic valve insufficiency usually accompanies subaortic stenosis. Mild aortic valve regurgitation is visualized by colour flow Doppler from the right parasternal long-axis outflow tract view and the left apical 5-chamber view (Figure 6.35; see also **Subaortic stenosis (1)** and **(2)** clips on DVD). Echocardiography may also reveal subaortic narrowing and post-stenotic dilatation of the ascending aorta. A fibrous ridge may be visualized as a discrete linear echo within the left ventricular outflow tract (Figure 6.36). The membrane is detected more

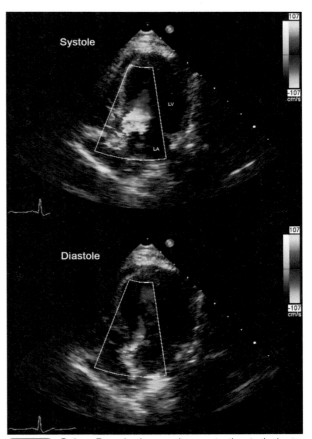

6.35 Colour Doppler image demonstrating turbulent systolic flow in the left ventricular outflow tract of a dog with subaortic stenosis. A mild degree of aortic valve regurgitation was visualized in diastole. LA = left atrium, LV = left ventricle.

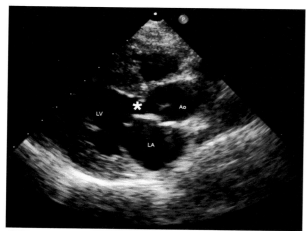

6.36 Right parasternal long-axis outflow view showing a ridge of fibrous tissue (*) just below the aortic valve (Ao). LA = left atrium; LV = left ventricle.

easily from an apical view because it is perpendicular to the ultrasound beam. However, small lesions may not be visible on 2D echocardiography.

The severity of the subaortic gradient is determined by CW Doppler from the left apical 5-chamber view. The subcostal window (Figure 6.37) can also be used because it allows perfect alignment of the ultrasound beam with blood flow in the left ventricular outflow tract, and has been shown to provide the maximal velocity values. A low frequency transducer is often required because of the increased distance (depth) between the transducer and the heart from this window. The severity of the stenosis is based on the magnitude of the peak systolic pressure gradient across the stenosis (Bussadori *et al.*, 2000).

- Mild stenosis corresponds to a peak gradient of 20–49 mmHg (velocity of 2.25–3.5 m/s).
- Moderate stenosis is defined as a peak gradient of 50–80 mmHg (velocity of 3.5–4.5 m/s).
- Severe stenosis corresponds to a peak gradient >80 mmHg (velocity >4.5 m/s).

Concentric hypertrophy is present with moderate to severe subaortic stenosis (see **Subaortic stenosis (3)** and **(4)** clips on DVD). This is confirmed by measuring left ventricular and interventricular wall thickness on a 2D or M-mode image (Figure 6.38).

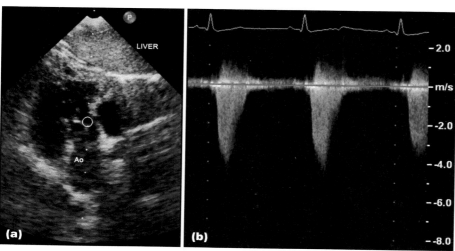

6.37 **(a)** The ascending aorta (Ao) visualized from a subcostal window. Blood flow is perfectly aligned with the ultrasound beam. **(b)** CW Doppler image demonstrating a peak velocity of 4 m/s, consistent with a peak pressure gradient of 64 mmHg across the stenosis.

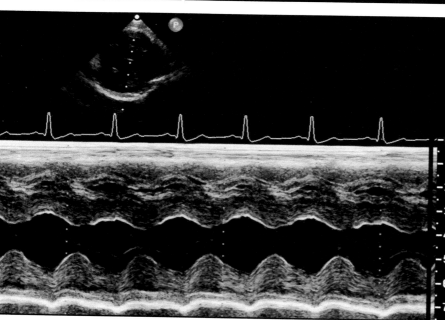

6.38 M-mode echocardiogram of a dog with severe subaortic stenosis demonstrating concentric hypertrophy of the interventricular septum and left ventricular free wall.

Pulmonic stenosis

Pulmonic stenosis is an obstruction of the right ventricular outflow tract. It may occur at subvalvular, valvular or supravalvular levels. Subvalvular stenosis is rare, and is always associated with valvular lesions (Figure 6.39; see also **Pulmonic stenosis (1)** clip on DVD). A coronary artery anomaly (R2A) is found in some breeds, mainly Bulldogs and Boxers. In these dogs, coronary supply to the left ventricle originates from the right coronary artery. The artery circles in front of the pulmonary outflow tract in the subvalvular region. Rupture of the vessel may occur when balloon valvuloplasty is performed to treat the valvular stenosis (Figure 6.40).

Valvular stenosis is the most common form of pulmonic stenosis. It is more common in small-breed dogs, and is known to be hereditary in Beagles. Two forms of valvular stenosis are described. In the most common form, there is commissural fusion of the cusps, which gives the valve a dome-like shape with a narrowed orifice. The valve annulus is normal in size. There is marked post-stenotic dilatation with moderate to severe disease (see **Pulmonic stenosis (2)** clip on DVD). The dysplastic form is associated with thick leaflets and hypoplasia of the pulmonary valve annulus. Post-stenotic dilatation of the pulmonary artery is usually absent. Supravalvular stenosis is extremely rare.

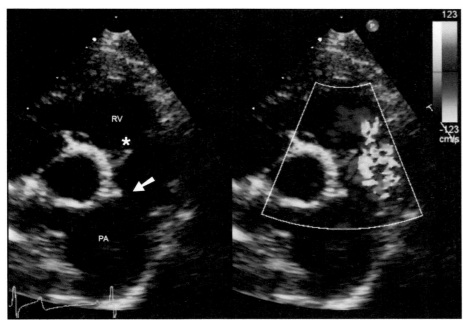

6.39 Subvalvular and valvular stenosis in a dog. A fibromuscular area of stenosis (∗) is visible in the right ventricular outflow tract region from a right parasternal short-axis view. Valvular stenosis (arrowed) is also present. There is marked post-stenotic dilatation of the main pulmonary artery (PA). The colour Doppler image shows the turbulent blood flow originating at the level of the subaortic region. RV = right ventricle.

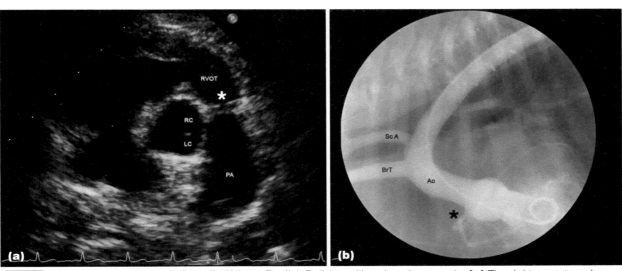

6.40 Coronary artery anomaly (type R2A) in an English Bulldog with pulmonic stenosis. **(a)** The right parasternal short-axis view at the level of the aorta (Ao) reveals a large coronary artery, originating at the level of the right coronary cusp (RC) and travelling in from the right ventricular outflow tract (RVOT), just below the valve. This may be an echocardiographic sign of a coronary anomaly. However, it is common for dogs with severe pulmonic stenosis to have a dilated right coronary artery. An angiogram is usually necessary to confirm the suspicion. Note the post-stenotic dilatation of the main pulmonary artery (PA). **(b)** Aortic root angiogram showing the main left coronary artery (∗) branching from the origin of the right coronary artery. No artery is seen originating from the left sinus of Valsalva. BrT = brachiocephalic trunk; LC = left coronary cusp; ScA = subclavian artery.

The haemodynamic effects of pulmonic stenosis result in concentric hypertrophy of the right ventricular free wall and ventricular papillary muscles in response to a fixed right ventricular outflow tract obstruction. Right ventricular and right atrial volume overload may occur in older animals, when the obstruction is extreme, or if concurrent tricuspid valve insufficiency is present. The severity of the stenosis does not worsen during the first year of life.

In the case of valvular stenosis, 2D echocardiography is used to determine whether the stenosis results from fused cusps or a dysplastic valve. This is best visualized in a right parasternal short-axis view at the level of the pulmonary artery (Figure 6.41). To determine whether annular hypoplasia is present,

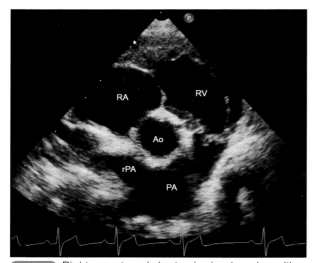

6.41 Right parasternal short-axis view in a dog with valvular pulmonic stenosis. There is mild thickening of the valvular cusps. A post-stenotic bulge of the main pulmonary artery (PA) is present. The dog was diagnosed with severe pulmonic stenosis. However, the right ventricular (RV) hypertrophy is only moderate. The right atrium (RA) is mildly dilated. Ao = aorta; rPA = right pulmonary artery.

the diameter of the pulmonary annulus is measured and compared with the aortic annulus. Normally, the pulmonary valve annulus is similar in size to the aortic annulus (ratio of 1).

Doppler echocardiography is essential to determine the severity of the stenosis. CW Doppler is used to determine the peak systolic pressure gradient across the stenosis (Figure 6.42). Good alignment of the Doppler beam with blood flow can usually be obtained from the right parasternal short-axis view at the level of the pulmonary artery, or from a left cranial window along the sternum. The severity of the stenosis is based on peak systolic pressure gradient.

- Mild stenosis corresponds to a peak gradient of 20–49 mmHg (velocity of 2.25–3.5 m/s).
- Moderate stenosis is defined as a peak gradient of 50–80 mmHg (velocity of 3.5–4.5 m/s).
- Severe stenosis corresponds to a peak gradient of >80 mmHg (velocity >4.5 m/s).

Right ventricular size and function is assessed qualitatively by 2D echocardiography.

Importantly, right ventricular wall thickness does not always correlate well with the severity of the stenosis; therefore, Doppler echocardiography is essential to determine the severity of the stenosis.

Atrioventricular valve dysplasia

Tricuspid valve
Tricuspid valve dysplasia is a malformation of the tricuspid valve leaflets, chordae tendinae and right ventricular papillary muscles. Labradors and Boxers are most commonly affected. Tricuspid valve dysplasia is associated with variable degrees of tricuspid valve regurgitation. Right ventricular and atrial volume overload occur in dogs with severe disease.

On echocardiography, tricuspid valve dysplasia is best assessed from the right parasternal long-axis 4-chamber view (Figure 6.43) and the left apical

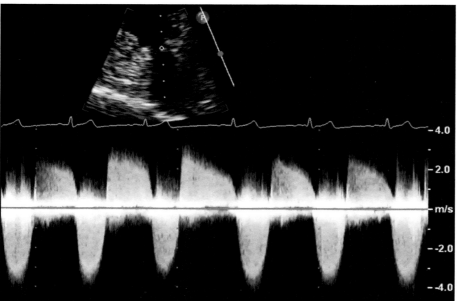

6.42 CW Doppler image through the right ventricular outflow tract and the pulmonic valve of a dog with pulmonic stenosis. The peak pressure gradient in systole is approximately 64 mmHg (peak velocity of 4 m/s). Note that pulmonic valve insufficiency is also present.

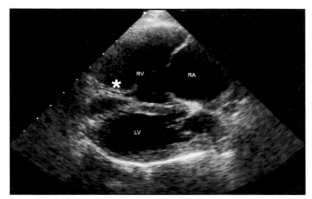

6.43 Right parasternal long-axis 4-chamber view, revealing severe dilatation of the right atrium (RA) and right ventricle (RV) in a dog with tricuspid valve dysplasia. The anterior leaflet of the valve is elongated. Note the hypertrophied moderator band (∗). LV = left ventricle.

4-chamber view. A dysplastic valve is characterized by elongated and redundant leaflets with abnormal chordal attachment. Ebstein anomaly describes a form of tricuspid valve dysplasia characterized by apical displacement of the tricuspid valve annulus. This is best assessed from the apical 4-chamber view. It is important to note that the tricuspid valve annulus is normally positioned more apically than the mitral valve. 2D echocardiography is also used to qualitatively assess the dimensions of the right ventricle (see **Tricuspid valve dysplasia (1)** clip on DVD). Severity of the disease is based on the degree of enlargement of the right atrium. The right atrium is severely dilated when it appears significantly larger than the left atrium.

Tricuspid valve regurgitation is always present with tricuspid valve dysplasia. Colour and CW Doppler are used to evaluate its severity and peak velocity (see **Tricuspid valve dysplasia (2)** clip on DVD). The severity of tricuspid valve regurgitation can be assessed by comparing the size of the colour jet to the area of the atrium on a 2D image. The regurgitation is severe if it covers >50% of the surface of the atrium (Figure 6.44). The peak velocity of tricuspid valve regurgitation may be decreased if right atrial pressures are markedly increased.

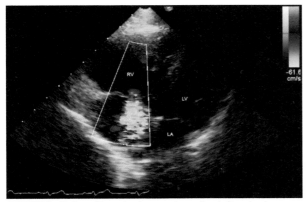

6.44 Colour Doppler image from the left apical 4-chamber view in a dog with tricuspid valve dysplasia. A large jet of tricuspid valve regurgitation covers approximately 50% of the area of the right atrium. LA = left atrium; LV = left ventricle; RV = right ventricle.

Mitral valve

Mitral valve dysplasia is a term used in veterinary cardiology to describe primary mitral valve regurgitation in the absence of signs of mitral valve endocardiosis or endocarditis. Secondary mitral valve regurgitation as a result of annular dilatation or papillary muscle displacement, which is commonly associated with dilated cardiomyopathy, should also be ruled out. 2D imaging of the mitral valve apparatus may reveal short and thick leaflets, long and thin chordae tendinae, or an abnormal attachment of the leaflets to the chordae (Figure 6.45). Moderate to severe mitral valve regurgitation is usually present on colour Doppler imaging. Finally, decreased left ventricular systolic function may be observed from the right parasternal approach in large-breed dogs with severe mitral valve insufficiency.

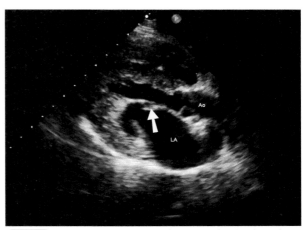

6.45 2D echocardiogram of the mitral valve in a dog with mitral valve dysplasia. The elongated septal leaflet (arrowed) is connected to the papillary muscle by short and thick chordae tendinae. Ao = aorta; LA = left atrium.

Complex diseases

Tetralogy of Fallot

Tetralogy of Fallot is the most common cyanotic congenital cardiac disorder in small animals. It is rarely diagnosed and has been reported more frequently in dogs than cats. It is a hereditary disorder in Keeshonds. The defects that make up the complex anomaly include a large non-restrictive VSD, right ventricular outflow tract obstruction, rightward displacement of the aorta (dextroposition) and secondary right ventricular concentric hypertrophy. In this condition, the large VSD offers no resistance to blood flow. The direction of blood flow is determined by the resistance of the pulmonary *versus* the systemic circulation. Due to the presence of pulmonic stenosis, right-to-left shunting is normally present, and this is responsible for central cyanosis and polycythaemia.

On echocardiography, the VSD and the overriding of the aorta are visualized from the right parasternal long-axis view. Up to 50% of the aorta overlies the right ventricle. If >50% of the aorta overlies the right ventricle, the disorder is called double-outlet right ventricle. The right ventricular outflow tract is best assessed from the right parasternal short-axis view.

The stenosis is usually subvalvular as a result of the displacement of the infundibular septum. Valvular stenosis may also be present. CW Doppler interrogation of flow in the right ventricular outflow tract is used to determine the pressure gradient across the stenosis. Right ventricular concentric hypertrophy and septal flattening are assessed from 2D views. Direction of blood flow across the VSD can be determined by injection of agitated saline. However, the animal's haematocrit is a better indicator of the degree and chronicity of the right-to-left shunting.

Persistent truncus arteriosus

Persistent truncus arteriosus is characterized by a single great vessel originating from the base of the heart, which then divides into pulmonary and systemic vessels. The unique vessel overrides a large non-restrictive VSD. This condition has rarely been described in dogs and cats. Visualization of a large VSD and a single large vessel that overlies the septum is usually obtained from a right parasternal long-axis view. The posterior wall of the great artery is continuous with the septal leaflet of the mitral valve. The pulmonary vessels originate from the unique vessel. If they arise from the vessel as a pulmonary trunk, which then bifurcates into the left and right pulmonary arteries, the defect is described as a type 1 truncus. The defect is classified as a type 2 truncus if the left and right pulmonary arteries originate independently, but in close proximity, from the posterior wall of the unique vessel. The defect is classified as a type 3 truncus if the pulmonary arteries originate independently from the lateral sides of the vessel.

Atrioventricular canal defect

Atrioventricular canal (endocardial cushion) defects combine an ostium primum septal defect, an inlet VSD and structural abnormalities of the atrioventricular valves. The defect is described as partial (or incomplete) if there are two distinct atrioventricular orifices. It is called complete if there is one large orifice and an atrioventricular valve made up of multiple leaflets, including two large leaflets bridging the VSD. 2D echocardiography is used to identify the structural abnormalities. Colour Doppler imaging commonly reveals significant atrioventricular valve insufficiency. Saline injection is used to determine the direction of flow across the septal defects. The degree of cardiac chamber enlargement depends upon the severity of the atrioventricular valve regurgitation, blood shunting and the presence of pulmonary hypertension.

Cor triatriatum

Cor triatriatum is the partition of the left or right atrium by a fibrous membrane. Partition of the left atrium, or cor triatriatum sinister, occurs in cats. Partition of the right atrium, or cor triatriatum dexter, occurs in dogs. Identification of the membrane, as a hyperechoic line within the atrium, is usually readily made using 2D echocardiography. On the left side, the membrane divides the atrium into a superior chamber that receives blood from the pulmonary veins, and a bottom chamber that communicates

with the mitral valve. On the right side, the caudal chamber receives blood from the caudal vena cava and usually the coronary sinus. The cranial vena cava enters the cranial chamber that communicates with the tricuspid valve. Colour Doppler imaging is used to identify blood shunting between the two atrial chambers. In the left atrium the membrane is usually perforated; however, in the case of cor triatriatum sinister, the membrane is occasionally not perforated. Venous blood from the caudal half of the body usually reaches the heart via the azygous vein.

Acquired valvular diseases

Endocardiosis

Valvular endocardiosis, also known as chronic degenerative mitral valve disease or myxomatous valvular disease, is the most common acquired cardiovascular disease in small dogs. Moreover, it is the most common cause of left-sided congestive heart failure in dogs. Valvular endocardiosis is a chronic disease that develops with age. Its rate of progression from mild to severe varies markedly between dogs. It is known that Cavalier King Charles Spaniels develop the disease at a younger age than other breeds. The disease is also more common in males than females.

Myxomatous thickening of the mitral valve leaflets allows regurgitation of blood from the left ventricle into the left atrium during systole. This regurgitation results in volume overload of the left-sided cardiac chambers and subsequent dilatation of the left ventricle and left atrium. Elevated left atrial pressure promotes pulmonary congestion and secondary pulmonary hypertension. Tricuspid valve leaflet prolapse and lesions of endocardiosis on the tricuspid valve are commonly present at the same time. Tricuspid valve insufficiency is also frequently present (see **Tricuspid valve prolapse** and **Tricuspid valve regurgitation** clips on DVD).

Echocardiography is performed to describe the structure of the mitral valve apparatus. Mitral valve prolapse is generally present in dogs with endocardiosis. It is best visualized from the right parasternal long-axis 4-chamber view or the left apical 4-chamber view. There is prolapse when one or two leaflets break the plane of the mitral annulus and bulge into the left atrium (Figure 6.46). In addition, mitral valve thickening secondary to myxomatous degeneration may affect one or two leaflets (Figure 6.47a). In some dogs, it may resemble a mass and can be confused with a vegetative lesion of endocarditis. Special attention should be paid to chordae tendinae thickening and rupture, which is best visualized in the right parasternal long-axis 4-chamber view. Rupture of small, second order chordae tendinae, which are attached to the mid-ventricular surface of the leaflets, is usually of no clinical significance. However, the tips of the mitral valve leaflets are anchored to the papillary muscles by large, first order chordae tendinae; their disruption may lead to acute heart failure. A flail leaflet is identified by the chaotic motion of its tip, which extends beyond the mitral annular plane and points toward the left atrium in systole (Figure 6.47b). In

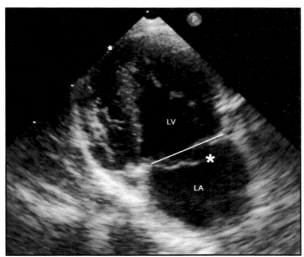

6.46 Early systolic right parasternal long-axis 4-chamber view showing the prolapse of the septal leaflet (∗) of the mitral valve behind the plane of the annulus. LA = left atrium; LV = left ventricle.

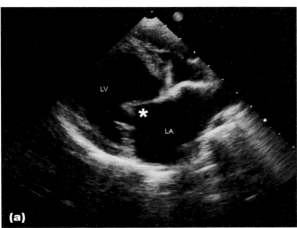

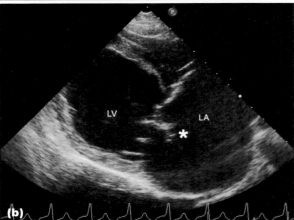

6.47 **(a)** Right parasternal long-axis 4-chamber view in a dog with chronic degenerative valve disease. The left atrium is markedly enlarged and the interatrial septum is bowing towards the right atrium. Myxomatous lesions (∗) are visualized on the mitral valve leaflets. **(b)** Right parasternal long-axis 4-chamber view in a dog with a flail septal leaflet (∗). Note that the leaflet and attached chordae are positioned above the mitral valve annulus, and that the tip of the leaflet is pointing away from the left ventricular apex. LA = left atrium; LV = left ventricle.

diastole, the leaflet is thrust into the left ventricle and towards the left ventricular outflow tract. Thickened chordae tendinae, which are detached from the papillary muscles, can be seen as bright hyperechoic filaments moving freely between the left ventricle and the left atrium. Rupture of chordae tendinae anchored to the septal leaflet of the mitral valve is more common. When this occurs colour Doppler reveals a large jet of mitral valve insufficiency.

The severity of valvular disease is based on the degree of left atrial and left ventricular enlargement. Qualitative evaluation of left atrial dilatation is undertaken from the right parasternal long-axis 4-chamber view (see **Mitral valve regurgitation (1)** clip on DVD). Calculation of the ratio between the left atrial diameter and aortic diameter, usually from a right parasternal short-axis view at the aortic level, is used to semi-quantify the severity of the disease as mild, moderate or severe (Figure 6.48). In addition, linear measurements of the left ventricular internal diameter in diastole and systole give information on the degree of left ventricular eccentric hypertrophy (Figure 6.49). The shortening fraction is typically increased in dogs with valvular endocardiosis. Myocardial failure may occur in dogs with end-stage disease; however, this is difficult to assess on 2D echocardiography.

Doppler echocardiography is used to describe the direction and size of the regurgitant jet across the mitral valve. This is undertaken from the right parasternal long-axis view (Figure 6.50) and left apical 4-chamber view. The orientation of the jet of mitral valve regurgitation is described as central or eccentric, single or multiple. Usually, the direction of an eccentric jet is opposite to the leaflet with the lesion at the origin of the regurgitation. For example, a lesion of the septal leaflet results in a posterior jet of regurgitation. The severity of the mitral valve regurgitation can be determined by comparing the surface covered by the colour Doppler jet to the area of the left atrium on a left apical 4-chamber view (Gouni *et al.*, 2007).

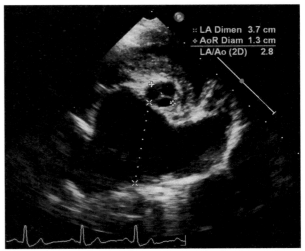

6.48 The left atrial diameter to aortic diameter ratio (LA/Ao) is determined from the right parasternal short-axis view at the level of the aortic valve. In this case the ratio is 2.8, which indicates severe atrial enlargement secondary to chronic mitral valve disease. Normal LA/Ao ratio is approximately 1.4.

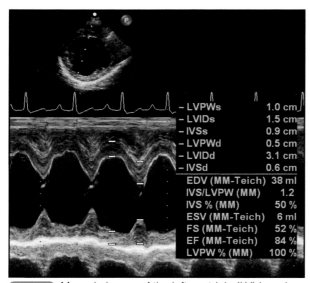

– LVPWs	1.0 cm
– LVIDs	1.5 cm
– IVSs	0.9 cm
– LVPWd	0.5 cm
– LVIDd	3.1 cm
– IVSd	0.6 cm
EDV (MM-Teich)	38 ml
IVS/LVPW (MM)	1.2
IVS % (MM)	50 %
ESV (MM-Teich)	6 ml
FS (MM-Teich)	52 %
EF (MM-Teich)	84 %
LVPW % (MM)	100 %

6.49 M-mode image of the left ventricle (LV) in a dog with chronic mitral valve disease. The left ventricular contraction is hyperdynamic, as demonstrated by the shortening fraction (FS) at 52%. This is a result of the low resistance to blood ejection during systole created by the large volume of regurgitation into the low pressure left atrium. Note that the motion of the interventricular septum (IVS) is more pronounced than the motion of the left ventricular free wall (LVPW). This is common in dogs with chronic mitral valve disease.

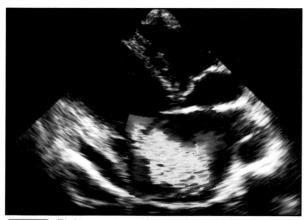

6.50 Right parasternal long-axis view in a dog with moderate to severe mitral valve regurgitation. The colour flow covers approximately 50% of the total left atrial surface. This is consistent with moderate mitral valve regurgitation. Note that the size of the left atrium is another parameter used to define the severity of the disease, and this may be a stronger predictor of the risk of developing congestive heart failure than the size of the mitral valve regurgitation jet.

- Mild mitral valve regurgitation corresponds to a jet area <30% of the area of the left atrium.
- Moderate mitral valve regurgitation is defined as a jet area ≥30% but <70% of the area of the left atrium (see **Mitral valve regurgitation (2)** clip on DVD).
- Severe mitral valve regurgitation is defined as a jet area ≥70% of the area of the left atrium (see **Mitral valve regurgitation (3)** clip on DVD).

The maximal velocity of the mitral valve regurgitant jet is measured by CW Doppler from the left apical 4-chamber view (Figure 6.51). By estimating left atrial pressure and using the simplified Bernoulli equation, peak systolic left ventricular pressure can be calculated. It may be increased in dogs with systemic hypertension. On occasion, it is decreased in dogs with elevated left atrial pressure and severe left ventricular myocardial failure.

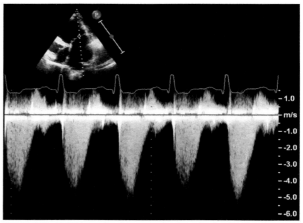

6.51 CW Doppler image of a jet of mitral valve regurgitation. The peak velocity of the jet is approximately 5 m/s and corresponds to a pressure gradient of 100 mmHg between the left ventricle and the left atrium.

Left atrial rupture is an uncommon complication of severe chronic mitral valve disease. It results from chronic trauma to the endocardial surface of the left atrium by a high velocity jet of mitral valve regurgitation. Left atrial rupture leads to cardiac tamponade. Dogs are presented with signs of low cardiac output, extreme weakness and collapse. On echocardiography, an atrial tear is not directly visible. However, pericardial effusion is present in association with signs of severe mitral valve disease, such as thickened mitral valve leaflets, a severely dilated left atrium, and a large jet of mitral valve regurgitation. A clot may also be seen in the pericardial space.

Endocarditis

Endocarditis is suspected in medium to large-breed dogs with signs of an acute ongoing infection and a new murmur or a change in intensity of a previously diagnosed murmur. However, endocarditis does not always cause a cardiac murmur, and it is only diagnosed after an extensive investigation that includes a full cardiology work-up. Vegetative lesions are most likely to be seen on the mitral valve; less commonly, they develop on the aortic valve. A vegetative lesion visualized by echocardiography supports the diagnosis of endocarditis. Vegetations usually appear as irregularly shaped, highly mobile masses attached to the free edge of a leaflet. The absence of mobility argues against the diagnosis of endocarditis. The lesion usually develops on the atrial side of the mitral valve and on the ventricular side of the aortic valve (Figure 6.52; see also **Endocarditis (1)** and **(2)** clips on DVD). In addition, the mass is usually

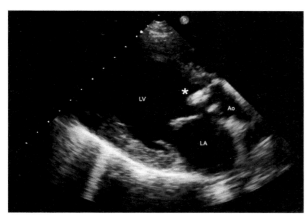

6.52 A large aortic valve vegetation (∗) is seen in diastole from the right parasternal long-axis outflow tract view. Ao = aorta; LA = left atrium; LV = left ventricle.

homogeneous with echogenicity similar to that of the myocardium. Mitral valve endocarditis is commonly associated with mild to severe mitral valve regurgitation, and aortic valve endocarditis with aortic valve insufficiency. It is important that images are taken from all echocardiographic windows to increase the probability of detecting vegetations. It

should also be remembered that myxomatous mitral valve disease may mimic lesions of endocarditis.

Myocardial diseases

Dilated cardiomyopathy

Dilated cardiomyopathy (DCM) is characterized by left ventricular dilatation and systolic dysfunction. It is more common in large-breed dogs. It may result from infection or cardiotoxic agents but it is usually idiopathic. In cats, DCM was frequently associated with a deficiency in the essential amino acid taurine until this was added to commercial feline diets.

Echocardiographic diagnosis of DCM is based on visualization of left ventricular dilatation associated with systolic dysfunction. M-mode imaging of the left ventricle is used to determine the left ventricular internal diameter in diastole and in systole, and thus calculate the shortening fraction (Figure 6.53). However, because of the variability in the echocardiographic parameters, it is difficult to use fractional shortening to monitor response to inotropic therapy. Echocardiography can be used to decide whether therapy with inotropes is indicated, but only clinical response determines whether they should be continued.

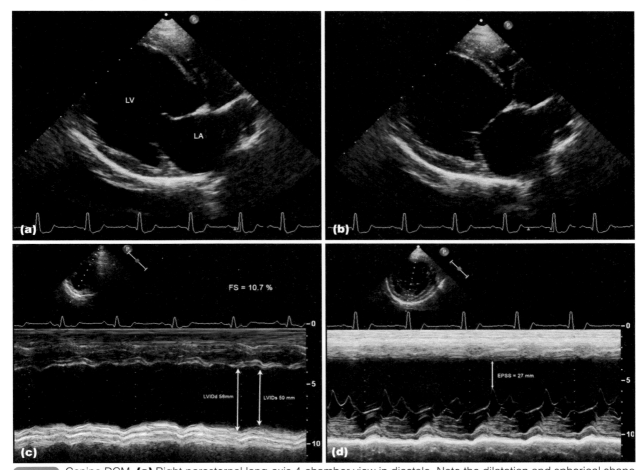

6.53 Canine DCM. **(a)** Right parasternal long-axis 4-chamber view in diastole. Note the dilatation and spherical shape of the left ventricle (LV). **(b)** Systolic frame demonstrating the generalized hypokinesis of the myocardium. **(c)** M-mode echocardiogram demonstrating that the shortening fraction (FS) is approximately 10.7%. **(d)** M-mode echocardiogram recorded at the level of the mitral valve. The increased E-point to septal separation (EPSS) is an indication of decreased ejection fraction. LA = left atrium; LVIDd = left ventricular internal diameter in diastole; LVIDs = left ventricular internal diameter in systole.

Parameters, such as the index of sphericity and the E-point to septum separation (EPSS) can be determined to further quantify the degree of systolic dysfunction. The index of sphericity is the ratio between the length of the left ventricle and its diameter. With chamber enlargement, the left ventricle takes a more spherical shape and the index of sphericity decreases. It contributes to papillary muscle displacement, causing mitral valve regurgitation. EPSS is measured as the distance between the tip of the septal leaflet of the mitral valve at maximal opening (E wave) and the interventricular septum on an M-mode right parasternal short-axis view at the level of the mitral valve. EPSS is correlated with systolic function. Normal EPSS is <6 mm.

In dogs with DCM, colour Doppler evaluation of the mitral valve frequently reveals mild to moderate regurgitation, which results from mitral valve annulus dilatation. In addition, pulmonary hypertension is a common complication of left heart disease, resulting from passive pulmonary venous congestion, active pulmonary arterial vasoconstriction and vascular remodelling. Echocardiographic features of pulmonary hypertension include right ventricular dilatation, right ventricular free wall thickening and tricuspid valve insufficiency.

Hypertrophic cardiomyopathy

Hypertrophic cardiomyopathy (HCM) is characterized by inappropriate left ventricular concentric hypertrophy. Primary HCM is sporadic or familial. It is more common in cats, with breed predispositions including Maine Coons and Ragdolls; it is rare in dogs. Importantly, cardiac changes similar to HCM are commonly seen secondary to hyperthyroidism in cats. The degree of left ventricular hypertrophy is variable as well as the location, which can be equally distributed or limited to portions of the interventricular septum or left ventricular free wall.

HCM results in diastolic dysfunction (i.e. impaired filling, secondary to left ventricular hypertrophy). In some animals, dynamic left ventricular obstruction in systole (SAM) is secondary to systolic anterior motion of the mitral valve. Displacement of the septal leaflet of the mitral valve and chordae towards the region of the left ventricular outflow tract in systole. It occurs in response to changes in left ventricle geometry in combination with increased outflow tract velocities in systole, which are associated with septal hypertrophy and a decreased left ventricular outflow tract diameter. SAM results in obstruction of the outflow tract and a small jet of mitral valve regurgitation. It is important to note that this is a dynamic phenomenon, which is dependent on heart rate and the contractility of the left ventricle, and is usually observed with elevated heart rates.

On echocardiography, feline HCM is defined as a diastolic left ventricular free wall (Figure 6.54) or an interventricular septal thickness >6 mm. In some cats, hypertrophy is limited to only small regions of the left ventricular wall. Papillary muscle hypertrophy is usually evident (Figure 6.55). Systolic left ventricular cavity obliteration due to hypertrophy can be demonstrated from a right parasternal short-axis view of the left ventricle (see **Hypertrophic cardiomyopathy (1)** clip on DVD). Repeated contact between the septal leaflet of the mitral valve and the hypertrophied septal base may result in a hyperechoic lesion on the endocardial surface of the interventricular septum, which can be seen on a right parasternal long-axis view. Moreover, in cats with congestive heart failure, a small amount of pericardial effusion, identified on an echocardiogram as an echolucent line surrounding the ventricles, may be present (Figure 6.56; see also **Hypertrophic cardiomyopathy (2)** clip on DVD).

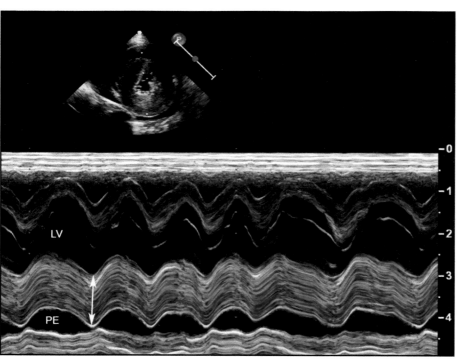

6.54 M-mode echocardiogram in a cat with HCM. The left ventricular free wall is markedly thickened. Note that the hypertrophy of the interventricular septum is less pronounced. An echo-free space, consistent with pericardial effusion (PE) is seen below the left ventricular free wall. LV = left ventricle.

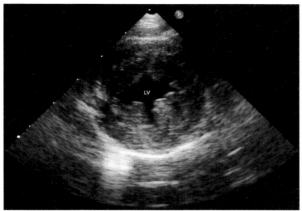

6.55 Right parasternal short-axis view at the papillary muscle level in a cat with HCM. This view allows the distribution of hypertrophy between the interventricular septum and the wall of the left ventricle (LV) to be appreciated. Note the two prominent papillary muscles. This is a finding consistent with HCM.

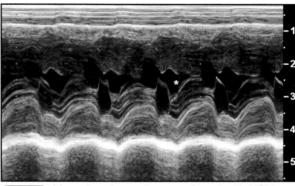

6.57 M-mode echocardiogram of a cat with HCM showing SAM of the mitral valve (*). During systole there is anterior displacement of the mitral valve, which results in contact with the interventricular septum, and provides evidence of left ventricular outflow tract obstruction.

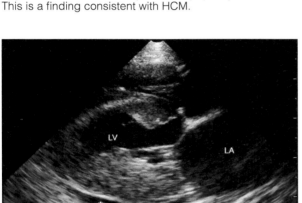

6.56 Right parasternal long-axis 4-chamber view recorded in early systole in a cat with HCM (same cat as in Figure 6.52). The left atrium (LA) is markedly enlarged. There is massive hypertrophy of the left ventricular free wall. Note the hypertrophy at the base of the septum in the region of the left ventricular outflow tract. A small amount of pericardial effusion (*) is present. LV = left ventricle.

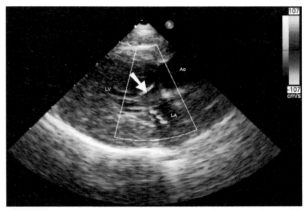

6.58 Right parasternal long-axis 4-chamber view with colour flow Doppler of the left ventricular outflow tract and mitral valve areas. On this systolic image, turbulent blood flow (arrowed) is identified in the outflow tract secondary to SAM of the mitral valve. There is secondary mitral valve regurgitation resulting from the abnormal coaptation of the leaflets. Note the small eccentric jet of mitral valve regurgitation. Ao = aorta; LA = left atrium; LV = left ventricle.

Other important parameters to assess using Doppler echocardiography include the presence of dynamic left ventricular obstruction (SAM) and signs of diastolic dysfunction. Dynamic left ventricular outflow tract obstruction can be demonstrated on an M-mode image from a right parasternal long-axis view at the level of the mitral valve. In the presence of SAM, displacement of the septal leaflet of the mitral valve towards the septum is visualized in systole (Figure 6.57; see also **Systolic anterior motion of the chordae** clip on DVD). In addition, colour Doppler imaging of the left ventricular outflow tract region and mitral valve from a right parasternal long-axis view demonstrates turbulent flow in the outflow tract region associated with a small eccentric jet of mitral valve regurgitation (Figure 6.58; see also **Systolic anterior motion of the mitral valve** clip on DVD). From a left

apical 5-chamber view, CW Doppler imaging of the left ventricular outflow tract provides information on the severity of the obstruction; the flow has a typical 'dagger' shaped appearance (Figure 6.59).

Diastolic dysfunction can be demonstrated by assessing mitral valve inflow with PW Doppler from a left apical 4-chamber view. The normal E wave to A wave ratio is >1. Abnormal left ventricular relaxation results in an inversion of the ratio (E/A <1) (Figure 6.60). As the disease progresses, volume overload of the left atrium and elevated filling pressures are responsible for a normalization of the ratio (pseudonormalization). E and A wave fusion occurs when the heart rate reaches 160–180 beats/minute, which limits the clinical use of this parameter to assess the degree of left ventricular diastolic dysfunction.

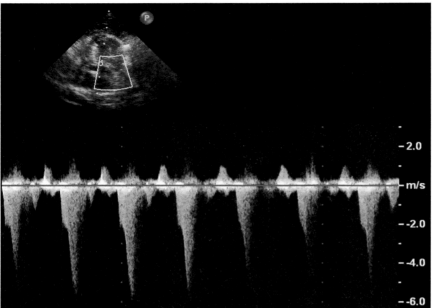

6.59 CW Doppler image of the flow in the left ventricular outflow tract in a cat with obstructive HCM. Note the late peaking 'dagger' shaped contour of the spectral display. This CW Doppler profile reflects the occurrence of the obstruction during mid- to late systole.

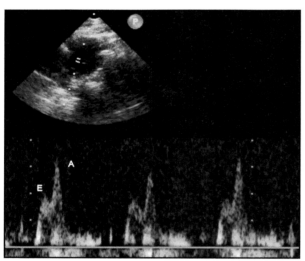

6.60 PW Doppler image of mitral valve inflow in a cat with HCM. The sample window is placed at the level of the tip of the mitral valve leaflets in diastole. There is an E/A wave ratio reversal, indicating an abnormal relaxation pattern of the left ventricle.

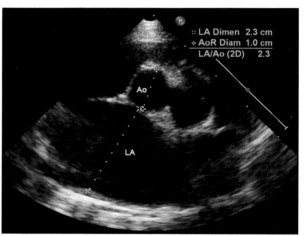

6.61 Left atrial (LA) to aortic (Ao) diameter ratio of 2.3 measured from a right parasternal short-axis view at the aortic valve level in a cat with HCM. Note the enlargement of the left auricular appendage.

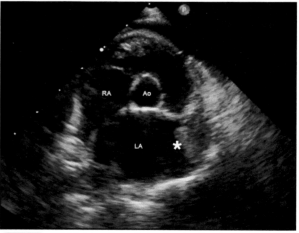

6.62 Right parasternal short-axis view in a cat with HCM showing a thrombus (*) in the left auricular appendage. Ao = aorta; LA = left atrium; RA = right atrium.

Echocardiographic parameters can also be used to assess the severity of the disease. The diameter of the left atrium and the left atrial to aortic diameter ratio are used to determine the severity of disease. In cats, enlargement of the left auricular appendage may occur without significant dilatation of the main chamber of the left atrium. Therefore, the left atrial to aortic diameter ratio does not always correlate well with the qualitative assessment of atrial enlargement made from the right parasternal short-axis view (Figure 6.61). The degree of left ventricular hypertrophy may also suggest a higher risk of complications, including arrhythmias, and a more rapid progression of the disease. Careful examination of the left auricular appendage region is important to detect the presence of a thrombus in cats with a severely enlarged left atrium (Figure 6.62). Spontaneous echo contrast is also seen in the markedly dilated left atrium of cats with HCM. This may be an indicator of an increased risk for systemic thromboembolism.

Arrhythmogenic right ventricular cardiomyopathy

Arrhythmogenic right ventricular cardiomyopathy (ARVC) is most commonly identified in Boxers. It is characterized by fibrofatty replacement of the right ventricular myocardium and severe ventricular arrhythmias. Dogs may be presented as an emergency after an episode of collapse or with signs of cardiogenic shock due to rapid sustained ventricular tachycardia. Echocardiography is frequently unremarkable in these dogs. Some patients show signs of myocardial failure secondary to the extension of the disease to the left side of the heart. It is important to know about cardiac function before using antiarrhythmic drugs, as some of them have negative inotropic effects.

Echocardiographic evaluation of a dog with ARVC may reveal isolated right ventricular enlargement, localized aneurysms (identified as outpouchings of the right ventricular free wall) and increased echogenicity of the myocardium, reflecting adipose infiltration. However, these reported findings in humans are not usually seen in dogs. Many dogs with ARVC have a normal echocardiographic evaluation. Left ventricular myocardial failure may also occur with left ventricular dilatation in diastole and systole, and with decreased fractional shortening.

ARVC is also reported in cats. It is associated with ventricular arrhythmias, and most cats have signs of congestive heart failure. Marked right ventricular and right atrial dilatation, and tricuspid valve regurgitation are the main echocardiographic findings; these abnormalities are best seen from the right parasternal acoustic window.

Restrictive cardiomyopathy

Restrictive cardiomyopathy (RCM) occurs in cats; however, it is rare compared with HCM. Diagnosis is challenging because there is significant impairment of ventricular diastolic function without significant changes in the morphology of the ventricles. Moreover, non-invasive diagnosis of diastolic dysfunction is difficult to perform and interpret.

A myocardial form and an endomyocardial variant of the disease have been described. Suspicion of the myocardial form of feline RCM is based on the presence of atrial enlargement without evidence of left ventricular concentric hypertrophy (which would raise suspicion for HCM) and in the presence of normal systolic function. In the endomyocardial form of the disease, large areas of fibrosis cover the endocardial surface of the ventricle, forming bridges between the free wall and the interventricular septum.

On echocardiography, left and right atrial dilatation is usually obvious, and the size and systolic function of the left ventricle is normal in the myocardial

form of the disease. Echocardiography also reveals hyperechoic lesions of fibrosis covering the endocardial surface of the left ventricle in the endomyocardial form of the disease. Doppler echocardiography of the mitral valve inflow may suggest diastolic dysfunction. In the endomyocardial form of the disease, turbulent blood flow may be detected within the left ventricle where fibrous bands bridging between the free wall and the interventricular septum cause mid-ventricular stenosis.

Pericardial diseases

Pericardial effusion

Pericardial effusion is the accumulation of fluid within the pericardial space, which can be acute or chronic. Acute cases result from haemorrhage within the pericardial space. Most commonly, haemopericardium is associated with atrial haemangiosarcoma, but other causes include diffuse neoplasia (such as mesothelioma), rupture of the left atrium secondary to chronic valvular disease and trauma.

Echocardiography is an important tool to confirm suspicion of cardiac tamponade, a situation which occurs when the accumulation of pericardial fluid impairs cardiac function. Acute tamponade is characterized by the accumulation of a small amount of fluid within a non-compliant pericardial sac, causing clinical signs of low cardiac output. Chronic tamponade results from the slow accumulation of a large volume of fluid, which slowly stretches the pericardium. Right intracardiac pressure rises until it causes right heart failure with ascites. Chronic tamponade may be associated with a cardiac tumour, but commonly the cause for tamponade is not found (see **Pericardial effusion** clip on DVD).

On echocardiography, pericardial effusion appears as an echo-free (black) space around the ventricles. A small effusion can be seen as a very small echo-free space in the left atrioventricular groove on a right parasternal long-axis view. Due to the fact that the pericardium adheres to the large vessels, there is no accumulation of fluid at the base of the heart. This can be used to differentiate pericardial effusion from pleural effusion, which accumulates homogeneously around the heart unless marked inflammation results in loculated effusion. The identification of the tip of the right auricular appendage moving freely within the pericardial fluid on a right parasternal long-axis view, or the tip of the left auricular appendage surrounded by fluid on a right parasternal short-axis view, are two very helpful signs to discriminate between pericardial effusion and pleural effusion. It should also be noted that a markedly dilated left auricular appendage may mimic pericardial effusion in some echocardiographic views. This is because, in dogs and cats with severe left atrial dilatation, the left auricular appendage expands along the lateroposterior side of the left ventricle, creating an echo-free space on the side of the left ventricle (Figure 6.63).

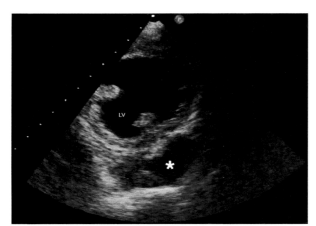

6.63 Right parasternal short-axis view at the level of the papillary muscles in a dog with a severely enlarged left atrium (∗). The left atrium is visualized on the lateral wall of the left ventricle (LV), mimicking pericardial effusion.

Additional echocardiographic parameters are used to establish the diagnosis of cardiac tamponade. Signs of cardiac tamponade include:

- Right atrial collapse during atrial diastole following atrial contraction
- Right ventricular collapse during ventricular diastole
- Underfilling of the left side of the heart.

The echocardiographic signs of tamponade are best appreciated on a right parasternal long-axis view (Figure 6.64); their presence indicates that intrapericardial pressure exceeds intracardiac pressure.

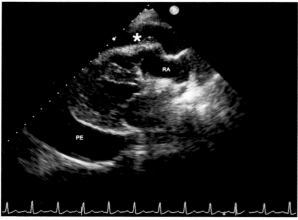

6.64 Right parasternal long-axis 4-chamber view in a dog with cardiac tamponade. There is a large amount of pericardial effusion (PE) and a small mass is visible at the right atrioventricular junction (∗). Note the collapse of the wall of the right atrium (RA) in diastole. This is a sensitive sign for cardiac tamponade.

Echocardiography is the most sensitive diagnostic test to identify the cause of the effusion. It is important to thoroughly examine the area of the right atrium, right auricular appendage and right atrioventricular junction for the presence of an echogenic

mass. An atrial mass is usually a haemangiosarcoma (see **Right atrial mass** clip on DVD) but blood clots can have a similar ultrasonographic appearance. Pericardial fluid around the heart facilitates the detection of an atrial mass. It is the preference of the author to perform the echocardiogram before pericardiocentesis, if possible. The heart base should also be examined for the presence of a mass. Most heart base masses are chemodectomas. On echocardiography, chemodectomas are usually located caudal to the ascending aorta and above the left atrium (Figures 6.65 and 6.66; see also **Heart base mass** clip on DVD).

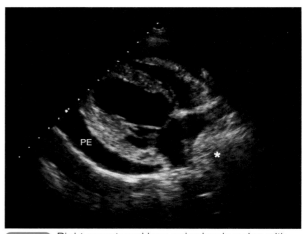

6.65 Right parasternal long-axis view in a dog with cardiac tamponade. Pericardial effusion is visible (PE). There is also a mass above the left atrium (∗); this is usually consistent with a chemodectoma.

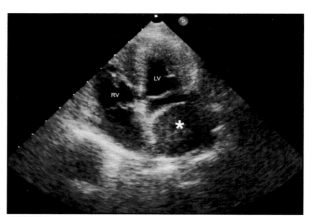

6.66 A large heart base mass (∗), compressing the dorsal wall of the left atrium, is visible on the left apical 4-chamber view. LV = left ventricle; RV = right ventricle.

Constrictive pericarditis

In dogs, constrictive pericarditis has been reported. It is more common in large-breed dogs. Diagnosis is based on clinical findings of right-sided heart failure in the presence of normal cardiac structures on echocardiography. A small amount of pericardial effusion and a thickened pericardium may be visible in some cases. However, thickening of the pericardium is difficult to evaluate.

Screening programmes for cardiac diseases

Hereditary cardiac disease may be present at birth (congenital) or become apparent later in life (acquired). Common congenital diseases include subaortic stenosis, pulmonic stenosis and PDA. Common acquired diseases include atrioventricular valve endocardiosis, DCM and HCM. Currently, there is no consensus on the diagnostic work-up that should be performed prior to breeding dogs of breeds that have a high prevalence of inherited cardiac diseases. However, recommendations are available for a few disorders. Recommendations between dog breeding clubs may vary.

Subaortic stenosis

As the disease is known to progress until 12 months of age, screening of dogs prior to breeding should be performed after their first year of life. An echocardiogram should be performed in dogs with a heart murmur. However, it may be difficult to differentiate dogs with mild subaortic stenosis from normal dogs. With mild disease, structural cardiac changes are usually not present on 2D echocardiography. Doppler imaging of the left ventricular outflow tract is performed from the left apical view and the subcostal window to determine the pressure gradient below the aortic valve. There is no consensus on the maximal blood velocity in the left ventricular outflow tract that differentiates normal dogs with flow murmurs from dogs with mild subaortic stenosis. An aortic peak velocity >2 m/s as determined by CW Doppler usually indicates stenosis. Boxers have been shown to have a narrower outflow tract than other breeds. Innocent murmurs are common in this breed, and it is possible that normal Boxers have a peak velocity >2 m/s. The American Boxer club has raised the cut-off value for mild subaortic stenosis to 2.4 m/s and recommends screening at 24 months of age. Trivial to mild aortic valve insufficiency, detected by Doppler imaging, is common in dogs with subaortic stenosis. It is likely that dogs with an aortic peak velocity between 1.5 and 2 m/s and aortic valve insufficiency have mild subaortic stenosis.

Endocardiosis

Cavalier King Charles Spaniels have a higher incidence of endocardiosis than other breeds of dog. Breed clubs have developed guidelines to decrease the prevalence of the disease. The dogs should be ≥5 years old and have a normal cardiac examination prior to breeding. Alternatively, they should be at least 2.5 years old with documentation of both parents having a normal cardiac examination at ≥5 years of age. Dogs should be evaluated every year and importantly within a year of being bred. Endocardiosis is usually diagnosed by auscultation. 2D echocardiography and Doppler imaging are used to confirm the presence of the disease.

Dilated cardiomyopathy

The non-clinical phase of DCM may last up to 3–4 years. It is challenging to identify this occult phase of the disease. In Dobermanns, the prevalence of the disease is high. Diagnosis of cardiomyopathy is based on the detection of structural and functional cardiac changes on echocardiography and arrhythmias on 24-hour Holter recording. Echocardiographic criteria to diagnose DCM include increased end-diastolic and end-systolic left ventricular dimensions, increased left ventricular sphericity, a shortening fraction <20–25% and an increased EPSS.

References and further reading

Abbott JA and MacLean HN (2003) Comparison of Doppler-derived peak aortic velocities obtained from subcostal and apical transducer sites in healthy dogs. *Veterinary Radiology and Ultrasound* **44**, 695–698

Abbott JA and MacLean HN (2006) Two-dimensional echocardiographic assessment of the feline left atrium. *Journal of Veterinary Internal Medicine* **20**, 111–119

Arndt JW and Oyama MA (2008) Agitated saline contrast echocardiography to diagnose a congenital heart defect in a dog. *Journal of Veterinary Cardiology* **10**, 129–132

Baumwart RD, Meurs KM, Atkins CE *et al.* (2005) Clinical, echocardiographic and electrocardiographic abnormalities in Boxers with cardiomyopathy and left ventricular systolic dysfunction: 48 cases (1985–2003). *Journal of the American Veterinary Medical Association* **226**, 1102–1104

Beardow AW and Buchanan JW (1993) Chronic mitral valve disease in Cavalier King Charles Spaniels: 95 cases (1987–1991). *Journal of the American Veterinary Medical Association* **203**, 1023–1029

Berry CR, Lombard CW, Hager DA, Ackerman N and King RR (1988) Echocardiographic evaluation of cardiac tamponade in dogs before and after pericardiocentesis: four cases (1984–1986). *Journal of the American Veterinary Medical Association* **192**, 1597–1603

Bonagura JD (2000) Feline echocardiography. *Journal of Feline Medicine and Surgery* **2**, 147–151

Bonagura JD and Miller MW (1998) Doppler echocardiography. II. Color Doppler imaging. *Veterinary Clinics of North America: Small Animal Practice* **28**, 1361–1389

Bonagura JD, Miller MW and Darke PG (1998) Doppler echocardiography. I. Pulsed-wave and continuous-wave examinations. *Veterinary Clinics of North America: Small Animal Practice* **28**, 1325–1359

Bonagura JD and Schober KE (2009) Can ventricular function be assessed by echocardiography in chronic canine mitral valve disease? *Journal of Small Animal Practice* **50 (Suppl 1)**, 12–24

Borgarelli M, Santilli RA, Chiavegato D *et al.* (2006) Prognostic indicators for dogs with dilated cardiomyopathy. *Journal of Veterinary Internal Medicine* **20**, 104–110

Borgarelli M, Savarino P, Crosara S *et al.* (2008) Survival characteristics and prognostic variables of dogs with mitral regurgitation attributable to myxomatous valve disease. *Journal of Veterinary Internal Medicine* **22**, 120–128

Brown DJ, Knight DH and King RR (1991) Use of pulsed-wave Doppler echocardiography to determine aortic and pulmonary velocity and flow variables in clinically normal dogs. *American Journal of Veterinary Research* **52**, 543–550

Bussadori C, Amberger C, Le Bobinnec G *et al.* (2000) Guidelines for the echocardiographic studies of suspected subaortic and pulmonic stenosis. *Journal of Veterinary Cardiology* **2**, 15–22

Chetboul V, Charles V, Nicolle A *et al.* (2006) Retrospective study of 156 atrial septal defects in dogs and cats (2001–2005). *Journal of Veterinary Medicine: Series A – Physiology, Pathology, Clinical Medicine* **53**, 179–184

Chetboul V, Concordet D, Pouchelon JL *et al.* (2003) Effects of inter- and intra-observer variability on echocardiographic measurements in awake cats. *Journal of Veterinary Medicine: Series A – Physiology, Pathology, Clinical Medicine* **50**, 326–331

Chetboul V, Tidholm A, Nicolle A *et al.* (2005) Effects of animal position and number of repeated measurements on selected two-dimensional and M-mode echocardiographic variables in healthy dogs. *Journal of the American Veterinary Medical Association* **227**, 743–747

Cornell CC, Kittleson MD, Della Torre P *et al.* (2004) Allometric scaling of M-mode cardiac measurements in normal adult dogs. *Journal of Veterinary Internal Medicine* **18**, 311–321

Cunningham SM, Rush JE, Freeman LM, Brown DJ and Smith CE (2008) Echocardiographic ratio indices in overtly healthy Boxer dogs screened for heart disease. *Journal of Veterinary Internal Medicine* **22**, 924–930

Dukes McEwan J, Borgarelli M, Tidholm A, Vollmar AC and Haggstrom J (2003) Proposed guidelines for the diagnosis of canine idiopathic dilated cardiomyopathy. *Journal of Veterinary Cardiology* **5**, 7–19

Dukes McEwan J, French AT and Corcoran BM (2002) Doppler echocardiography in the dog: measurement variability and reproducibility. *Veterinary Radiology and Ultrasound* **43**, 144–152

Ferasin L (2009) Feline myocardial disease 2: diagnosis, prognosis and clinical management. *Journal of Feline Medicine and Surgery* **11**, 183–194

Ferasin L, Sturgess CP, Cannon MJ *et al.* (2003) Feline idiopathic cardiomyopathy: a retrospective study of 106 cats (1994–2001). *Journal of Feline Medicine and Surgery* **5**, 151–159

Fox PR, Liu SK and Maron BJ (1995) Echocardiographic assessment of spontaneously occurring feline hypertrophic cardiomyopathy: an animal model of human disease. *Circulation* **92**, 2645–2651

Fox PR, Maron BJ, Basso C, Liu SK and Thiene G (2000) Spontaneously occurring arrhythmogenic right ventricular cardiomyopathy in the domestic cat: a new animal model similar to the human disease. *Circulation* **102**, 1863–1870

Gordon SG, Miller MW, Roland RM *et al.* (2009) Transcatheter atrial septal defect closure with the Amplatzer atrial septal occluder in 13 dogs: short and mid-term outcome. *Journal of Veterinary Internal Medicine* **23**, 995–1002

Gouni V, Serres FJ, Pouchelon JL *et al.* (2007) Quantification of mitral valve regurgitation in dogs with degenerative mitral valve disease by use of the proximal isovelocity surface area method. *Journal of the American Veterinary Medical Association* **231**, 399–406

Hall DJ, Cornell CC, Crawford S and Brown DJ (2008) Meta-analysis of normal canine echocardiographic dimensional data using ratio indices. *Journal of Veterinary Cardiology* **10**, 11–23

Hansson K, Haggstrom J, Kvart C and Lord P (2002) Left atrial to aortic root indices using two-dimensional and M-mode echocardiography in Cavalier King Charles Spaniels with and without left atrial enlargement. *Veterinary Radiology and Ultrasound* **43**, 568–575

Jacquet J, Nicolle AP, Chetboul V, Behr L and Pouchelon JL (2005) Echocardiographic and Doppler characteristics of postoperative ductal aneurysm in a dog. *Veterinary Radiology and Ultrasound* **46**, 518–520

Jenni S, Gardelle O, Zini E and Glaus TM (2009) Use of auscultation and Doppler echocardiography in Boxer puppies to predict development of subaortic or pulmonary stenosis. *Journal of Veterinary Internal Medicine* **23**, 81–86

Johnson L, Boon J and Orton EC (1999) Clinical characteristics of 53 dogs with Doppler-derived evidence of pulmonary hypertension (1992–1996). *Journal of Veterinary Internal Medicine* **13**, 440–447

Kittleson MD and Brown WA (2003) Regurgitant fraction measured by using the proximal isovelocity surface area method in dogs with chronic myxomatous mitral valve disease. *Journal of Veterinary Internal Medicine* **17**, 84–88

Loureiro J, Smith S, Fonfara S *et al.* (2008) Canine dynamic left ventricular outflow tract obstruction: assessment of myocardial function and clinical outcome. *Journal of Small Animal Practice* **49**, 578–586

MacDonald KA, Cagney O and Magne ML (2009) Echocardiographic and clinicopathologic characterization of pericardial effusion in dogs: 107 cases (1985–2006). *Journal of the American Veterinary Medical Association* **235**, 1456–1461

Meurs KM, Spier AW, Miller MW, Lehmkuhl L and Towbin JA (1999) Familial ventricular arrhythmias in Boxers. *Journal of Veterinary Internal Medicine* **13**, 437–439

Nakayama T, Wakao Y, Ishikawa R and Takahashi M (1996) Progression of subaortic stenosis detected by continuous wave Doppler echocardiography in a dog. *Journal of Veterinary Internal Medicine* **10**, 97–98

O'Sullivan ML, O'Grady MR and Minors SL (2007) Assessment of diastolic function by Doppler echocardiography in normal Doberman Pinschers and Doberman Pinschers with dilated cardiomyopathy. *Journal of Veterinary Internal Medicine* **21**, 81–91

Oyama MA (2004) Advances in echocardiography. *Veterinary Clinics of North America: Small Animal Practice* **34**, 1083–1104

Oyama MA, Sisson DD, Bulmer BJ and Constable PD (2004) Echocardiographic estimation of mean left atrial pressure in a canine model of acute mitral valve insufficiency. *Journal of Veterinary Internal Medicine* **18**, 667–672

Oyama MA and Thomas WP (2002) Two-dimensional and M-mode echocardiographic predictors of disease severity in dogs with congenital subaortic stenosis. *Journal of the American Animal Hospital Association* **38**, 209–215

Oyama MA, Weidman JA and Cole SG (2008) Calculation of pressure half-time. *Journal of Veterinary Cardiology* **10**, 57–60

Paige CF, Abbott JA and Pyle RL (2007) Systolic anterior motion of the mitral valve associated with right ventricular systolic hypertension in 9 dogs. *Journal of Veterinary Cardiology* **9**, 9–14

Pariaut R, Sydney Moise N, Kraus MS *et al.* (2004) Use of transesophageal echocardiography for visualization of the patent ductus arteriosus during transcatheter coil embolization. *Journal of Veterinary Cardiology* **6**, 32–39

Peddle G and Sleeper MM (2007) Canine bacterial endocarditis: a review. *Journal of the American Animal Hospital Association* **43**, 258–263

Pion PD, Kittleson MD, Skiles ML, Rogers QR and Morris JG (1992) Dilated cardiomyopathy associated with taurine deficiency in the domestic cat: relationship to diet and myocardial taurine content. *Advances in Experimental Medicine and Biology* **315**, 63–73

Rishniw M and Erb HN (2000) Evaluation of four 2-dimensional echocardiographic methods of assessing left atrial size in dogs. *Journal of Veterinary Internal Medicine* **14**, 429–435

Santilli RA, Bontempi LV, Perego M, Fornai L and Basso C (2009) Outflow tract segmental arrhythmogenic right ventricular cardiomyopathy in an English Bulldog. *Journal of Veterinary Cardiology* **11**, 47–51

Saunders AB, Miller MW, Gordon SG and Bahr A (2007) Echocardiographic and angiographic comparison of ductal dimensions in dogs with patent ductus arteriosus. *Journal of Veterinary Internal Medicine* **21**, 68–75

Schneider M, Hildebrandt N, Schweigl T and Wehner M (2007) Transthoracic echocardiographic measurement of patent ductus arteriosus in dogs. *Journal of Veterinary Internal Medicine* **21**, 251–257

Schober KE (2005) Doppler echocardiographic assessment of ventricular function – time to move to the right? *Journal of Veterinary Internal Medicine* **19**, 785–787

Schober KE and Baade H (2000) Comparability of left ventricular M-mode echocardiography in dogs performed in long-axis and short-axis. *Veterinary Radiology and Ultrasound* **41**, 543–549

Schober KE and Baade H (2006) Doppler echocardiographic prediction of pulmonary hypertension in West Highland White Terriers with chronic pulmonary disease. *Journal of Veterinary Internal Medicine* **20**, 912–920

Schober KE and Luis Fuentes V (2001) Mitral annulus motion as determined by M-mode echocardiography in normal dogs and dogs with cardiac disease. *Veterinary Radiology and Ultrasound* **42**, 52–61

Schober KE, Luis Fuentes V, Dukes McEwan J and French AT (1998) Pulmonary venous flow characteristics as assessed by transthoracic pulsed Doppler echocardiography in normal dogs. *Veterinary Radiology and Ultrasound* **39**, 33–41

Schober KE, Stern JA, DaCunha DN *et al.* (2008) Estimation of left ventricular filling pressure by Doppler echocardiography in dogs with pacing-induced heart failure. *Journal of Veterinary Internal Medicine* **22**, 578–585

Serres F, Chetboul V, Gouni V *et al.* (2007) Diagnostic value of echo-Doppler and tissue Doppler imaging in dogs with pulmonary arterial hypertension. *Journal of Veterinary Internal Medicine* **21**, 1280–1289

Serres FJ, Chetboul V, Tissier R *et al.* (2006) Doppler echocardiography-derived evidence of pulmonary arterial hypertension in dogs with degenerative mitral valve disease: 86 cases (2001–2005). *Journal of the American Veterinary Medical Association* **229**, 1772–1778

Serres F, Chetboul V, Tissier R *et al.* (2008) Comparison of 3 ultrasound methods for quantifying left ventricular systolic function: correlation with disease severity and prognostic value in dogs with mitral valve disease. *Journal of Veterinary Internal Medicine* **22**, 566–577

Serres F, Chetboul V, Tissier R *et al.* (2009) Quantification of pulmonary to systemic flow ratio by a Doppler echocardiographic method in the normal dog: repeatability, reproducibility and reference ranges. *Journal of Veterinary Cardiology* **11**, 23–29

Simpson KE, Devine BC, Gunn-Moore DA *et al.* (2007) Assessment of the repeatability of feline echocardiography using conventional echocardiography and spectral pulse-wave Doppler tissue imaging techniques. *Veterinary Radiology and Ultrasound* **48**, 58–68

Simpson KE, Gunn-Moore DA, Shaw DJ *et al.* (2009) Pulsed-wave Doppler tissue imaging velocities in normal geriatric cats and geriatric cats with primary or systemic diseases linked to specific cardiomyopathies in humans, and the influence of age and heart rate upon these velocities. *Journal of Feline Medicine and Surgery* **11**, 293–304

Terzo E, Di Marcello M, McAllister H *et al.* (2009) Echocardiographic assessment of 537 dogs with mitral valve prolapse and leaflet involvement. *Veterinary Radiology and Ultrasound* **50**, 416–422

Teshima K, Asano K, Iwanaga K *et al.* (2007) Evaluation of left ventricular Tei index (index of myocardial performance) in healthy dogs and dogs with mitral regurgitation. *Journal of Veterinary Medicine and Science* **69**, 117–123

Thomas WP, Gaber CE, Jacobs GJ *et al.* (1993) Recommendations for standards in transthoracic two-dimensional echocardiography in the dog and cat. Echocardiography Committee of the Specialty of Cardiology, American College of Veterinary Internal Medicine. *Journal of Veterinary Internal Medicine* **7**, 247–252

Tou SP, Adin DB and Estrada AH (2006) Echocardiographic estimation of systemic systolic blood pressure in dogs with mild mitral regurgitation. *Journal of Veterinary Internal Medicine* **20**, 1127–1131

Vollmar AC (1999) Use of echocardiography in the diagnosis of dilated cardiomyopathy in Irish Wolfhounds. *Journal of the American Animal Hospital Association* **35**, 279–283

Video extras

- Atrial septal defect
- Bubble study
- Endocarditis (1)
- Endocarditis (2)
- Heart base mass
- Hypertrophic cardiomyopathy (1)
- Hypertrophic cardiomyopathy (2)
- Left cranial view of the right atrium
- Mitral valve regurgitation (1)
- Mitral valve regurgitation (2)
- Mitral valve regurgitation (3)
- Patent ductus arteriosus
- Patent ductus arteriosus viewed from a transoesophageal approach
- Patent ductus arteriosus viewed from the left cranial window

- Pericardial effusion
- Pulmonic stenosis (1)
- Pulmonic stenosis (2)
- Right atrial mass
- Subaortic stenosis (1)
- Subaortic stenosis (2)
- Subaortic stenosis (3)
- Subaortic stenosis (4)
- Systolic anterior motion of the chordae
- Systolic anterior motion of the mitral valve
- Tricuspid valve dysplasia (1)
- Tricuspid valve dysplasia (2)
- Tricuspid valve prolapse
- Tricuspid valve regurgitation
- Ventricular septal defect (1)
- Ventricular septal defect (2)

Access via QR code or bsavalibrary.com/ultrasound_6

7

Abdomen

Jennifer Kinns

Indications

Ultrasonography of the abdomen is indicated in the evaluation of many conditions, and can be categorized as either emergency evaluation or elective abdominal ultrasonography. In many cases ultrasonography will be used as an adjunct to radiographic evaluation.

Emergency evaluation

Ultrasonography of the acute abdomen is performed primarily to determine whether surgery is indicated. In addition, the underlying disease process may be determined. It may have to be performed before the results of bloodwork are available. If the animal is unstable a rapid scan protocol (see below) may be employed to look for free fluid. Portable ultrasound systems can allow evaluation of the patient in the treatment room, limiting the need to move an unstable animal or one undergoing emergency treatment. The main aims of ultrasonography of the acute abdomen are to:

- Identify and sample free fluid
- Identify free gas
- Evaluate the intestines for evidence of mechanical obstruction
- Evaluate the pancreatic region for evidence of acute inflammation
- Evaluate the biliary tract for evidence of obstruction or perforation
- Evaluate the urinary tract for evidence of obstruction or rupture
- Look for evidence of neoplasia.

Elective evaluation

The majority of abdominal ultrasonographic procedures are performed as an elective part of the work-up of surgical or medical conditions for which abdominal involvement is suspected. Although the indications vary widely, the scanning techniques recommended (see below) are applicable to all cases.

Staging of neoplasia is a specific and common indication for elective abdominal ultrasonography in animals that may not have clinical signs referable to abdominal disease. Malignant neoplasms that typically metastasize to the abdominal organs, or disseminated round cell neoplasia, may be staged prior to instituting therapy. Draining and sentinel lymph node evaluation is also performed transabdominally for tumours such as perianal adenocarcinoma or prostatic neoplasia, which can spread to the sublumbar lymph nodes. Ultrasonography is also widely used for identifying, describing and staging primary tumours of the intra-abdominal organs.

Ultrasonography alone does not provide a definitive diagnosis, but can be used to guide fine-needle or tissue core biopsy procedures. In all cases a thorough evaluation of the abdomen is necessary.

Certain indications for elective abdominal ultrasonography may be evaluated by examination of a single system. Reproductive system examination and serial examinations to monitor progression of organ-specific disease are indications for a focused evaluation.

Value of ultrasonography compared with radiography and advanced imaging modalities

Ultrasonography is currently the best modality for small animal abdominal evaluation. Unlike with radiography, there is no superimposition of structures and the contrast is superior. Ultrasonography allows evaluation of organ parenchymal characteristics and can be used to accurately sample specific lesions. For certain conditions, such as mechanical obstruction of the small intestines, ultrasonography can be more sensitive than survey radiographs. Surgical planning may also be enhanced as more specific lesion localization and details of vascular and lymph node involvement are possible. From a safety perspective, there is no ionizing radiation involved and, therefore, no risk to personnel. In many cases the animal can be evaluated without the need for sedation or anaesthesia, as manual restraint is possible. Ultrasonography is widely available and less costly than computed tomography (CT) or magnetic resonance imaging (MRI). However, ultrasonography is strongly operator-dependent, and the value of the study will therefore increase with the expertise of the ultrasonographer.

Imaging technique

Patient preparation

Appropriate patient preparation can improve the diagnostic quality of a scan. Withholding food for 12 hours prior to examination is recommended for elective ultrasound studies, as the presence of air or food in the gastrointestinal tract decreases the visibility of certain organs. Standard skin preparation should be employed (see Chapter 3). The area of hair to be clipped varies according to the scanning position. For scanning in dorsal recumbency, the animal should be clipped from the pubis to the xiphoid following the costal arch on both sides. For scanning in lateral recumbency, the area clipped should extend further laterally. To examine the pylorus, pancreas, duodenum, right kidney and right adrenal gland it is often necessary to use an intercostal approach, for which the clipped area should be extended cranially.

Positioning

Abdominal ultrasonography may be performed with the animal in dorsal or lateral recumbency (Figure 7.1a). The method chosen is largely determined by the prior experience of the operator, but can also be influenced by the clinical presentation. Animals with haemodynamic or respiratory compromise may better tolerate lateral recumbency. If lateral recumbent scanning is performed, it is recommended that the animal be turned on to its other side part-way through the examination for complete evaluation. Dorsal recumbency is best maintained with the animal in a padded trough (Figure 7.1b). It may be necessary to change the position of the animal to answer certain questions.

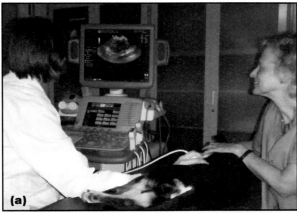

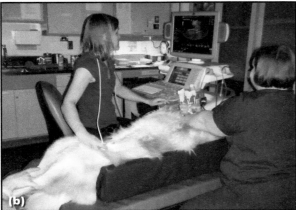

7.1 **(a)** Positioning for lateral recumbent abdominal ultrasonography. It is recommended that the animal be scanned from both sides and therefore turned part-way through the examination. **(b)** Positioning for dorsal recumbent abdominal ultrasonography. A padded trough makes positioning easier and more comfortable for the animal.

The presence of gravity-dependent material, such as bladder stones, can be confirmed by moving the animal. Conversely, free gas will accumulate in the non-dependent abdomen.

Protocol

Whichever position is chosen, a systematic approach is recommended for thorough and consistent evaluation. A protocol that images each organ in turn is recommended, the order of which may be determined by the scanning position. It is not always possible to visualize every part of a normal organ or every lymph node, but a thorough examination and good knowledge of the anatomical location of each structure will increase the likelihood of detecting abnormalities.

Lateral recumbent ultrasonography
Start with the patient in right lateral recumbency and image:

1. Left liver.
2. Gastric fundus and body.
3. Spleen.
4. Left pancreas.
5. Left kidney and ovary.
6. Left adrenal gland.
7. Small intestines.
8. Colon.
9. Left medial iliac lymph nodes.
10. Urinary bladder and prostate gland or uterus.

Turn the patient so that they are in left lateral recumbency and image:

11. Right liver.
12. Biliary system.
13. Pylorus.
14. Duodenum.
15. Right pancreas.
16. Ileocolic region.
17. Right kidney and ovary.
18. Right adrenal gland.
19. Jejunal and colic lymph nodes.
20. Right medial iliac lymph nodes.

Dorsal recumbent ultrasonography
With the patient in dorsal recumbency, image:

1. Liver and biliary system.
2. Spleen.
3. Left kidney and ovary.
4. Left adrenal gland.
5. Left medial iliac lymph nodes.
6. Urinary bladder.
7. Prostate gland or uterus.
8. Right medial iliac lymph nodes.
9. Right kidney and ovary.
10. Right adrenal gland.
11. Duodenum.
12. Right and left pancreas.
13. Stomach.
14. Small intestines.
15. Colon.

Rapid scan protocols have been developed to look for free fluid in animals that present as an emergency with clinical signs referable to an acute abdomen. These FAST (**F**ocused **A**ssessment with **S**onography for **T**rauma) protocols are similar to those used in human emergency departments (Boysen *et al.*, 2004). The technique is designed for trauma patients, but can be used in any animal suspected of having free fluid, and can be performed adequately by clinicians with little previous ultrasonography experience.

FAST scan for identifying free fluid

With the animal in lateral recumbency, obtain transverse and longitudinal images at four sites:

1. Caudal to the xiphoid.
2. Midline over the urinary bladder.
3. Right flank.
4. Left flank.

Equipment

Appropriate use of machine settings (see Chapter 2) is imperative in obtaining a diagnostic scan. Many machines allow the operator to use established presets for different sized animals, such as 'large abdomen' or 'cat abdomen'. Depth, gain and focal zone location should all be adjusted throughout the scan to maximize image quality for each structure. The abdomen should be scanned with the transducer in a longitudinal orientation, with additional transverse images used to verify findings and complete measurements as necessary. Consistent orientation of the image will enable interpretation. The cranial part of a dorsal or sagittal scan plane image should be on the left of the screen. For transverse images the standard radiographic protocol should be followed, with the right side of the animal on the left side of the screen. Labelling of the image, particularly for oblique scan planes, can assist in understanding of the orientation.

The choice of transducer will be determined by the size of the animal. In general, a curvilinear 8 MHz transducer will provide adequate penetration for most canine abdomens. The exceptions are broad-chested and obese large-breed dogs for which a lower frequency transducer may be necessary for complete evaluation of the cranial abdomen. Cats and toy breed dogs may also be examined using a higher frequency linear transducer, such as 12 MHz. This improves spatial resolution, but the larger footprint of the linear transducer can limit access to some areas of the abdomen. In general, when a higher frequency transducer is available it is recommended for evaluation of superficial organs (such as the spleen) in all animals.

When the abdominal vessels are evaluated they may be interrogated with Doppler ultrasonography. Colour Doppler can help rule out filling defects such as those due to tumour invasion or thrombosis. Colour or power Doppler can also be used to determine the presence of blood flow within lesions suspected to be either neoplastic or ischaemic. Tissue harmonics, when available, can be used to increase the contrast and therefore conspicuity of tissue interfaces. Compounding, available on newer machines, can be used to decrease the noise on the image and thus improve border definition of structures such as lymph nodes (Whatmough *et al.*, 2007).

Normal ultrasonographic appearance

The normal appearance of the major abdominal organs is covered in other Chapters. Thus, only certain features of the abdomen, the peritoneal and retroperitoneal spaces, and the lymph nodes are discussed here.

Diaphragm

The normal diaphragm is seen as a curved hyperechoic line at the cranial aspect of the liver. Certain common artefacts can be mistaken for diaphragmatic rupture. Depth misregistration occurs when the ultrasound beam traverses a volume of falciform fat rather than soft tissue. As the speed of sound waves in soft tissue is used to calculate depth, those that have travelled more slowly through fat will be misplaced on the image as being further from the skin surface. When this occurs on an image of the diaphragm it can appear as a sharply demarcated defect (Figure 7.2a). Scanning the same area from a different approach will determine whether the perceived lesion is real. The 'mirror image' artefact is associated with the curved highly reflective nature of the gas interface. The sound wave is reflected in a different direction before it returns to the transducer. As the system assumes that all echoes arise from points in a straight line, this results in the liver being artefactually placed within the thorax on the image (Figure 7.2b).

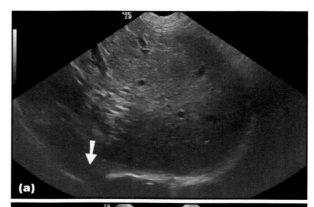

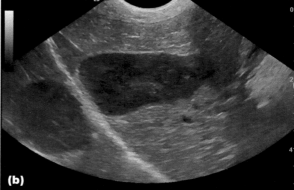

7.2 **(a)** Depth misregistration due to falciform fat. There is an artefactual discontinuity of the diaphragm (arrowed). **(b)** Mirror image artefact, giving the appearance of the liver and gallbladder on the thoracic side of the diaphragm.

Peritoneal space and general abdomen

The normal peritoneal cavity is a potential space between the thin membranes that line the parietal and visceral components of the abdomen. A scant amount of fluid within this space lubricates the serosal surfaces, but it is not usually detected ultrasonographically, except in very young animals. There is a variable amount of fat within the abdomen located in the falciform ligament, mesentery and omentum. These are not visualized as separate structures unless there is a large volume effusion. In general, the mesentery appears mildly hypoechoic to the adjacent organs, with hyperechoic linear scatter throughout (Figure 7.3; see also **Normal mesentery** clip on DVD).

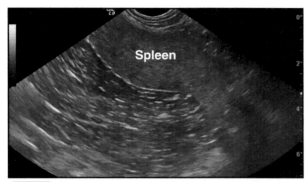

7.3 Normal appearance of the mesentery. The spleen is superficially in this image and has normal mesentery adjacent to it.

Lymph nodes

Many normal lymph nodes are now seen routinely on small animal abdominal ultrasonograms. The location of these lymph nodes and the organs drained by them is shown in Figure 7.4. Normal nodes are characteristically smooth in outline, oval or fusiform in shape, uniform in echogenicity and isoechoic or mildly hypoechoic to the adjacent mesentery. The short- to long-axis ratio of the nodes should be <0.5 in normal dogs (Llabres-Diaz, 2004; Nyman et al., 2004). A hyperechoic linear hilus may be seen in normal lymph nodes, and blood flow, if identified, is hilar in distribution. It is recommended that the anatomical location of certain lymph nodes be routinely evaluated, even if the nodes themselves are not always seen. The drainage characteristics of these nodes are summarized in Figure 7.5.

Jejunal lymph nodes are the most easily identified of the mesenteric group. They are markedly fusiform in shape and lie either side of the mesenteric artery and vein (Figure 7.6a). They are generally easiest to locate when the animal is in left lateral recumbency, using an acoustic window on the right mid-abdomen. The size of the nodes is positively correlated with bodyweight and age in dogs, with the reported median maximum height and width being 3.9 mm and 7.5 mm, respectively (Agthe et al., 2009), although there is a wide size range. The colic nodes are more easily seen in cats than in dogs. They are found

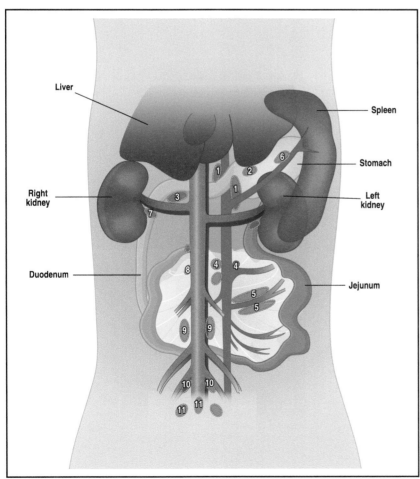

7.4 Abdominal lymph nodes. 1 = hepatic; 2 = gastric; 3 = pancreaticoduodenal; 4 = colic; 5 = jejunal; 6 = splenic; 7 = renal; 8 = lumbar aortic; 9 = medial iliac; 10 = hypogastric; 11 = sacral.

Lymph node group	Location	Normal lymph nodes seen?	Drainage
Hepatic	Either side of the portal vein adjacent to the porta hepatis	Variable	Stomach; duodenum; pancreas; liver
Gastric	Between the stomach and liver in the lesser omentum	Variable	Oesophagus; stomach; liver; diaphragm; peritoneum
Pancreaticoduodenal	Adjacent to the cranial duodenal flexure	Variable	Duodenum; pancreas; omentum
Colic	Adjacent to the ileocolic junction	Yes (cats)	Ileum; caecum; colon
Jejunal	Either side of the mesenteric artery and vein	Yes	Jejunum; ileum; pancreas
Splenic	Adjacent to the splenic vein	No	Oesophagus; stomach; pancreas; spleen; liver; omentum; diaphragm
Renal	Adjacent to the renal vessels	No	Kidneys
Lumbar aortic	Along the aorta and caudal vena cava	No	Lumbar vertebrae; ribs; lumbar, intercostal and abdominal muscles; aorta; nervous system; mediastinum and pleura; diaphragm and peritoneum; adrenal glands; urogenital system
Medial iliac, hypogastric and sacral	Medial iliac: between the deep circumflex and external iliac arteries Hypogastric: between the internal iliac and median sacral artery Sacral: along the median sacral artery	Medial iliac	Pelvic limb and pelvis; caudal urogenital system

7.5 Position, conspicuity and drainage characteristics of the abdominal lymph nodes (Bezuidenhout, 1993).

adjacent to the ileocaecocolic junction in the right mid-abdomen, cranial to the jejunal nodes, and typically appear as a cluster of two or more nodes that are more oval in shape. The hepatic nodes (Figure 7.6b) are located either side of the portal vein, immediately caudal to the hepatic hilus, but are not often seen when normal. The gastric node is located between the stomach and liver, whilst the pancreaticoduodenal node lies in front of the cranial duodenal flexure. These are also more often identified in the cat.

The medial iliac nodes (Figure 7.6c) are the largest nodes of the parietal group and are located between the deep circumflex iliac and external iliac arteries. There is usually one node on each side, although more may be present. They are most easily seen with the patient in lateral recumbency, using a window on the flank ventral to the epaxial muscles. They are seen cranial and superficial to the aortic and caval bifurcation. The more caudal nodes of the parietal chain (the hypogastric and sacral nodes) are rarely seen unless enlarged.

Abdominal vessels

Imaging of the abdominal vessels is indicated to rule out vascular invasion by neoplastic tissue, to diagnose the presence of suspected vascular anomalies, and to identify clinically suspected intravascular emboli. Vascular evaluation is also indicated in any animal presented with a condition that is likely to produce a hypercoagulable state, such as immune-mediated haemolytic anaemia. In addition, the abdominal vessels serve as important landmarks for identifying, amongst others, lymph nodes, the adrenal glands and pancreas. The normal vascular anatomy of the abdomen is shown in Figure 7.7. Complete evaluation of the vasculature requires experience as well as an understanding of both anatomy and Doppler techniques.

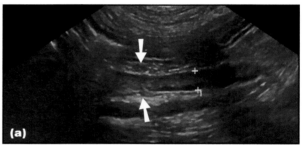

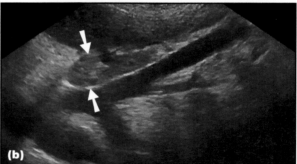

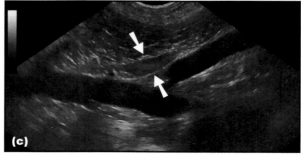

7.6 **(a)** Normal jejunal lymph node (arrowed) demonstrating the fusiform shape. **(b)** Hepatic lymph node (arrowed) seen adjacent to the portal vein. This node has a small cyst-like area within it. **(c)** Normal medial iliac lymph node (arrowed) in a 5-year-old Cocker Spaniel. The caudal vena cava is seen deep to the node.

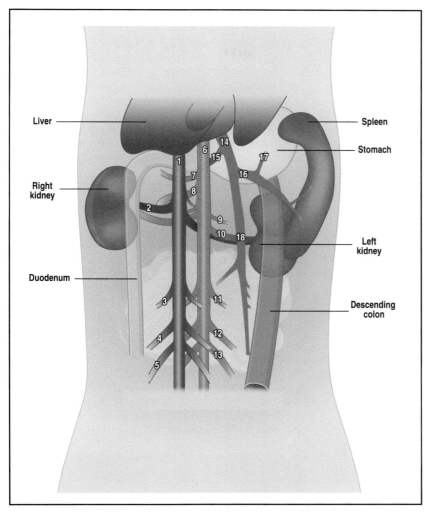

Liver

Right
kidney

Duodenum

Spleen

Stomach

Left
kidney

Descending
colon

7.7 Major abdominal vessels.
1 = caudal vena cava;
2 = renal vein; 3 = circumflex iliac vein;
4 = external iliac vein; 5 = internal iliac
vein; 6 = aorta; 7 = coeliac artery;
8 = cranial mesenteric artery;
9 = phrenicoabdominal artery;
10 = renal artery; 11 = circumflex iliac
artery;12 = external iliac artery;
13 = internal iliac artery; 14 = portal
vein; 15 = gastroduodenal vein;
16 = splenic vein; 17 = left gastric vein;
18 = cranial mesenteric vein.

Certain ultrasonographic features pertain to all vessels. On greyscale images the vessel lumen should be anechoic (Figure 7.8). Slice thickness artefacts may result in spurious echoes within the lumen, but interrogation of the vessel in both transverse and longitudinal planes permits differentiation of the artefact from an abnormality. Colour Doppler imaging of vessels, when performed with the correct machine settings, should result in a solid colour within the lumen representative of flow in the expected direction towards (red) or away from (blue) the transducer. It should be noted that, depending on the direction of

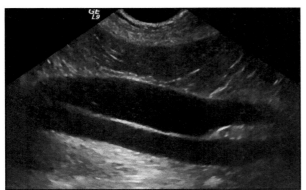

7.8 Normal caudal vena cava and aorta at their bifurcation.

the ultrasound beam, flow in both arteries and veins may be shown as either red or blue. A mosaic effect will result if there is turbulent flow within a vessel, such as that caused by narrowing, intraluminal disease or abnormal vascular anatomy. Such an effect can be created in normal vessels if the pulse repetition frequency (PRF) or wall filter settings are too low, or if the Doppler gain is set too high.

On routine abdominal ultrasonography the caudal vena cava, aorta, renal vessels, splenic vein and portal system may be visualized. The caudal vena cava can be seen most easily in the caudodorsal abdomen where it runs parallel and close to the aorta, and in the mid-cranial abdomen where it traverses the liver before crossing the diaphragm. Cranially, pulsed wave (PW) Doppler of the normal vena cava demonstrates a waveform characteristic of the change in pressure within the right atrium into which it flows, as well as the intra-abdominal and intrathoracic pressure changes associated with ventilation (Figure 7.9a). This is in contrast to the portal vein, which has an almost flat characteristic venous profile (Figure 7.9b). The difference in pulsed waveform can be used in addition to anatomical location, and the straighter course of the caudal vena cava, to differentiate the two vessels. The portal system is discussed in more detail in Chapter 8.

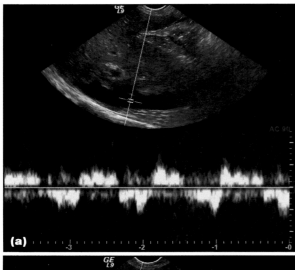

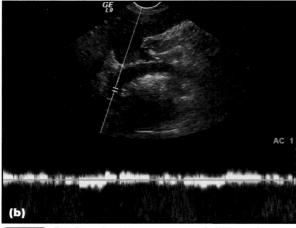

7.9 PW Doppler ultrasonograms. **(a)** Normal caudal vena cava at the diaphragm. **(b)** Normal portal vein.

The aorta is also best visualized in the caudo-dorsal abdomen, where it runs parallel to the caudal vena cava, and can then be followed forward. The cranial mesenteric and coeliac arteries can be identified as they leave the aorta cranial to the renal artery; their location is important for identification of the right adrenal gland.

Abdominal conditions

Abdominal wall rupture and herniation

Abdominal wall defects can be congenital or traumatic in origin. A suspected hernia or rupture is often identified on clinical examination, and ultrasonography can then be used to determine whether there is organ displacement through the defect. The small intestine is the most commonly displaced structure. Loops of bowel adjacent to the abdominal wall defect should be carefully followed to detect displacement into the area. Herniated bowel may become entrapped and then dilated. The associated ischaemia that may occur appears as thickening of the intestinal wall and pos-sible loss of wall layering and corrugation. Abdominal wall defects can also occur secondary to breakdown of surgical closure (see **Postsurgical hernia** clip on DVD).

Traumatic body wall ruptures are most often caused by bite wounds and can lead to herniation with the small intestine being the most commonly displaced organ. These ruptures can occur in any location and there is often significant trauma to the adjacent subcutaneous tissues, which can make evaluation of the wall itself difficult. Continuity of fluid between the peritoneal cavity and the subcutaneous tissues may be seen, along with displacement of the intestine or other organs into the defect. Such hernias are often closed and free gas is therefore not necessarily present.

Abdominal wall masses

Ultrasonography can assist in the evaluation of palpable abdominal wall masses, but such masses may also be identified during a routine abdominal ultrasound examination. The appearance of the mass is determined by its tissue composition. The most commonly identified abdominal wall mass is a lipoma. These characteristically appear well defined with a thin hyperechoic capsule and internal hyperechoic striations (Figure 7.10). Most occur within the fascial planes or in the subcutaneous tissues, but invasive lipomas disrupt the normal contours of the abdominal wall musculature. Liposarcomas have a much greater soft tissue component and are likely to appear more heterogeneous, but it is not possible to differentiate invasive lipomas from liposarcomas ultrasonographically.

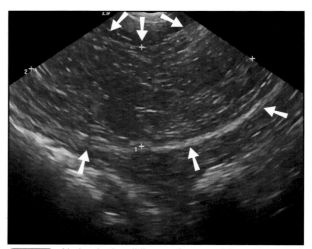

7.10 Abdominal wall lipoma (arrowed) in a 12-year-old Labrador Retriever.

Other neoplastic masses of the abdominal wall include fibrosarcomas, haemangiosarcomas and caudal rib associated osteosarcomas or chondrosarcomas. Malignant lesions generally have a heterogeneous or complex appearance, and irregular or poorly defined margins (Figure 7.11); although, sarcomas can have a well defined wall, which belies the finger-like extensions of the tumour that characteristically occur. Mast cell tumours often have a homogeneous echotexture with well defined margins and subcapsular vessels. Abdominal ultrasonography can also be used to identify invasion into the peritoneal cavity by any abdominal wall mass.

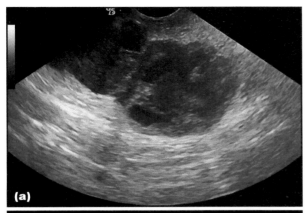

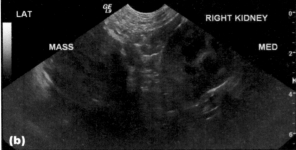

7.11 **(a)** Heterogeneous cavitated mass in the inguinal region of an 11-year-old mixed-breed dog. This was diagnosed as an undifferentiated sarcoma. **(b)** Cutaneous haemangiosarcoma in a 9-year-old Labrador Retriever. The lesion crossed the abdominal wall and displaced the right kidney.

Abdominal wall sinus tracts

Sinus tracts within the abdominal wall may occur due to penetrating trauma, foreign body migration or drainage of a body wall abscess. The tract itself is typically linear and hypoechoic to anechoic, with surrounding hyperechoic tissue due to inflammation. Following draining tracts requires appropriate re-orientation of the transducer for thorough evaluation, as clinically important extensions of the tract can be missed. Pockets of fluid are often present at the origin of the tract and appear hypoechoic, frequently with internal echoes due to the cellularity of purulent material. Gas within an abscess appears as hyperechoic foci with associated reverberation artefacts, which are often moving within the fluid pocket. The presence of distal acoustic enhancement can be used to confirm fluid content, but purulent material is frequently seen to swirl around when pressure is applied with the transducer.

Diaphragmatic rupture and herniation

Animals with clinical signs that raise suspicion for diaphragmatic rupture should always have abdominal radiographs performed prior to the ultrasonographic examination. Disruption of the diaphragm can occur congenitally or secondary to blunt trauma. True disruption must be differentiated from artefact (see above). Peritoneopericardial diaphragmatic hernias (PPDHs) are always congenital. Peritoneal structures can be identified adjacent to the heart within the pericardial sac. For further information, see Chapter 5.

Peritoneal fluid

Free fluid accumulates in the dependent part of the abdomen, and its location may therefore depend on the position of the patient. Small volumes of fluid tend to accumulate adjacent to the urinary bladder or between liver lobes. Ultrasonography is more sensitive than radiography for detection of small volumes of fluid. In 1989 Henley *et al.* were able to detect 1 ml/kg of peritoneal free fluid, and with advances in technology it is very likely that smaller volumes can now be reliably identified.

The echogenicity of the fluid gives some information about its composition. Increased echogenicity generally indicates increased cellularity (Figure 7.12a; see also **Peritoneal effusion** clip on DVD), but the smaller the volume of fluid, the more difficult it is to accurately judge echogenicity. Fluid adjacent to the urinary bladder can be compared with urine, which should be anechoic (Figure 7.12bc). Increasing the gain setting when imaging free fluid can improve characterization of the echogenicity.

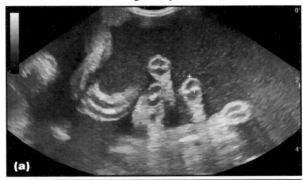

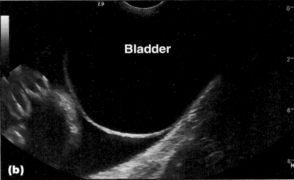

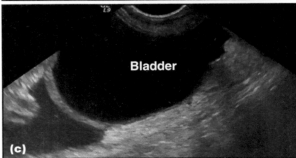

7.12 **(a)** Echogenic effusion surrounding the small intestines in a 10-year-old Golden Retriever with a haemoabdomen secondary to a splenic haemangiosarcoma. **(b)** Anechoic fluid adjacent to the urinary bladder in a dog with ascites secondary to cirrhosis and portal hypertension. **(c)** Echogenic effusion adjacent to the urinary bladder in a dog with peritonitis.

Pneumoperitoneum

Pneumoperitoneum can be spontaneous or traumatic. The most common cause of spontaneous pneumoperitoneum is rupture of the gastrointestinal tract, but it may also be due to bacterial peritonitis, splenic necrosis or bladder rupture. Iatrogenic pneumoperitoneum may be seen following abdominocentesis, needle biopsy or percutaneous gastrotomy tube placement. Therefore, it is recommended that a complete ultrasound evaluation be performed prior to such procedures. Abdominal radiography is an important screening method for pneumoperitoneum. Ultrasonography can be used in conjunction with radiography (including horizontal beam radiography) to increase the chances of detection of peritoneal gas.

Small amounts of free gas appear as floating hyperechoic foci or lines that may be recognized by the associated reverberation artefacts (Figure 7.13). This should not be confused with gas within the lumen of the small intestines. Free peritoneal gas bubbles move when the position of the animal is adjusted. Gas typically accumulates in the non-dependent part of the abdomen adjacent to the wall, although focal gas accumulation may occur with a local gastrointestinal perforation.

Large volumes of free gas, such as may be present postoperatively, can theoretically limit evaluation of the abdomen due to reflection and reverberation. In practice there is very rarely enough to limit the examination, and a different approach to each organ can bypass the problem. As free gas can persist for several days after surgery, pneumoperitoneum alone is not sufficient for a diagnosis of dehiscence.

Diffuse peritoneal disease

Steatitis

Inflammation of fat is referred to as steatitis. Idiopathic omental and mesenteric steatitis has been described in the dog, where the ultrasonographic appearance was of mesenteric and omental masses between the stomach and spleen and around the small intestines (Komori *et al.*, 2002). In contrast to steatitis, nodular fat necrosis is a benign and incidental finding, most common in obese animals. It appears as well defined hyperechoic nodules in the mesenteric and omental fat. These nodules tend to be hyperattenuating and thus produce distal shadows.

Peritonitis

Peritonitis refers to diffuse inflammation of the peritoneum and can occur due to infectious (e.g. feline coronavirus) or non-infectious causes (Figure 7.14). It leads to increased attenuation of sound waves by the mesenteric fat and variable amounts of effusion. The ultrasonographic appearance is characterized by the hyperechoic mesentery (Figure 7.15; see also **Changes to the mesentary** clip on DVD) and variable shadowing, which may obscure visualization of local organs. Small volumes of non-inflammatory peritoneal effusion can also lead to hyperechogenicity of the mesentery, without histopathological evidence of inflammation; therefore, evidence of peritoneal inflammation should be interpreted in relation to other findings, such as corrugation of adjacent small intestines.

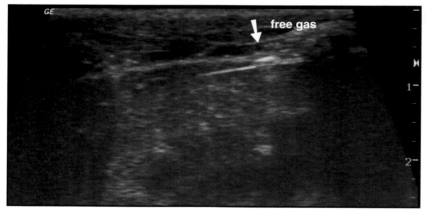

7.13 Focal peritoneal free gas (labelled) in a dog with duodenal perforation secondary to ulceration. The gas bubble (arrowed) is associated with a reverberation artefact.

Cause	Ultrasonographic findings
Rupture of the biliary tract	Inflammation localized in the cranial abdomen; evidence of biliary disease (e.g. mucocele)
Gastrointestinal perforation	Free peritoneal gas; gastrointestinal lesion
Pancreatitis	Inflammation in the region of the pancreas; associated pancreatic changes
Penetrating trauma	Evidence of fistula; free peritoneal gas
Feline coronavirus	Large volumes of anechoic fluid (wet form); may find enlargement of multiple organs
Foreign body	Focal hyperechoic mesentery and possible focal free fluid; shadowing object not associated with any known anatomical structure

7.14 Causes of peritonitis and the associated ultrasonographic findings.

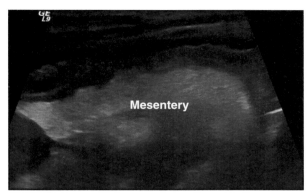

7.15 Hyperechoic mesentery adjacent to the duodenum in a dog with localized peritonitis due to pancreatitis. The inflamed pancreas is seen deep to the duodenum, but is poorly defined due to shadowing from the inflamed mesentery.

Abdominal carcinomatosis

Abdominal carcinomatosis refers to the dissemination of neoplasia along the peritoneal surfaces (Figure 7.16). The term includes peritoneal invasion by epithelial, mesenchymal or haemopoietic tumours. Free peritoneal fluid and masses in the connecting peritoneum are the most common finding in cats with carcinomatosis. There may also be concurrent pleural effusion, lymph node enlargement and masses in the abdominal organs. In some cases, peritoneal effusion may be the only ultrasonographic finding.

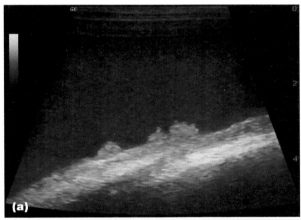

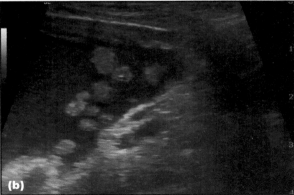

7.16 Abdominal carcinomatosis secondary to ovarian carcinoma in a 7-year-old Shih Tzu bitch. The echogenic fluid is characteristic of carcinomatosis. **(a)** Focal peritoneal masses. **(b)** Masses along the median ligament of the bladder.

Abdominal masses

Certain neoplastic masses can arise within the mesentery without an identifiable organ of origin (Figure 7.17). Intra-abdominal lipomas are similar in echogenicity to the mesenteric and omental fat, and appear hyperechoic to the spleen and renal cortex. They may have internal hypoechoic streaks and, if necrotic, can have a hypoechoic to anechoic centre. Mesenteric haemangiosarcoma is similar to other haemangiosarcoma lesions, with marked heterogeneity, irregular margination and cavitated regions. It cannot be ultrasonographically differentiated from a mesenteric haematoma (such as those that may result following trauma). Intra-abdominal abscesses most often appear as irregularly defined, hypoechoic masses, often with echogenic fluid in the centre. Gas within the abscess appears as hyperechoic foci with associated reverberation artefacts. Mesenteric granulomas are rare, but may occur with foreign bodies.

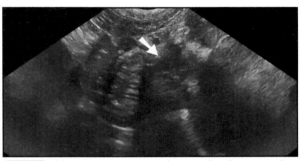

7.17 Mass in the omentum (arrowed) adjacent to the gastric fundus in a 7-year-old Bernese Mountain Dog. The mass was diagnosed as a histiocytic sarcoma by ultrasound-guided fine-needle aspiration.

Foreign bodies

Abdominal foreign bodies can occur through penetrating injury (including direct penetration of the abdominal wall), penetration of the gastrointestinal tract by ingested foreign bodies, and penetration of the diaphragm by inhaled foreign material. The other origin of abdominal foreign bodies is iatrogenic, with retained surgical sponges being most common.

Foreign material can be directly visualized ultrasonographically, although the ability to do so is dependent on the size of the object. The ultrasonographic appearance of a structure depends on its acoustic impedance, which varies with physical density.

- Wooden foreign bodies have a moderate surface echo with complete or 'dirty' distal shadowing.
- Grass awns have a double or triple spindle-shaped echogenic surface and a variable distal shadow, which is more often seen in the transverse plane.
- Retained surgical sponges characteristically appear as a hypoechoic mass with an irregular hyperechoic centre.

Peritonitis often results from the presence of a foreign body, and this may be easier to identify than the object itself. Chronic foreign bodies may be associated with abscesses, granulomas or sinus tracts.

Abnormal lymph nodes

Lymph node enlargement may occur due to reactivity or malignant infiltration. Whilst ultrasonographic changes in lymph nodes are not specific, certain features are more likely to occur with malignant rather than benign processes (Figure 7.18; see also **Enlarged abdominal lymph nodes (1)** and **(2)** clips on DVD). A lymph node short- to long-axis ratio of >0.5, peripheral rather than hilar blood flow, and increased resistive and pulsatility indices have all been associated with malignancy in dogs (Nyman *et al.*, 2004; Prieto *et al.*, 2009). Abdominal lymph node heterogeneity has also been associated with malignancy in dogs, but not cats (Kinns and Mai, 2007); although, normal younger animals may also have nodes with a heterogeneous echotexture.

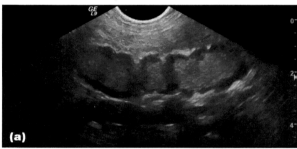
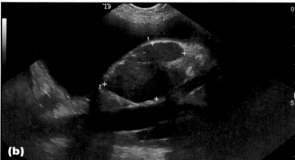

7.18 **(a)** An enlarged and irregular jejunal lymph node with a hypoechoic rim in a 9-year-old Rottweiler with lymphosarcoma. The adjacent mesentery is hyperechoic. **(b)** An enlarged, rounded and hypoechoic right medial iliac lymph node in an 11-year-old mixed-breed dog with prostatic carcinoma. The lymph node was aspirated under ultrasound guidance and confirmed to be infiltrated with metastatic neoplasia.

Vascular abnormalities

Embolic disease can affect any of the intra-abdominal vessels. Thrombi appear as echogenic tissue within the lumen of the vessel (Figure 7.19a; see also **Splenic thrombi** clip on DVD), causing partial or complete obstruction to visualized blood flow. Within the first few hours thrombi can be difficult to visualize as they are poorly echoic, but they then remain echogenic for at least a week or more. Where thrombi are suspected Doppler interrogation is recommended (Figure 7.19b) and any lesion should be confirmed by imaging in both longitudinal and transverse planes. Animals presenting in a hypercoagulable state may have slow or turbulent blood flow that can be recognized prior to thrombus formation. On greyscale images this can appear as echogenic 'smoke' within the abdominal vessels (Figure 7.20; see also **'Smoke' in the caudal vena cava** clip on DVD).

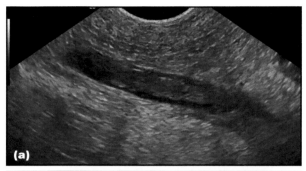
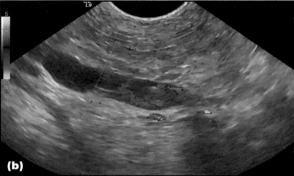

7.19 **(a)** Thrombus in the splenic vein of a 7-year-old Dobermann with renal failure. **(b)** Splenic vein thrombus in an 8-year-old Shih Tzu with immune-mediated haemolytic anaemia. Note the echogenic filling defect in the lumen of the vessel.

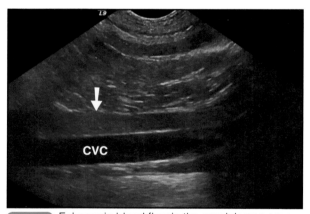

7.20 Echogenic blood flow in the caudal vena cava (CVC) of an 8-year-old Shih Tzu with immune-mediated haemolytic anaemia. Thrombi (arrowed) were located in the portal and splenic veins, but blood flow was continuous in the cava.

Caudal vena cava abnormalities are most commonly seen in association with neoplasia of the right adrenal gland (see Chapter 13), but can occur with invasion of hepatic, lymph node (Figure 7.21) or renal neoplasia, or due to extension of femoral or iliac thrombosis. It is difficult to differentiate between thrombosis, which can occur secondary to compromise or compression of the wall, and overt neoplastic invasion. Both appear as echogenic structures within the lumen of the vessel. Colour Doppler imaging shows a filling defect within the vessel. Complete occlusion will result in absence of flow beyond the lesion. Partial occlusion may result in turbulence adjacent to the lesion, which will appear as a mosaic of colour.

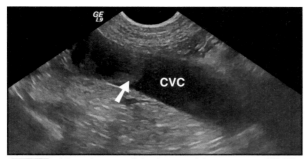

7.21 Mass (arrowed) in the caudal vena cava (CVC) of an 8-year-old Golden Retriever with lymphosarcoma. On necropsy the mass was confirmed to be an extension of a lymph node malignancy into the vessel.

Aortic and iliac arterial thromboembolism is most commonly seen in cats with hypertrophic cardiomyopathy, but can also be found in dogs secondary to neoplasia, cardiac disease or hypercoagulable states. The ultrasonographic appearance is similar to that of venous thrombi.

Vascular anomalies, other than those arising from the portal system, are rare. Lesions such as segmental caudal vena cava aplasia may be recognized ultrasonographically, although other modalities such as CT angiography are usually required for a definitive diagnosis.

Retroperitoneal conditions

The retroperitoneal space is bound by the vertebrae and sublumbar muscles dorsally, the parietal surface of the peritoneum ventrally, the diaphragm cranially and the anus caudally. Thus, lesions within the retroperitoneal space can originate from the adjacent structures, as well as from the retroperitoneal contents. The retroperitoneal space contains blood vessels, fat, small muscle bundles, nerves and lymphatic tissue in addition to the great vessels, kidneys, adrenal glands, ureters and sublumbar lymph nodes. Retroperitoneal ultrasonography can be very useful in determining the origin of a retroperitoneal mass effect or loss of retroperitoneal detail identified radiographically.

Retroperitoneal effusion

Retroperitoneal free fluid can be an ultrasonographic feature of haemorrhage, neoplasia, inflammation and urine extravasation. As with peritoneal effusion, the echogenicity of the free retroperitoneal fluid can help to determine its cellularity. Ultrasonography may also be used to guide sampling of localized pockets of effusion.

Retroperitoneal haemorrhage may be associated with neoplasia, trauma or coagulopathy. Adrenal gland phaeochromocytomas, in addition to renal and retroperitoneal sarcomas, can cause acute retroperitoneal haemorrhage. Trauma-associated haemorrhage may arise from the kidney or retroperitoneal vessels. Renal artery avulsion is difficult to visualize directly, but Doppler interrogation demonstrates a lack of renal perfusion and may reveal the presence of an arterial thrombus.

The leakage of urine into the retroperitoneal space is most often associated with blunt trauma and consequent ureteral rupture. Iatrogenic ureteral tearing or transection also results in uroretroperitoneum. Counter intuitively, when ureteral rupture occurs, the renal pelvis may appear dilated. Proximal urethral and bladder trigone tears can also result in retroperitoneal urine accumulation, due to tracing of urine along tissue planes. Ultrasonographically, the acute appearance is of anechoic fluid.

Perirenal fluid accumulation can occur in dogs and cats with acute renal failure (see **Retroperitoneal effusion** clip on DVD). It is most often bilateral and is not specific for any underlying cause, having been seen with obstructive, neoplastic, toxic and infectious aetiologies. Other ultrasonographic features of acute renal disease (see Chapter 10) may also be present.

Retroperitonitis

Inflammation of the retroperitoneal space can occur secondary to urinary extravasation, surgery, trauma or infection.

Retroperitoneal masses

Retroperitoneal neoplasia may occur due to local spread from organs within the retroperitoneal space or from the structures bordering to the retroperitoneum, or may arise from the retroperitoneum itself. Soft tissue sarcomas, in particular haemangiosarcomas (Figure 7.22), are the most common type of spontaneous retroperitoneal tumour, although retroperitoneal carcinoma can occur.

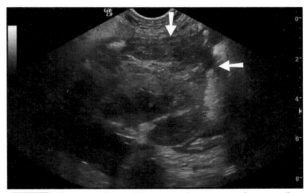

7.22 Retroperitoneal haemangiosarcoma (arrowed) adjacent to the kidney in a 10-year-old mixed-breed dog.

The most common clinical presentations are inappetence and abdominal pain, although these may also reflect the involvement of adjacent structures such as the spine. The retroperitoneal location can be difficult to determine, especially with large lesions. Secondary obstruction of the proximal ureters, invasion of the retroperitoneal structures or surrounding tissues, and displacement of the kidneys may be seen ultrasonographically, along with ventral displacement of the peritoneal organs that is more easily recognized radiographically. Differentiation of malignant from benign solid retroperitoneal masses is not possible using ultrasonography alone. Ultrasonography can be used to direct biopsy or fine-needle aspiration of mass lesions.

Foreign bodies

Retroperitoneal foreign bodies have a similar ultrasonographic appearance and aetiology to those in the peritoneal cavity (see above). Due to the association of the retroperitoneal space with the diaphragm and sublumbar musculature, the incidence of migrating foreign bodies (such as grass awns) may be higher in this location than in the peritoneal cavity.

Particular considerations for sampling

Abdominocentesis is commonly performed for sampling of peritoneal effusion. Ultrasound guidance can assist in needle placement, particularly where only small volumes of fluid are present.

References and recommended further reading

Agthe P, Caine AR, Posch B and Herrtage M (2009) Ultrasonographic appearance of jejunal lymph nodes in dogs without clinical signs of gastrointestinal disease. *Veterinary Radiology and Ultrasound* **50**(2), 195–200

Armbrust LJ, Biller DS, Radlinsky MG and Hoskinson JJ (2003) Ultrasonographic diagnosis of foreign bodies associated with chronic draining tracts and abscesses in dogs. *Veterinary Radiology and Ultrasound* **44**(1), 66–70

Barberet V, Schreurs E, Rademacher N, Nitzl D, Taeymans O *et al.* (2008) Quantification of the effect of various patient and image factors on ultrasonographic detection of select canine abdominal organs. *Veterinary Radiology and Ultrasound* **49**(3), 273–276

Boswood A, Lamb CR and White RN (2000) Aortic and iliac thrombosis in six dogs. *Journal of Small Animal Practice* **41**(3), 109–114

Boysen SR, Rozanski EA, Tidwell AS, Holm JL, Shaw SP and Rush JE (2004) Evaluation of a focused assessment with sonography for trauma protocol to detect free abdominal fluid in dogs involved in motor vehicle accidents. *Journal of the American Veterinary Medical Association* **225**(8), 1198–1204

Boysen SR, Tidwell AS and Penninck DG (2003) Ultrasonographic findings in dogs and cats with gastrointestinal perforation. *Veterinary Radiology and Ultrasound* **44**(5), 556–564

Finn-Bodner ST and Hudson JA (1998) Abdominal vascular sonography. *Veterinary Clinics of North America: Small Animal Practice* **28**(4), 887–942

Fowlkes JB, Strieter RM, Downing LJ, Brown SL, Saluja A *et al.* (1998) Ultrasound echogenicity in experimental venous thrombosis. *Ultrasound in Medicine and Biology* **24**(8), 1175–1182

Gnudi G, Volta A, Bonazzi M, Gazzola M and Bertoni G (2005) Ultrasonographic features of grass awn migration in the dog. *Veterinary Radiology and Ultrasound* **46**(5), 423–426

Henley RK, Hager DA and Ackerman N (1989) A comparison of two-dimensional ultrasonography and radiography for the detection of small amounts of free peritoneal fluid in the dog. *Veterinary Radiology and Ultrasound* **30**(3), 121–124

Holloway A and O'Brien R (2007) Perirenal effusion in dogs and cats with acute renal failure. *Veterinary Radiology and Ultrasound* **48**(6), 574–579

Kinns J and Mai W (2007) Association between malignancy and sonographic heterogeneity in canine and feline abdominal lymph nodes. *Veterinary Radiology and Ultrasound* **48**(6), 565–569

Komori S, Nakagaki K, Koyama H and Yamagami T (2002) Idiopathic mesenteric and omental steatitis in a dog. *Journal of the American Veterinary Medical Association* **221**(11), 1591–1593

Liptak JM, Dernell WS, Ehrhart EJ, Rizzo SA, Rooney MB *et al.* (2004) Retroperitoneal sarcomas in dogs: 14 cases (1992–2002) *Journal of the American Veterinary Medical Association* **224**(9), 1471–1477

Llabres-Diaz FJ (2004) Ultrasonography of the medial iliac lymph nodes in the dog. *Veterinary Radiology and Ultrasound* **45**(2), 156–165

Loh ZHK, Allan GS, Nicoll RG and Hunt GB (2009) Ultrasonographic characteristics of soft tissue tumours in dogs. *Australian Veterinary Journal* **87**(8), 323–329

Merlo M and Lamb CR (2000) Radiographic and ultrasonographic features of retained surgical sponge in eight dogs. *Veterinary Radiology and Ultrasound* **41**(3), 279–283

Monteiro CB and O'Brien RT (2004) A retrospective study on the sonographic findings of abdominal carcinomatosis in 14 cats. *Veterinary Radiology and Ultrasound* **45**(6), 559–564

Nyman HT, Kristensen AT, Flagstad A and McEvoy FJ (2004) A review of the sonographic assessment of tumor metastases in liver and superficial lymph nodes. *Veterinary Radiology and Ultrasound* **45**(5), 438–448

Prieto S, Gomez-Ochoa P, De Blas I, Gascon M, Acena C *et al.* (2009) Pathologic correlation of resistive and pulsatility indices in canine abdominal lymph nodes. *Veterinary Radiology and Ultrasound* **50**(5), 525–529

Saunders WB and Tobias KM (2003) Pneumoperitoneum in dogs and cats: 39 cases (1983–2002). *Journal of the American Veterinary Medical Association* **223**(4), 462–468

Schwarz T, Morandi F, Gnudi G, Wisner E, Paterson C *et al* (2000) Nodular fat necrosis in the feline and canine abdomen. *Veterinary Radiology and Ultrasound* **41**(4), 335–339

Schwarz T, Rossi F, Wray JD, Ablad B, Beal MW *et al.* (2009) Computed tomographic and magnetic resonance imaging features of canine segmental caudal vena cava aplasia. *Journal of Small Animal Practice* **50**(7), 341–349

Shaw SR, Rozanski EA and Rush JE (2003) Traumatic body wall herniation in 36 dogs and cats. *Journal of the American Animal Hospital Association* **39**(1), 35–46

Spaulding KA (1997) A review of sonographic identification of abdominal blood vessels and juxtavascular organs. *Veterinary Radiology and Ultrasound* **38**(1), 4–23

Szatmari V, Sotonyi P and Voros K (2001) Normal duplex Doppler waveforms of major abdominal blood vessels in dogs: a review. *Veterinary Radiology and Ultrasound* **42**(2), 93–107

Tyrrell D and Beck C (2006) Survey of the use of radiography vs. ultrasonography in the investigation of gastrointestinal foreign bodies in small animals. *Veterinary Radiology and Ultrasound* **47**(4), 404–408

Volta A, Bonazzi M, Gnudi G, Gazzola M and Bertoni G (2006) Ultrasonographic features of canine lipomas. *Veterinary Radiology and Ultrasound* **47**(6), 589–591

Whatmough C, Guitian J, Baines E, Benigni L, Mahoney PN *et al.* (2007) Ultrasound image compounding: effect on perceived image quality. *Veterinary Radiology and Ultrasound* **48**(2), 141–145

Video extras

- Changes to the mesentery
- Enlarged abdominal lymph nodes (1)
- Enlarged abdominal lymph nodes (2)
- Normal mesentery

- Peritoneal effusion
- Postsurgical hernia
- Retroperitoneal effusion
- 'Smoke' in the caudal vena cava
- Splenic thrombi

Access via QR code or bsavalibrary.com/ultrasound_7

8

Liver

Nathalie Rademacher

Indications

Ultrasonography is an essential imaging and screening method in animals with suspected liver disease, including vascular anomalies. Indications include:

- Clinical signs or biochemical changes associated with liver disease
- Icterus
- Ascites
- Pyrexia of unknown origin
- Cranial abdominal mass
- Cranial abdominal pain
- To search for metastatic disease when a primary tumour has been found elsewhere.

A complete abdominal ultrasound examination is recommended for each animal. Normal findings do not rule out liver disease and abnormal findings are not pathognomonic for a specific disease. Therefore, fine-needle aspiration (FNA) or ultrasound-guided core tissue biopsy of the liver is required for a final diagnosis. Doppler ultrasonography adds important information about blood flow and vascular patterns.

Value of ultrasonography compared with radiography and computed tomography

Radiography
Radiography is widely available and recommended in cases of suspected liver disease, but is more sensitive for focal or multifocal disease than diffuse disease. Radiographs provide valuable information for the assessment of liver size and whether enlargement is generalized or focal. Radiography also gives an overview of the entire abdomen and the extra-skeletal structures, which is not possible with ultrasonography.

Ultrasonography
Ultrasonography is complementary to abdominal radiography and provides more detailed evaluation of the inner structure of the liver and surrounding organs. Ultrasonography has replaced radiography in most instances as an imaging tool for the evaluation of liver disease due to its non-invasive nature, ease of examination and higher sensitivity. Hepatic parenchymal abnormalities are characterized as being diffuse, focal or multifocal. Ultrasonography is sensitive at detecting focal and multifocal disease, but can be poor at detecting diffuse changes. A definitive diagnosis should be based on a combination of features such as ultrasound examination findings, blood test results, clinical examination and tissue sampling.

Contrast-enhanced ultrasonography is a new imaging technique, utilizing intravenously injected microscopic gas bubbles that are between 2 and 6 µm in diameter. It allows non-invasive assessment of the perfusion of organs and has been used in veterinary medicine in the liver, spleen and kidney. The underlying principle is the detection of the non-linear oscillation or harmonic frequencies, which are generated when the ultrasound beam interacts with the contrast media (see Chapter 1). Therefore, specialized equipment (such as transducers and software) is needed for this technique. The liver is the most common organ investigated with contrast-enhanced ultrasonography. The technique seems to be accurate in differentiating benign from malignant nodules in the liver of dogs, with no reported complications or morbidity (O'Brien et al., 2004; Kanemoto et al., 2009; Kensuke et al., 2010). Contrast-enhanced ultrasonography may be a promising new method of detecting increased arterial blood flow, which is an indicator of portosystemic shunting in dogs.

Computed tomography
Computed tomography (CT) of the liver in dogs and cats has been mainly used for identification of hepatic shunts and vascular abnormalities. The contrast medium can be injected into a peripheral vein, eliminating the need for invasive radiographic angiography procedures. Other advantages include excellent anatomical depiction of the origin, determination and course of the anomalous vessel, and the possibility of three-dimensional (3D) reconstructions. In comparison with ultrasonography, this technique is less operator-dependent. Disadvantages include the need for general anaesthesia and access to CT scanners being limited to academic institutions and specialty practices. CT has been used as an aid for surgical planning, especially for liver masses >2 cm in diameter, as this technique provides better information on the relationship between the hepatic mass and other anatomical structures, in order to determine resectability. In humans, differentiation of benign and malignant hepatic lesions is commonly made with magnetic resonance imaging (MRI) or CT. However, no studies in veterinary medicine are available to this date.

Imaging technique

Patient preparation

The ability to visualize the liver is dependent upon body conformation, liver size and gastrointestinal content. Gas in the stomach is a barrier to successful ultrasonographic imaging; therefore, procedures that result in aerophagia should be avoided. In addition, food should be withheld prior to the examination. Hair should be clipped from the cranial ventral abdomen, along the costal arch, to the last two intercostal spaces, especially in deep-chested dogs and those with microhepatica.

Positioning

Animals can be scanned in dorsal, left lateral or right lateral recumbency, after acoustic gel application, depending on the preference of the ultrasonographer. Most commonly, a 7.5 MHz sector or curvilinear transducer is used in small to medium-sized dogs and cats. In large to giant-breed dogs, a ≤5 MHz transducer may be necessary to visualize the entire liver. Linear transducers are usually not ideal due to their large footprints and the linear field of view, which limit evaluation of the intracostally located liver.

Subxiphoid and intercostal windows should be used for complete evaluation of the liver and gallbladder. In small dogs and cats, the subxiphoid or subcostal window can usually be used to visualize the entire liver. The transducer should be placed immediately caudal to the xiphoid process, and oriented in both transverse and longitudinal directions whilst fanning through the entire liver. The transverse colon can limit hepatic visibility, especially when filled with gas or faecal material, or if the liver is small. In these cases, the intercostal approach provides a useful alternative. The right intercostal approach is especially useful for evaluation of the biliary tract and portal vasculature (e.g. in cases of suspected portosystemic shunts (PSSs)).

Normal ultrasonographic appearance

In dogs and cats the liver is located within the ribcage, just cranial to the stomach, with its cranial margins against the diaphragm and lung interface. The diaphragm appears as a curved hyperechoic line, sometimes associated with a 'mirror image' artefact caused by multiple echoes at the highly reflective interface with the air-filled lung. This artefact results in the liver being displayed beyond the diaphragm on ultrasonograms (Figure 8.1a). Caudally, the liver is in contact with the spleen on the left, the stomach centrally (Figure 8.1b) and with the kidney on the right side at the level of the renal fossa of the caudate lobe. The falciform ligament, filled with a variable amount of fat, is located ventral to the liver and dorsal to the xiphoid process. This poorly defined structure is usually isoechoic to hyperechoic with a coarse echotexture relative to the liver, and can be separated from it by a hyperechoic capsule (Figure 8.2). The falciform ligament may be mistaken for an enlarged liver, especially in cats.

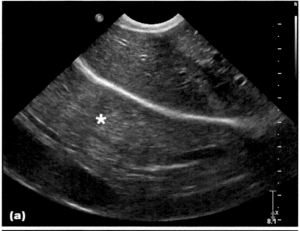

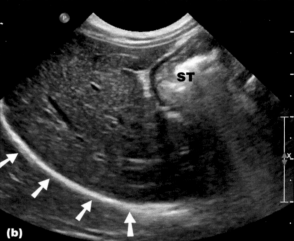

8.1 **(a)** Longitudinal image of the normal liver in a dog. Note the liver parenchyma (∗) is displayed distal to the hyperechoic diaphragm as a result of a 'mirror image' artefact. **(b)** Longitudinal image of the left side of the normal liver in a dog. Note the caudal location of the stomach (ST) and the hyperechoic interface of the diaphragm (arrowed).

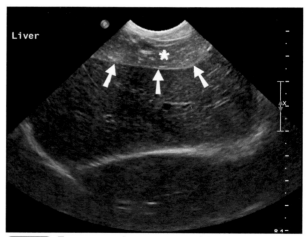

8.2 Transverse ultrasonogram of the normal liver in a dog showing the coarse echotexture of the falciform fat (∗) compared with the liver. Note the hyperechoic interface (arrowed) marking the separation between the liver and ventrally located falciform fat, which can be mistaken for an enlarged liver. The liver is of normal size and echogenicity.

The liver is divided into left, quadrate, right and caudate lobes. The separation of liver lobes is not well seen ultrasonographically unless abdominal fluid is present. The normal hepatic parenchyma has a uniform medium level of echogenicity, with interruption caused by the hepatic and portal veins. The echotexture is coarser and more hypoechoic compared with the spleen (Figure 8.3). The echogenicity in comparison with the renal cortex is more variable, although the liver is usually more hyperechoic. Hepatic echogenicity must be evaluated in comparison with neighbouring organs at the same depth and preferably within the same image. Portal veins have echogenic walls (see Figure 8.4c) and can be traced back to the porta hepatis in cases where Doppler ultrasonography is not available. Hepatic veins lack these echogenic walls and may be seen entering the caudal vena cava.

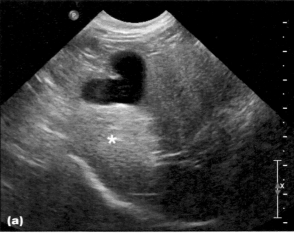

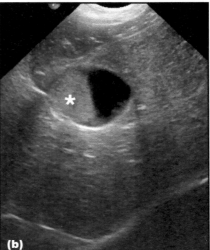

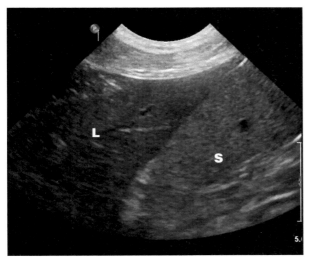

8.3 Longitudinal ultrasonogram of the normal liver (L). The liver appears more hypoechoic and coarse in echotexture compared with the spleen (S). This is due to the presence of the hepatic and portal veins.

The intrahepatic biliary tree is not seen in normal patients. The gallbladder, occasionally bilobed in cats (Figure 8.4a), is a pear-shaped anechoic structure, located between the quadrate and right medial liver lobes in the dog and between two parts of the right medial liver lobe in the cat. The gallbladder functions as a bile reservoir and can vary in size, becoming enlarged in anorexic or fasted animals. It can also contain a variable amount of sludge (Figure 8.4b). The wall of the gallbladder is thin and smooth (Figure 8.4c), measuring <1 mm in cats and up to 2–3 mm in dogs. Acoustic enhancement is commonly observed. The gallbladder must be differentiated from a focal hepatic lesion.

Diffuse parenchymal disease

Diffuse parenchymal disease generally affects all lobes, which may appear isoechoic, hypoechoic or hyperechoic to the expected appearance. A large group of diseases exist that can infiltrate the liver, without disrupting the architecture, and cause only subtle

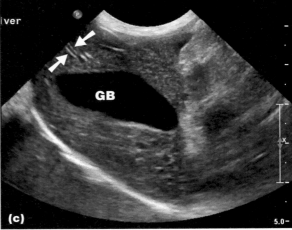

8.4 **(a)** Longitudinal ultrasonogram of the liver in a cat. The gallbladder is bilobed and appears heart-shaped. This is an incidental finding in cats. Note also the acoustic enhancement distal to the gallbladder (*), which is due to lower attenuation from the bile and should not be confused with a hyperechoic lesion. The liver is diffusely hyperechoic due to the presence of hepatic lipidosis. **(b)** Transverse ultrasonogram of a gallbladder in a dog. Note the hyperechoic sludge (*) in the dependent part of the gallbladder. **(c)** Ultrasonogram of the normal liver in a dog. The gallbladder (GB) is seen with anechoic content and thin walls, which are barely visible. Note the hyperechoic walls of the portal veins (arrowed).

changes, making disease difficult to detect. It can be challenging to differentiate diffuse parenchymal diseases from poorly defined multifocal diseases. It is also not uncommon to find more than two abnormalities in the same patient. Biopsy or FNA is almost always necessary to achieve a definitive diagnosis, even if the liver appears normal. The echogenicity of the liver must be compared with that of the right kidney and spleen at the same depth and image settings. Care must be taken to ensure that the organ being compared with the liver is not also diseased. Figure 8.5 summarizes the differential diagnoses for diffuse echogenic changes of the liver parenchyma.

Diffuse hypoechogenicity
• Passive congestion • Acute hepatitis or cholangiohepatitis • Lymphoma • Leukaemia • Histiocytic neoplasia • Amyloidosis • Liver lobe torsion
Diffuse hyperechogenicity
• Steroid hepatopathy • Lipidosis • Vacuolar hepatopathies • Fibrosis • Cirrhosis • Lymphoma • Mast cell tumour
Diffuse mixed echogenicity
• Steroid hepatopathy with benign hyperplasia or other combination of diseases • Chronic active hepatitis • Lymphoma • Hepatocellular carcinoma • Metastasis • Necrosis • Amyloidosis

8.5 Differential diagnoses for diffuse changes in echogenicity of the hepatic parenchyma.

The ultrasonographic assessment of liver size is subjective and changes may be focal or generalized. The caudal tips are usually rounded with hepatomegaly. Causes for generalized hepatomegaly include:

- Steroid hepatopathy
- Lipidosis
- Amyloidosis
- Diabetes mellitus
- Hepatitis
- Congestion
- Neoplasia (e.g. lymphoma, mast cell tumour, histiocytic sarcoma and hepatocellular carcinoma).

Inflammation

Diffuse hepatic inflammatory processes can show variable ultrasonographic features. In cases with acute hepatitis or cholangiohepatitis, the liver may appear diffusely hypoechoic with prominent hyperechoic portal vein walls or periportal tissue (Figure 8.6). Additional findings often include biliary abnormalities

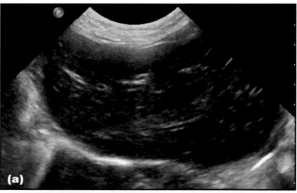

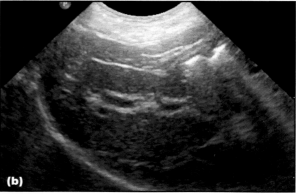

8.6 **(a)** Ultrasonogram of a dog with hypoglycaemia and in hypovolaemic shock. Note the diffusely hypoechoic liver with prominent hyperechoic portal vessel walls, consistent with hepatitis. **(b)** Ultrasonogram of a dog with pancreatitis and elevated liver enzymes. Note the thick-walled portal vessels and diffusely hypoechoic liver, consistent with cholangiohepatitis.

such as biliary sludge, cholelithiasis and gallbladder wall thickening, especially in cats. Decreased liver size with hyperechoic parenchyma, irregular margins, regenerative nodules and abdominal effusion is usually seen with chronic hepatitis. The presence of chronic active inflammation, consisting of inflammatory cells, oedema, fibrosis, necrosis and regenerative nodules can cause a severely heterogeneous liver with variable echogenicity (Figure 8.7). In addition, acquired PSSs may be present due to the developing portal hypertension.

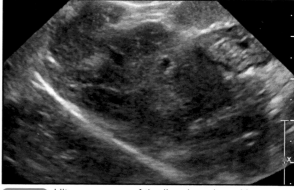

8.7 Ultrasonogram of the liver in a dog with chronically elevated liver enzymes for the past year. Note the irregular border of the liver and heterogeneous parenchyma. The surrounding mesentery appears hyperechoic. This finding is suggestive of liver fibrosis or cirrhosis.

Hepatocutaneous syndrome or canine superficial necrolytic dermatitis causes a unique Swiss-cheese or honeycomb appearance within the hepatic parenchyma (Figure 8.8) and characteristic skin lesions in older dogs.

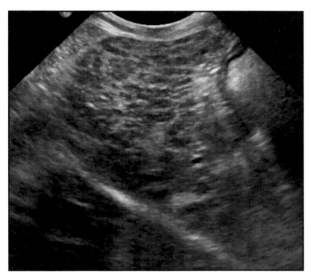

8.8 Hepatic ultrasonogram of a dog with chronic skin lesions. Note the diffusely hypoechoic foci surrounded by hyperechoic parenchyma resembling a honeycomb or Swiss-cheese pattern, commonly seen with hepatocutaneous syndrome.

Neoplasia
Neoplasia of the liver can manifest as diffuse, multifocal or focal disease. Lymphoma, histiocytic sarcoma and mast cell tumour are the most common neoplasms that may lead to diffuse changes and can remain ultrasonographically undetectable. Diffuse hypoechogenicity, hyperechogenicity or a mixed pattern may also occur (Figure 8.9). Generalized hepatomegaly is usually seen with neoplastic disease.

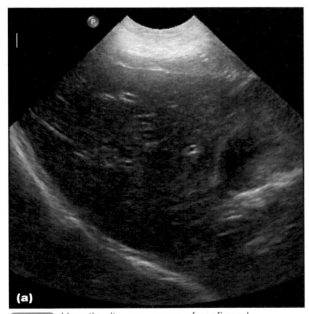

8.9 Hepatic ultrasonograms of confirmed lymphoma. **(a)** The liver appears diffusely hypoechoic with prominent portal markings. (continues) ▶

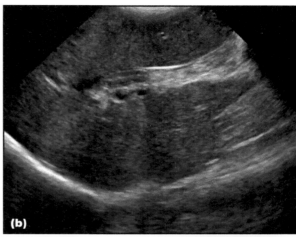

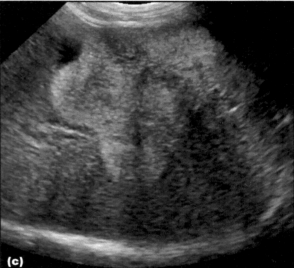

8.9 (continued) Hepatic ultrasonograms of confirmed lymphoma. **(b)** Diffuse hyperechoic liver with loss of vessel demarcation and irregular organ margins. **(c)** Hyperechoic well defined mass within the liver parenchyma.

Metabolic conditions
Vacuolar hepatopathy associated with steroid hepatopathy and hepatic lipidosis are common in small animals and often occur with other primary disorders. These hepatopathies usually present with hepatomegaly and an increase in echogenicity, making vessel walls indistinct and difficult to detect (Figure 8.10). The hepatic parenchyma can also cause increased beam attenuation, which results in a gradual decrease in echogenicity in the far-field of the image (Figure 8.11). In addition, the parenchyma can appear heterogeneous or contain hypoechoic foci (Figure 8.12), most likely due to concurrent nodular hyperplasia.

Hepatic amyloidosis can cause hepatic enlargement and parenchymal changes. Hepatic amyloidosis is commonly associated with inflammatory conditions in other organ systems and develops in the liver over the course of a chronic inflammatory disorder. In Shar Peis and Abyssinian, Siamese and other oriental cat breeds, a predisposition to amyloid deposition is known (Cullen, 2009). Ultrasonographically, diffusely heterogeneous liver parenchyma with mixed hyperechoic and hypoechoic foci may be present.

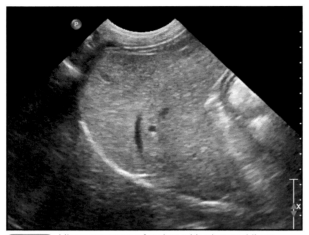

8.10 Ultrasonogram of a dog with elevated liver enzymes. The liver appears diffusely hyperechoic with loss of vessel wall distinction. Cytological diagnosis was hepatopathy with glycogen accumulation.

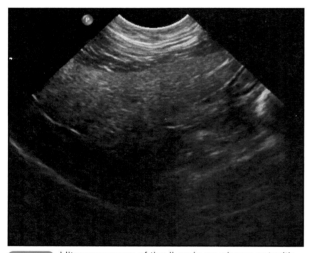

8.11 Ultrasonogram of the liver in an obese cat with diabetes mellitus and hepatic lipidosis diagnosed with FNA. The liver is markedly hyperechoic in the near-field. Note the decreased echogenicity in the far-field due to beam attenuation; this is commonly seen in cats with hepatic lipidosis.

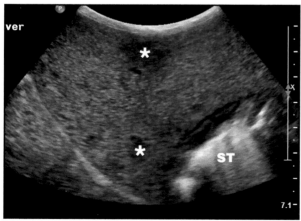

8.12 Ultrasonogram of a dog with histological confirmation of vacuolization and regeneration. The liver appears diffusely hyperechoic with loss of vessel wall distinction and multifocal hypoechoic lesions (*). The stomach (ST) is seen caudally.

Focal parenchymal disease

Focal or multifocal changes are easily identified on ultrasonography because of the uniform background of the liver parenchyma. Focal or lobar hepatomegaly can be caused by:

- Primary or metastatic neoplastic disease
- Cysts
- Haematomas
- Abscesses
- Granulomas
- Lobar torsion
- Thrombosis.

Small lesions on the serosal surface of the liver may be difficult to detect due to interference from gas in the stomach or surrounding fat, unless peritoneal effusion is present. Intraparenchymal lesions can also deform the capsule, causing irregular liver margins. These focal lesions may be isoechoic, hypoechoic, hyperechoic or of mixed echogenicity, and in some cases target lesions are seen. It is not possible to make a diagnosis based on the ultrasound appearance alone; tissue sampling is necessary for confirmation.

Target lesions (Figure 8.13) are a specific type of focal lesion consisting of a hyperechoic or isoechoic centre surrounded by a hypoechoic rim, resulting in a bullseye effect. They are usually associated with malignancy (primary or metastatic neoplasia), especially if more than one lesion is present in an organ. However, they have also been reported with non-neoplastic conditions such as nodular hyperplasia, pyogranulomatous disease and cirrhosis. In dogs with PSSs, cirrhosis or fibrosis, the liver is usually small and the stomach appears closer to the diaphragm than usual (Figure 8.14).

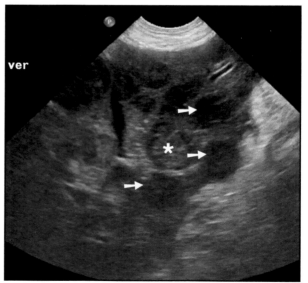

8.13 Ultrasonogram of a dog with histological confirmation of a hepatocellular carcinoma. Note the well defined hypoechoic nodules, partially protruding beyond the liver surface (arrowed). Multifocal target lesions (*) are seen with a hyperechoic centre and a hypoechoic rim.

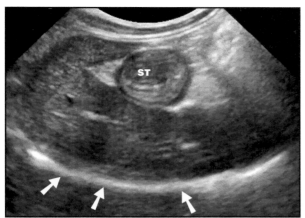

8.14 Longitudinal ultrasonogram of the liver in a dog with a congenital extrahepatic shunt and elevated bile acids. Note the small liver with the stomach (ST) being closer to the diaphragm (arrowed) than usual.

Inflammation

Hepatic abscesses occur rarely in small animals and may appear similar to primary tumours, granulomas or haematomas because of the highly variable ultra-sonographic features. Hepatic abscesses form either as isolated lesions or, more commonly, in association with infections elsewhere in the body. They may also form secondary to necrosis of hepatic neoplasia and can look similar to parasitic cystic structures. On ultrasonography, abscesses may appear as round or irregular with a hypoechoic centre or mixed echo-genicity (Figure 8.15). Central hyperechoic foci with reverberation artefacts consistent with gas can also be observed. Anechoic centres with distal acoustic enhancement also occur. Regional lymphadenopathy may be present with hepatic neoplasia or abscess-ation. Free peritoneal effusion and hyperechoic mes-entery may be seen with abscessation.

Hepatic granulomas may occur in a wide variety of diseases, but most are part of a generalized disease process. Infectious causes include *Mycobacterium* spp., *Bartonella* spp., systemic mycoses, *Leishmania* spp. and other parasitic infections. Ultrasonographically, granulomas may appear as multifocal hyperechoic and well marginated parenchymal lesions.

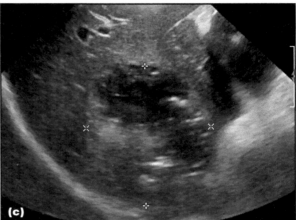

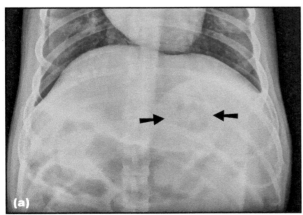

8.15 **(a)** Ventrodorsal radiograph of the cranial abdomen in a dog with lethargy, anorexia and fever. Radiolucent gas bubbles are present within the liver parenchyma cranial and medial to the stomach (between the arrows), consistent with a cavitary hepatic lesion such as a liver abscess. (continues) ▶

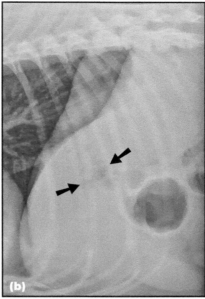

8.15 (continued) **(b)** Lateral radiograph showing the radiolucent gas bubbles (arrowed) in the liver. **(c)** Ultrasonogram of the lesion showing the well defined hypoechoic area (between the callipers) and the hyperechoic areas with dirty shadowing consistent with gas inclusion. The cytological diagnosis confirmed a liver abscess.

Neoplasia

Primary neoplasia is uncommon and accounts for <1.5% of all canine tumours and 1.0–2.9% of all feline tumours. Hepatocellular carcinoma is the most com-mon, although other malignant liver tumours include bile duct carcinomas, carcinoids and sarcomas (Liptak *et al.*, 2004). Metastasis to the liver from non-hepatic neoplasia is more common and occurs 2.5 times more frequently than primary hepatic tumours in dogs. These neoplasms originate mainly from the spleen, pancreas and gastrointestinal tract. Primary hepatobiliary tumours are more common than meta-static disease in cats (Liptak, 2007). Carcinomas tend to spread diffusely throughout the liver and often lead to a mixed pattern of echogenicity (Figure 8.16; see also **Hepatocellular carcinoma with contrast** clip on DVD). Often target lesions are evident, more com-monly with metastasis. With histiocytic sarcoma (Figure 8.17) and lymphoma, multifocal nodules or masses (hypoechoic or mixed in echogenicity) have been identified on ultrasound examination.

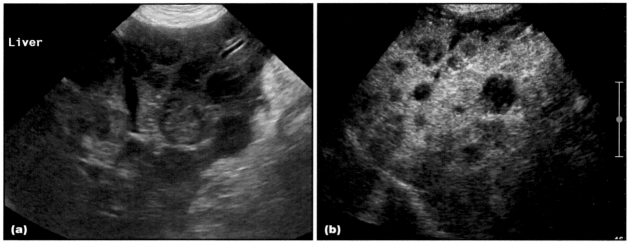

8.16 **(a)** Ultrasonogram of the liver in a dog with histological confirmation of a hepatocellular carcinoma. Note the multifocal hypoechoic lesions throughout the liver parenchyma. **(b)** Contrast-enhanced harmonic ultrasonogram of the liver following intravenous injection of contrast medium. Note the multifocal hypoperfused well defined areas consistent with a malignant hepatocellular carcinoma.

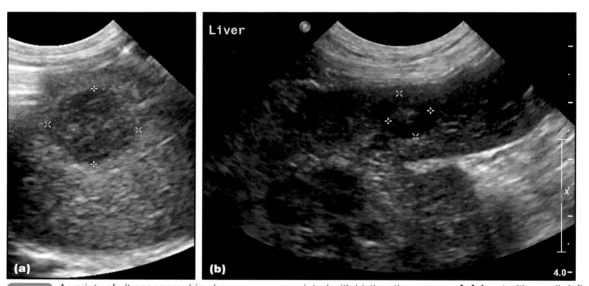

8.17 A variety of ultrasonographic changes are associated with histiocytic sarcoma. **(a)** A cat with a well defined hypoechoic nodule within the otherwise hyperechoic liver. **(b)** A dog with target lesions within the liver.

Regenerative nodular hyperplasia

Benign regenerative nodular hyperplasia is common in dogs, especially in older animals. These regenerative nodules vary in echogenicity and size, appear as hypoechoic nodules measuring <1 cm in diameter, and are detected often (Figure 8.18; see also **Hepatopathy with contrast** clip on DVD). The margins may be well or poorly defined. Benign hepatic adenomas or hepatomas are usually focal hyperechoic masses of variable size.

Cysts

Causes for anechoic cavitary structures in the liver include necrosis, neoplasms or cysts. Hepatic and biliary cysts are sometimes identified in dogs and cats as well defined regular or irregular, anechoic structures, typically with distal acoustic enhancement (Figure 8.19). Cysts are benign lesions surrounded by normal parenchyma. They may appear similar to biliary cystadenomas and cystadenocarcinomas.

Causes include congenital cysts, post-traumatic cavitations, biliary pseudocysts and parasites. Cats with polycystic kidney disease may also have cysts within the liver.

Peliosis hepatis

Peliosis hepatis is defined as a random distribution of dilated vascular spaces in the hepatic parenchyma. It occurs in aged cats, and occasionally in dogs, and can be mistaken for a vascular tumour such as haemangioma or haemangiosarcoma (Cullen *et al.*, 2006; Cullen, 2009).

Liver lobe torsion

Liver lobe torsion is rare in dogs, but can be the cause of acute abdomen and abdominal effusion. The torsion leads to congestion and necrosis of the affected lobe or lobes. Ultrasonographically, the affected lobe appears hypoechoic, with reduced or no blood flow on colour Doppler.

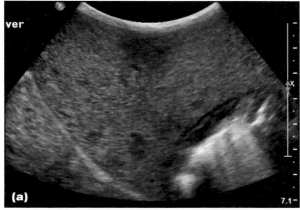

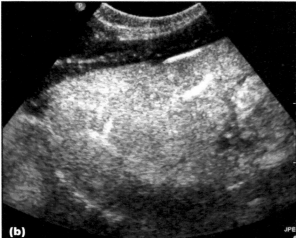

8.18 **(a)** Ultrasonogram of the liver in a dog with multifocal hypoechoic nodules. The liver is diffusely hyperechoic. Hepatopathy with vacuolization and regeneration was diagnosed on FNA. **(b)** Contrast-enhanced harmonic ultrasonogram following injection of microbubble contrast medium. The liver appears generally hyperechoic without evidence of nodules consistent with nodular hyperplasia.

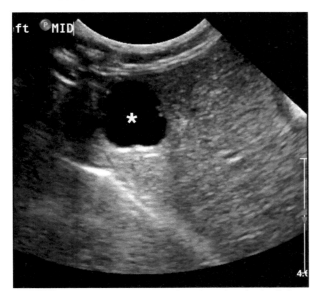

8.19 Ultrasonogram of the liver in a dog. In the left liver lobe an anechoic, round, thin-walled structure (∗) with distal acoustic enhancement was found. This was considered an incidental finding and a liver cyst was diagnosed.

Biliary tract conditions

Biliary sludge and cholelithiasis

Sludge is routinely identified in cats and dogs and is composed of a complex mixture of cholesterol crystals, precipitated bile pigments, mucin and bile salts. It appears as echogenic debris, is usually mobile and changes with body position, causing swirling and redistribution. It is usually considered non-significant, especially in dogs. In cats, it has been associated with elevated serum liver parameters and could predict hepatobiliary disease (Harran *et al.*, 2009).

Sludge balls are accumulations of thick or inspissated bile and can be found in the gallbladder lumen or within the bile duct. They are round, mobile, non-shadowing structures of moderate echogenicity (Figure 8.20). Mineralized and non-mineralized material can also be found in the bile ducts. Choleliths can occur, more commonly in dogs, and appear as hyperechoic structures of variable size, number and shape, which can produce acoustic shadowing (Figure 8.21). They may also be associated with cholecystitis.

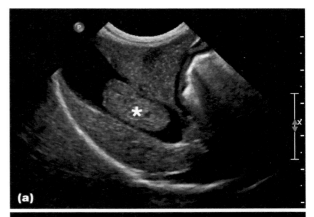

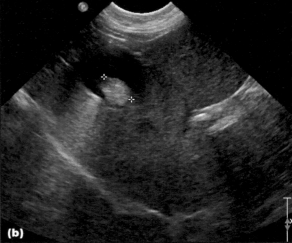

8.20 **(a)** Ultrasonogram of the liver in a dog showing accumulation of a round structure (∗) within the gallbladder isoechoic to the liver parenchyma with no evidence of distal shadowing, indicating no mineralization (sludge ball). **(b)** Ultrasonogram of a sludge ball (between the callipers) in the lumen of the gallbladder in a dog. The structure is hyperechoic in comparison with the liver parenchyma. Note the lack of distal acoustic shadowing.

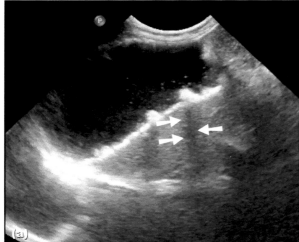

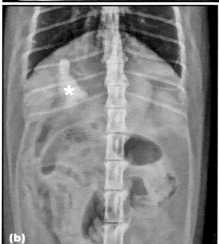

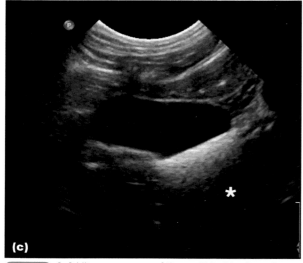

8.21 **(a)** Ultrasonogram of the gallbladder in a dog. The curvilinear structures with distal shadowing (arrowed) in the gallbladder lumen representing choleliths. Note the diffuse thickening of the gallbladder wall. **(b)** Ventrodorsal radiograph of a cat. Note the mineral opaque material (*) consistent with sand in the gallbladder. **(c)** Ultrasonogram of the gallbladder of the cat in (b). Note the hyperechoic line with marked distal shadowing (*) in the gallbladder lumen representing accumulation of dense sludge, likely containing crystals. The material was swirling and mobile with positional changes of the patient.

Biliary obstruction

Ultrasonography has become a routine diagnostic tool for assessing icteric dogs and cats with biliary obstruction. Cholestasis can be caused by extra-hepatic and intrahepatic diseases. Causes of extra-hepatic obstruction (affecting mainly the distal common bile duct) include luminal obstruction by bile duct calculi, inspissated bile and extraluminal compression due to neoplasia or inflammation, especially of the pancreas or duodenum. Dilatation of the duct depends on the degree and duration of the obstruction. The normal diameter of the common bile duct can be up to 3 mm in dogs and up to 4 mm in cats. Long-standing obstruction (3–7 days) of the common bile duct may lead to dilatation of the extrahepatic and intrahepatic ducts. Anechoic tubular structures at the porta hepatis or throughout the parenchyma are seen (Figure 8.22; see also **Obstructive cholestasis** clip on DVD), which follow the more linear portal veins and lack blood flow on colour Doppler examination. Gallbladder dilatation was seen in <50% of cats in a retrospective study (Gaillot *et al.*, 2007). Therefore, absence of gallbladder dilatation does not rule out extrahepatic biliary obstruction.

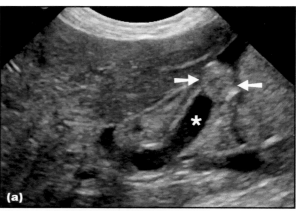

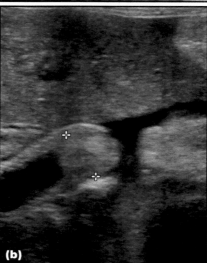

8.22 Ultrasonograms of the liver in an icteric cat with elevated liver enzymes. **(a)** Note the anechoic free fluid in the abdomen and the marked dilatation of the common bile duct (*). The common bile duct ends abruptly and a hyperechoic round mass is seen in between the arrows. **(b)** Magnified image of the mass in the common bile duct showing extrahepatic cholestasis.

Thickening of the gallbladder wall

Generalized gallbladder wall thickening can occur with cholecystitis, cholangiohepatitis, hepatitis and oedema (hypoproteinaemia, congestion). Moderate thickening can be mimicked by free peritoneal fluid accumulated around the gallbladder (Figure 8.23). The wall may have a double-layered appearance with an echogenic outer and inner rim. Cholecystitis occurs more frequently in cats than in dogs and is generally associated with bacterial infection. Neoplastic disease of the gallbladder wall resulting in focal thickening is less common than benign cystic hyperplasia of the mucous glands, which appear as broad-based or pedunculated hyperechoic structures. A similar ultrasonographic appearance has been described for polyps. Irregular or pinpoint-sized hyperechoic structures producing reverberation artefacts within the gallbladder lumen and/or liver parenchyma is consistent with gas and can be seen with cholecystitis (e.g. emphysema associated with diabetes mellitus or gas-producing bacteria such as *Escherichia coli* or *Clostridium perfringens*), cholangiohepatitis, choledochitis and abscess formation.

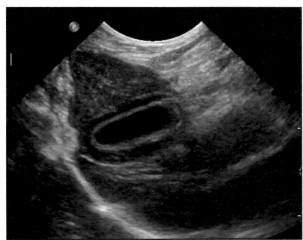

8.23 Ultrasonogram of the gallbladder in a dog. Note the concentric layered thickening of the gallbladder ('double gallbladder wall'), which can be observed in cases of peritoneal effusion, oedema or inflammation.

Gallbladder mucocele

Gallbladder mucoceles occur in dogs and are an important cause of icterus and obstructive disease. They are caused by cystic mucinous hyperplasia, leading to increased mucin production, which distends the gallbladder and can eventually cause wall necrosis and perforation. Ultrasonographically, they have a varied appearance. The classic finding is that of a 'kiwi fruit' pattern of hyperechoic striations radiating from a central point (Figure 8.24). Variations include irregular or striated non-gravitational dependent content, or content with a stellate pattern with a more or less prominent hypoechoic rim attributed to mucin between the gallbladder wall and the organized structure (Figure 8.25).

Gallbladder mucocele can also lead to extrahepatic biliary obstruction. Distension of either or both the intrahepatic and extrahepatic bile ducts may be

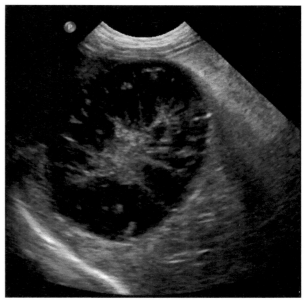

8.24 Ultrasonogram of the gallbladder in a dog showing a mucocele. The gallbladder contains hyperechoic striations in an organized pattern resembling the cut surface of a kiwi fruit. Note the hypoechoic rim representing mucin in between the wall and the mucocele.

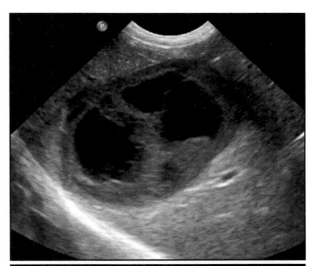

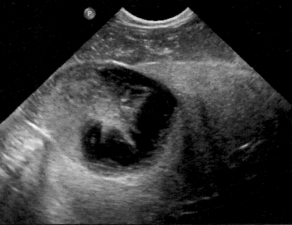

8.25 Gallbladder mucocele in different dogs showing the various types of pattern that can be observed on ultrasonographic examination.

seen. The therapeutic dilemma as to whether to perform cholecystectomy arises when a gallbladder mucocele is identified ultrasonographically but without signs of rupture. It has been shown that they can transform into an acute clinical condition. A breed predilection has been suggested in Cocker Spaniels, Shetland Sheepdogs and Miniature Schnauzers. In one study, a significant predisposition for gallbladder mucoceles in Shetland Sheepdogs was shown compared with the general hospital population.

Biliary tract rupture

Ultrasonographic signs of rupture include loss of gallbladder wall continuity, hyperechoic surrounding mesentery and free peritoneal fluid (Figure 8.26). A sensitivity of 94.4% and specificity of 44.4% for diagnosing gallbladder rupture on abdominal ultrasound examination has been reported, with echogenic reaction and effusion adjacent to the gallbladder as well as generalized echogenic abdominal effusion (Crews *et al.*, 2009). Biliary mucus or sludge filling the gallbladder was associated with an increased risk of gallbladder wall necrosis, regardless of the type of content (Uno *et al.*, 2009).

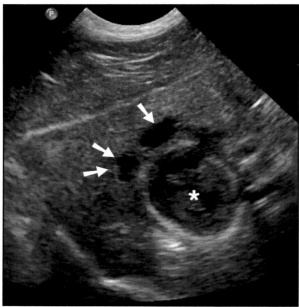

8.26 Ultrasonogram of the liver in a dog presented for vomiting. The gallbladder (*) contains some hyperechoic sludge and a thickened wall. Note the asymmetric fluid accumulation surrounding the gallbladder (arrowed). Gallbladder wall necrosis and rupture were diagnosed during surgery.

Vascular abnormalities

Hepatic venous congestion

Congestion usually occurs secondary to increased resistance to flow toward the right atrium by way of the caudal vena cava. Causes include obstruction due to a right atrial mass, pericardial effusion, invasion of the caudal vena cava by a tumour and right-sided cardiac failure. Enlargement of the hepatic veins and caudal vena cava is best visualized near the diaphragm (Figure 8.27; see also **Hepatic venous congestion** clip on DVD). Concurrent findings include a

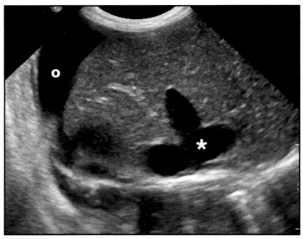

8.27 Ultrasonogram of the liver in a dog in right heart failure. Note the anechoic abdominal effusion (O). The liver is enlarged and the hepatic veins and caudal vena cava (*) are severely distended.

diffuse hypoechoic parenchyma, hepatomegaly and peritoneal effusion. On spectral Doppler examination a high-velocity retrograde flow, indicating high resistance to flow toward the right heart, can be identified.

Portosystemic shunts
Congenital

Congenital PSSs are single large calibre connections between the portal vein and systemic veins that allow blood from the intestine to bypass the liver. Congenital PSSs are more frequently seen in dogs than in cats. A congenital shunt can be intrahepatic or extrahepatic in location. Intrahepatic congenital shunts occur predominantly in large-breed dogs and are often attributable to a patent ductus venosus, originating from the left branch of the portal vein. If originating from the right branch of the portal vein, they drain directly into the caudal vena cava (Figure 8.28). Extrahepatic congenital PSSs occur more commonly in small-breed dogs (e.g. Yorkshire, Maltese and Cairn Terriers, Miniature Schnauzers) and connect the portal vein to the caudal vena cava or to another vein (e.g. the splenic, azygous, gastric or renal vein).

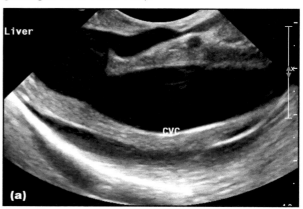

8.28 Ultrasonograms of the liver in a 9-month-old Labrador Retriever with elevated bile acids. **(a)** A large vessel connecting the portal vein with the caudal vena cava (CVC) is visible. The CVC is markedly distended. Diagnosis was a single congenital intrahepatic PSS. (continues) ►

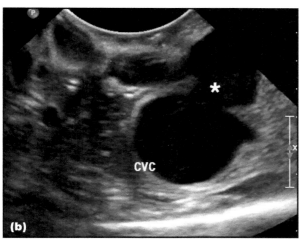

8.28 (continued) Ultrasonograms of the liver in a 9-month-old Labrador Retriever with elevated bile acids. **(b)** Transverse view of the liver showing the enlarged CVC with the termination of the large intrahepatic shunt (⋆).

In the cat both intrahepatic and extrahepatic shunts occur; extrahepatic shunts vary widely with respect to their origin and course.

Extrahepatic shunts typically originate from the splenic and left gastric vein and enter the caudal vena cava between the phrenicoabdominal vein and the liver. They are usually identified as tortuous appearing vessels with hepatofugal flow (Figure 8.29; see also **Portosystemic shunt** clip on DVD). The vena cava, portal vein and porta hepatis region should be scanned from the diaphragm to the level of the kidneys in search of an anomalous branching vessel entering the vena cava or travelling dorsally through the diaphragm toward the azygous vein adjacent to the aorta. Portocaval shunts terminate in the caudal vena cava, and their entrance is characterized by turbulent flow with colour and spectral Doppler ultrasonography.

Acoustic windows include the subxiphoid as well as a high right dorsal one. For the latter, the dog is placed in left lateral recumbency with the limbs positioned either toward or away from the ultrasonographer. A window is found in the intercostal spaces of the last three ribs, relatively close to the spine, until the liver is visualized cranial to the right kidney. In cross-section, the aorta, caudal vena cava and portal vein can be identified adjacent to one another. The shunting vessel can be identified coursing between the vena cava and portal vein. Furthermore, measurement of portal vein size can also be made in this window. The size of the portal vein cranial to the shunt is generally reduced in diameter. A portal vein: aortic ratio of ≤0.65 is predictive for the presence of an extrahepatic shunt, and a value of ≥0.8 excludes it. If the ratio is ≥0.80, other types of disease, such as microvascular dysplasia, intrahepatic shunt and portal hypertension attributable to chronic liver disease with secondary shunting, could still be present.

In addition, microhepatica, bilateral renomegaly, nephrocalcinosis, nephroliths and cystoliths attributable to urate crystals or stones may be identified. If portal hypertension is present, free fluid may be

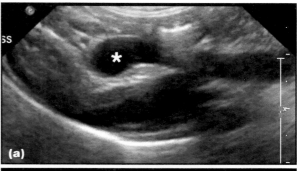

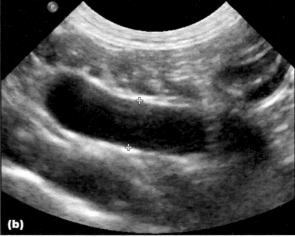

8.29 Ultrasonograms of the liver in a 10-month-old Maltese mixed-breed dog with central neurological signs. **(a)** A large tubular vessel (⋆) is visible originating from the portal vein. A single congenital extrahepatic shunt was diagnosed and confirmed on surgery. **(b)** The large vessel connecting to the caudal vena cava (between the callipers) is visible.

detected. The sensitivity and specificity of ultrasonography for the detection of extrahepatic PSSs have been reported to be 80.5% and 66.7%, respectively. A greater sensitivity of 100% was seen for intrahepatic PSSs alone. In a second study using ultrasonography for the diagnosis of congenital PSSs, results were improved by demonstrating a specificity of 98%, sensitivity of 95%, and an accuracy of 94% in 38 dogs.

Acquired

Multiple acquired PSSs (Figure 8.30a) develop secondary to chronic portal hypertension and result in reduced blood flow to the liver. Causes of portal hypertension are many and include chronic liver disease (see Figure 8.7), diffuse nodular regeneration, infiltrative neoplasia, congenital hypoplasia of the portal vein, arteriovenous fistula and portal vein thrombosis or extraluminal compression. Multiple small collateral tortuous vessels form connecting the portal vein or its tributaries to the caudal vena cava. Screening of the mid-abdomen is recommended to evaluate these vessels (Figure 8.30b). The vessels may develop collateral circulation by way of the renal vein and lead to clinical signs of PSS. Ascites is commonly found on ultrasonography in association with portal hypertension and the blood flow is reduced, seen on spectral Doppler ultrasonography, to mean velocities of ≤10 cm/s (Figure 8.30a).

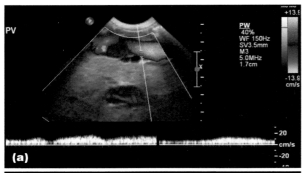

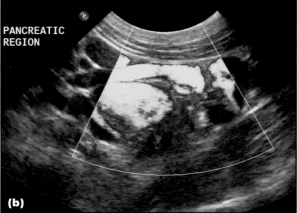

8.30 Spectral Doppler ultrasonograms of the liver in a 5-year-old Golden Retriever with a 4-month history of weight loss and lethargy after heartworm treatment. **(a)** Reduced blood flow velocity of 10 cm/s is evident in the portal vein consistent with portal hypertension. **(b)** Multiple enlarged tortuous vessels are identified caudal to the left kidney and outlined with power Doppler.

Arteriovenous fistula

Arteriovenous fistulas can be congenital or acquired and create connections between the portal vein and hepatic arteries. The resulting high pressure overloads the venous side and hypertension occurs. Acquired PSSs form because of the portal hypertension, and clinical signs of shunting occur. These animals usually present at a young age with marked ascites. Ultrasonographically, enlargement of the portal vein is seen. Intrahepatic tortuous and dilated branches may be difficult to detect ultrasonographically (Zwingenberger *et al.*, 2005).

Portal vein thrombosis

Thrombosis of the portal vein occurs with numerous diseases that are associated with the development of coagulopathies. They are recognized ultrasonographically as intraluminal structures of moderate to high echogenicity and the absence of colour Doppler signals within the lumen. Thrombosis can be focal or can extend into all branches of the portal venous system and cause acquired shunting. Free peritoneal fluid may develop.

Considerations for sampling

General principles are covered in Chapter 4. Percutaneous ultrasound-guided aspiration and biopsy of the liver have become routine in dogs and cats. Cytology or histopathology is often required to obtain a definitive diagnosis of most liver diseases, because the ultrasonographic appearance may be identical in different conditions. The decision to perform an aspiration or a tissue core biopsy is determined by the lesion to be sampled and the suspected abnormality. Ultrasound-guided FNA of the liver is a safe procedure that is usually performed on conscious animals, with sedation depending on the temperament of the dog or cat. Cats and dogs should preferably be placed under general anaesthesia for biopsy of the liver. A coagulation profile is an important screening test before tissue core biopsy procedures, especially considering that several coagulopathies may occur with liver disease.

FNA is generally performed with 20–22-gauge 1.5 inch needles for diffuse lesions (e.g. lymphoma, mast cell tumour and fatty infiltration), small nodules and cystic or highly vascular structures. A sector, curved or linear array transducer may be used depending on the location of the lesion. A superficial lesion can be well visualized with a high-frequency curved or linear array transducer, whereas deeper lesions may require low-frequency curved array or sector (phased array) transducers. Tissue core biopsy is generally recommended in most diffuse liver diseases (for chronic hepatitis, cirrhosis, amyloidosis, fibrosis, etc.) and larger masses (>2 cm). Tissue core biopsy needles with a 2 cm long sample notch should be used and are typically 16–18-gauge depending on the size of the animal. For medium to large dogs, 16-gauge needles are recommended; whereas 18-gauge needles are best for smaller dogs and cats. Manual, semiautomatic and automatic (spring-loaded gun) needles can be used, depending on the personal preferences of the ultrasonographer.

Generally, if a tissue core biopsy sample is being obtained, fine-needle aspirates can be collected at the same time, because a 'preliminary' cytological diagnosis can be made whilst waiting for the histopathology results, which usually take at least 24 hours. Touch preparations of the core biopsy sample can also be made for cytological analysis. Complications of ultrasound-guided tissue sampling are rare. After any tissue sampling procedure, the patient should be monitored directly with ultrasonography for the presence of free fluid. Small amounts of free fluid at the sampling site are not uncommon with tissue core biopsy, but are less frequent with FNA. Small amounts of fluid are generally self-limiting when the coagulation status of the patient is normal.

Ultrasound-guided percutaneous cholecystocentesis may be performed safely and can provide valuable cytological and bacteriological information to make a diagnosis of cholecystitis and apply appropriate antimicrobial therapy. The transhepatic approach is considered the safest method of bile aspiration, enabling the liver to seal off the area of gallbladder puncture (d'Anjou, 2008). The risk of complications is increased with a diseased wall or distended gallbladder, and include bile leakage and subsequent peritonitis, as well as haemorrhage.

References and further reading

Crews LJ, Feeney DA, Jessen CR, Rose ND and Matise I (2009) Clinical, ultrasonographic, and laboratory findings associated with gallbladder disease and rupture in dogs: 45 cases (1997–2007). *Journal of the American Veterinary Medical Association* **234**, 359–366

Cullen JM (2009) Summary of the World Small Animal Veterinary Association standardization committee guide to classification of liver disease in dogs and cats. *Veterinary Clinics of North America: Small Animal Practice* **39**, 395–418

Cullen JM, van den Ingh T, Bunch SE, Rothuizen J, Washabau RJ and Desmet VJ (2006) Morphological classification of circulatory disorders of the canine and feline liver. In: *Standards for Clinical and Histological Diagnosis of Canine and Feline Liver Diseases*, ed. Rothuizen et al., pp. 41–59. Saunders Elsevier, Philadelphia

d'Anjou M (2008) Liver. In: *Atlas of Small Animal Ultrasonography, 1st edn*, ed. D Penninck and M d'Anjou, pp. 217–262. Blackwell Publishing, Iowa

Gaillot HA, Penninck DG, Webster CR and Crawford S (2007) Ultrasonographic features of extrahepatic biliary obstruction in 30 cats. *Veterinary Radiology and Ultrasound* **48**, 439–447

Gaschen L (2009) Update on hepatobiliary imaging. *Veterinary Clinics of North America: Small Animal Practice* **39**, 439–467

Harran N, d'Anjou MA and Dunn M (2009) Gallbladder sludge in cats: prevalence and association with elevated serum liver parameters. *2009 Annual Scientific Meeting of the ACVR*. Memphis, TN. p. 31

Kanemoto H, Ohno K, Nakashima K, Takahashi M, Fujino Y, Nishimura R and Tsujimoto H (2009) Characterization of canine focal liver lesions with contrast-enhanced ultrasound using a novel contrast agent-sonazoid. *Veterinary Radiology and Ultrasound* **50**, 188–194

Kensuke N, Satoshi T, Noboru S, Wickramasekara Rajapakshage Bandula K, Masahiro M, Hiroshi O, Masahiro Y and Mitsuyoshi T (2010) Contrast-enhanced ultrasonography for characterization of canine focal liver lesions. *Veterinary Radiology and Ultrasound* **51**, 79–85

Liptak JM (2007) Hepatobiliary tumors. In: *Withrow's and MacEwen's Small Animal Clinical Oncology, 4th edn*, ed. SJ Withrow and DM Vail, pp. 483–491. Saunders Elsevier, St Louis

Liptak JM, Dernell WS, Monnet E, Powers BE, Bachand AM, Kenney JG and Withrow SJ (2004) Massive hepatocellular carcinoma in dogs: 48 cases (1992–2002). *Journal of the American Veterinary Medical Association* **225**, 1225–1230

Nyland T, Mattoon J, Herrgesell E and Wisner E (2002) Liver. In: *Small Animal Diagnostic Ultrasound, 2nd edn*, ed. TG Nyland and JS Mattoon, pp. 93–127. WB Saunders, Philadelphia

O'Brien RT, Iani M, Matheson J, Delaney F and Young K (2004) Contrast harmonic ultrasound of spontaneous liver nodules in 32 dogs. *Veterinary Radiology and Ultrasound* **45**, 547–553

Schwarz T (2009) The liver and gallbladder. In: *BSAVA Manual of Canine and Feline Abdominal Imaging*, ed. RT O'Brien and F Barr, pp. 144–156. BSAVA Publications, Gloucester

Uno T, Okamoto K, Onaka T, Fujita K, Yamamura H and Sakai T (2009) Correlation between ultrasonographic imaging of the gallbladder and gallbladder content in eleven cholecystectomised dogs and their prognoses. *Journal of Veterinary Medical Science* **71**, 1295–1300

Zwingenberger AL, McLear RC and Weisse C (2005) Diagnosis of arterioportal fistulae in four dogs using computed tomographic angiography. *Veterinary Radiology and Ultrasound* **46**, 472–477

Video extras

- **Hepatic venous congestion**
- **Hepatocellular carcinoma with contrast**
- **Hepatopathy with contrast**
- **Obstructive cholestasis**
- **Portosystemic shunt**

Access via QR code or bsavalibrary.com/ultrasound_8

9

Spleen

Paul Mahoney

Introduction

The spleen is an elongated, strap-like organ located adjacent to the left mid-abdominal wall, typically aligned in a dorsocranial–ventrocaudal plane. In describing the spleen, three regions are identified (the head, body and tail), although in practice there is no visible demarcation between each. In dogs without hepatomegaly or gastric distension, the head of the spleen is usually located deep to the 11th–13th ribs, cranial to the left kidney, and is often seen to fold medially on to itself (Figure 9.1a). The body continues just deep to the abdominal wall in a ventro-caudal direction, usually passing free of the rib shadows at a level midway between the vertebrae and the sternum. From there its continuation can be quite variable, and the tip of the tail may be found anywhere from alongside the left wall of the bladder to curving ventrally towards the right ventral mid-abdominal wall. In cats, the entire spleen is usually visible just deep to the left mid-abdominal wall, and the head of the spleen may be partly obscured by the 12th–13th ribs (Figure 9.1b).

The spleen acts as a blood reservoir, capable of storing up to 20% of the normal blood volume and 30% of the body's platelets. It has roles in haemo-poiesis, red blood cell filtration and phagocytosis, body immunity, storage of Factor VIII coagulant, regulation of angiotensin-converting enzyme (ACE), iron metabolism, and modulation of noradrenaline (norepinephrine) levels. Changes in size, shape and echogenicity may represent a normal response of the organ to these functions, and may be ultrasonographically indistinguishable from significant pathological processes.

In several recent large histopathology studies, approximately 35–50% of all spleen submissions had a non-neoplastic lesion, and 50–65% had a neoplastic lesion. Approximately half of the neoplastic lesions were haemangiosarcomas.

Indications

The spleen can be involved with many diseases, and clinical signs can be non-specific. Therefore, complete assessment of the spleen should form part of any routine abdominal ultrasound examination in clinical patients. Particular attention should be given to the spleen in animals presenting with:

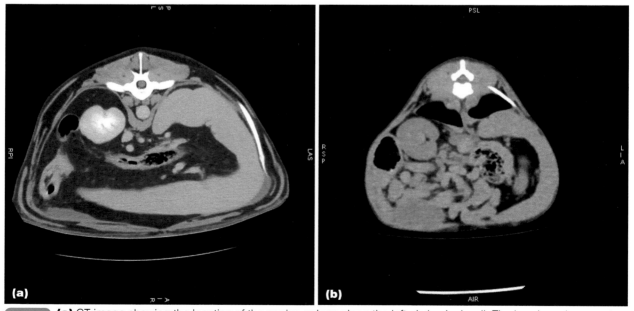

9.1 **(a)** CT image showing the location of the canine spleen along the left abdominal wall. The head can be seen to fold on to itself and the tail passes along the floor of the abdomen towards the right side. **(b)** CT image showing the location of the feline spleen along the left abdominal wall. The head of the spleen is partly overlain by the 13th rib.

- Haemoabdomen
- A palpable (or radiographically evident) mid-abdominal mass
- Palpable splenomegaly
- A history of abdominal trauma
- Deep-chested dogs with vague clinical signs that include abdominal discomfort.

Targeted assessment of the spleen may be considered in patients with known haemangiosarcoma elsewhere, and in dogs with a confirmed mast cell tumour where there is clinical suspicion of metastatic spread, or a histopathological grading where that may occur. Doppler ultrasonography is indicated in dogs suspected of having splenic torsion and in any patient with a coagulopathy or a predisposing disease process.

Value of ultrasonography compared with radiography and computed tomography

Ultrasonography should never be thought of as a replacement for abdominal radiography; the two procedures are often complementary. However, when specifically assessing the spleen, radiography can often be of limited benefit. Radiography will not detect many of the changes that are seen on ultrasonography and described later in this Chapter. As very little of the spleen is normally seen in most patients, occasionally an incorrect radiographic diagnosis of splenomegaly can be made when the normal spleen aligns along the floor of the abdomen such that the tail rests adjacent to the bladder, resulting in more spleen being visible on the lateral radiograph than is normal. Occasionally (particularly in cats) no spleen at all is seen on abdominal radiographs.

The presence of fluid within the abdomen can sometimes improve the quality of the ultrasound scan, but it invariably leads to reduced serosal detail on an abdominal radiograph. In animals with very large abdominal masses, it can be helpful to assess ab-dominal radiographs before starting the ultrasound scan; in many instances, the differential diagnoses list can be reduced quickly by starting with the radiographs (Figure 9.2). Ultrasound scans can sometimes prove quite time-consuming in such cases as very little of the original organ may remain, having been replaced by abnormal tissue, and presumptive diagnoses are instead made by ruling out normal organs one-by-one.

Computed tomography (CT) can be used to examine the spleen, but clinical experience in the veterinary setting is quite limited. It gives an improved view of the entire spleen in all animals, including those where the head of the spleen can be particularly difficult to image with ultrasonography. CT has been reported to be of value in dogs with splenic torsion. Fife *et al.* (2004) looked at the post-contrast enhancement characteristics of large splenic masses in 21 dogs, and found that haemangiosarcoma tended to have a lower Hounsfield unit (HU) when compared with non-malignant masses. However, although at the

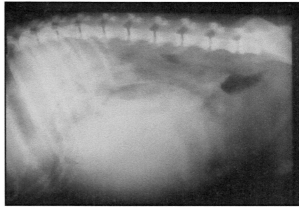

9.2 Lateral abdominal radiograph of a mid-abdominal mass showing displacement of intestines cranially, dorsally and caudally. The primary differential diagnosis for this would be a splenic mass.

cut-off (55 HU) it suggested to differentiate between the two types of mass, three of the 14 non-malignant masses would have been false-positives for malignancy. It is not known how the sensitivity and specificity of pre- and post-contrast CT scans of the spleen compare with those of ultrasonography.

Imaging technique

Patient preparation
A large area of skin needs to be clipped to view all of the spleen in many canine patients.

Positioning
In both dogs and cats the spleen can be examined with the patient in right lateral recumbency, and the organ visualized using a left flank approach. Not uncommonly in dogs, the tail of the spleen crosses the ventral midline as it arcs along the abdominal floor towards the right side, and this part of the spleen is then best visualized from the ventral right flank with the patient in left lateral recumbency.

It is surprising how far dorsal the head of the spleen can be located in dogs. The left kidney is a convenient landmark to find this part of the spleen, as it lies just cranial to the kidney's cranial pole. An intercostal approach is usually required, and if so, aligning the image plane parallel to the ribs and rocking the probe to sweep the image from cranial to caudal allows imaging of the head of the spleen without interference by the ribs (Figure 9.3a). This region should then be re-evaluated in a transverse (cross-sectional) imaging plane (Figure 9.3b), which is then continued caudoventrally following through the body and finally the tail. With some probes, the width of the spleen in the transverse plane can be greater than the width of the ultrasound beam. In such cases it is important to be sure that all of the spleen is visualized, and to ensure that this is done, the spleen should be scanned (in the transverse imaging plane) from head to tail with its cranial border kept within the field of view, and then scanned again from tail to head with its caudal border kept within the field of view.

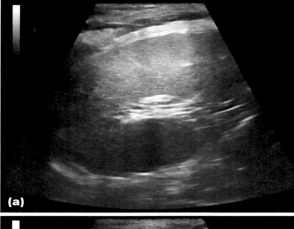

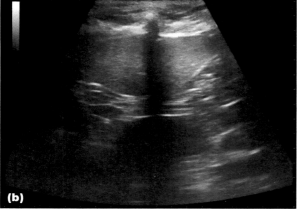

9.3 Ultrasonograms of the head of the spleen. **(a)** Intercostal approach with the probe aligned parallel to the ribs: the spleen is seen folding on to itself. **(b)** Transverse imaging plane: the tip of the head of the spleen is difficult to view and there is shadowing by an overlying rib.

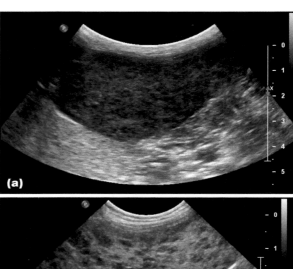

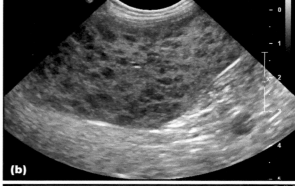

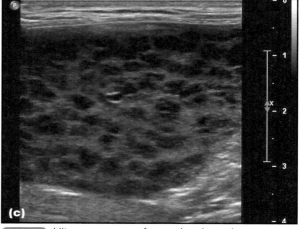

9.4 Ultrasonograms of a section through an enlarged canine spleen affected with lymphoma using different transducers. **(a)** 5 MHz curvilinear probe. The spleen has a variable echogenicity throughout and is less echogenic than a normal spleen. **(b)** 8 MHz microconvex probe. Numerous small hypoechoic nodules that were not clearly seen in (a) are now visible. **(c)** 15 MHz linear probe. The hypoechoic nodules are much more clearly seen and appear to be greater in number than in (b).

Equipment

There is no single transducer that would suit examination of the spleen in all canine and feline patients, and the choice depends upon the probes that are available at the practice as well as the patient size and conformation. As much of the spleen is relatively superficial, the use of higher frequency probes (>7 MHz) will improve image resolution. In feline and some canine patients, part of the spleen may be too close to the transducer to image well, and if there is no access to a linear probe, a stand-off may be required. However, it must be realized that the appearance of some spleen pathologies may alter depending on the type of probe and the frequency selected (Figure 9.4).

Normal ultrasonographic appearance

The size of the spleen in dogs and cats can be quite variable, and a diagnosis of splenomegaly is often made subjectively. Radiography may better demonstrate displacement of adjacent organs when the spleen is enlarged. The splenic parenchyma has a fine granular, relatively homogeneous echotexture throughout (Figure 9.5a; see also **Normal spleen in a cat** clip on DVD). In many dogs the splenic parenchyma is slightly more echogenic than the hepatic parenchyma, but this relationship is variable and changes do not necessarily represent pathology. The splenic parenchyma is generally more echogenic than the renal cortex. The spleen is surrounded by a thin hyperechoic capsule, which is only visible when the capsule and beam are at right angles to each other (Figure 9.5b; see also **Normal spleen in a dog** clip on DVD).

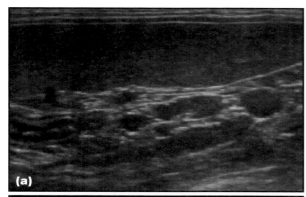

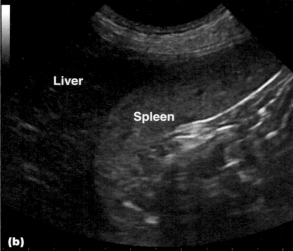

9.5 **(a)** The normal feline spleen has a fine evenly granular appearance. **(b)** The normal canine spleen has a fine evenly granular appearance. The hyperechoic line seen along the distal border of the spleen is the splenic capsule, which is at right angles to the beam in this region. In many normal dogs the splenic parenchyma is more echoic than the liver.

The blood supply to the spleen is via the splenic artery, a branch of the coeliac artery. Once it enters the spleen its branches are not generally visualized unless colour Doppler ultrasonography is used. Intrasplenic branches of the splenic vein can be readily visualized as anechoic tubular structures that drain towards the hilus. From here the splenic vein empties into the portal vein. Occasionally, hyperechoic invaginations can be seen around the splenic vein branches along the hilus (Figure 9.6). These represent myelolipidosis and have no clinical significance.

Thiopental and acepromazine can cause passive congestion of the spleen, resulting in an increase in size, reflectivity and attenuation, but often these changes are not noticed. Occasionally, dogs sedated with medetomidine show spontaneous echoes ('smoke') within the intra-abdominal veins (including the splenic vein), the degree of which is over-and-above the more subtle echogenic blood that can sometimes be seen within any slow-flowing vessel. A similar finding may be seen occasionally in dogs with anaemia (Figure 9.7). This should not be considered a precursor to intravascular thrombosis formation. Occasionally, accessory splenic tissue may be seen as nodules adjacent to the

spleen. Typically they have a similar echogenicity to spleen, and histologically they are identical to spleen (Figure 9.8).

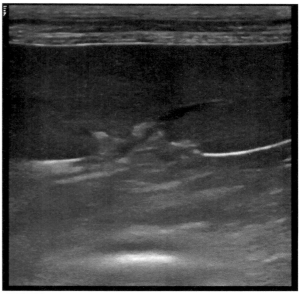

9.6 Hyperechoic invaginations along the splenic hilus are typical of myelolipidosis and are not felt to be clinically significant.

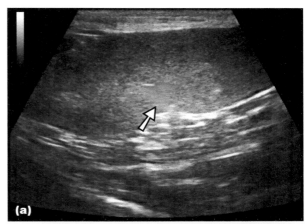

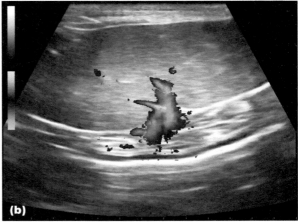

9.7 Ultrasonograms of a dog with immune-mediated haemolytic anaemia and a packed cell volume of 0.17. **(a)** Hyperechoic blood within a branch of the splenic vein (arrowed). The vessel is not clearly seen until demonstrated with colour Doppler. **(b)** Colour Doppler identifies the branch of the splenic vein not readily seen in (a).

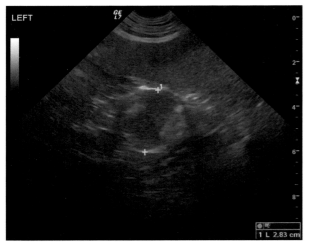

9.8 Ultrasonogram of an 8-year-old Rottweiler with a distal femoral osteosarcoma showing a rounded mass (between the callipers) deep to the spleen, most of which is isoechoic to the spleen. Fine-needle aspiration of the mass confirmed that this was accessory splenic tissue.

Diffuse parenchymal disease

Inflammation

The spleen has many functions, and its appearance may alter as a result of stimulation from a variety of sources. Examples in cats and dogs include extramedullary haemopoiesis, lymphoid hyperplasia, chronic inflammatory disease, immune-mediated disease, bacterial, fungal or rickettsial diseases, and blunt abdominal trauma. In each case the patient may develop an enlarged spleen that has a normal or altered echogenicity (Figure 9.9). Feline coronavirus has been reported to cause generalized splenomegaly without alteration to its echogenicity.

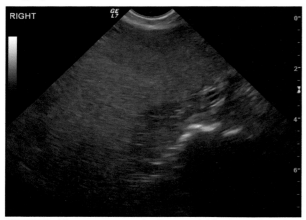

9.9 Ultrasonogram of a 5-year-old Springer Spaniel with immune-mediated anaemia showing a moderate degree of generalized splenomegaly without alteration of the parenchymal appearance.

Neoplasia

The neoplasms that can diffusely infiltrate the spleen can have variable effects on its appearance, none of which are specific. There may be no change at all in size, texture or echogenicity, there may be an increase in size, an increase in echogenicity, a reduction in echogenicity, the development of a diffuse

granulonodular texture, or a combination of these changes. A normal looking spleen does not rule out diffuse neoplastic infiltration. Tissue sampling of the spleen is therefore needed to obtain a definitive diagnosis. The most commonly reported infiltrative neoplasms affecting canine and feline spleens are lymphoma (Figure 9.10), mast cell tumour and histiocytic sarcoma. Less common differential diagnoses include leukaemic and myelomatous infiltrates.

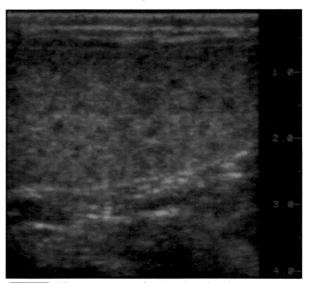

9.10 Ultrasonogram of a dog that developed a hyperechoic spleen with a diffuse granulonodular appearance to its parenchyma. The spleen was not significantly enlarged. Cytology of a fine-needle aspirate confirmed the presence of lymphoma.

Focal parenchymal disease

Inflammation

Splenic abscesses (Figure 9.11) may be solitary or multifocal, and can be hypoechoic, hyperechoic or have a mixed echogenicity. If gas is present within the lesion it is associated with reverberation or shadowing artefacts (see Chapter 1). The appearance of a splenic abscess may change over a relatively short period of time.

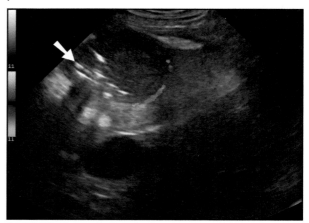

9.11 Hypoechoic splenic mass containing several small hyperechoic flecks (arrowed) indicating the presence of gas. Colour Doppler shows blood flow around but not within the mass. The mass was confirmed as a splenic abscess.

Neoplasia

Solitary lesions

The most common solitary splenic malignancy in dogs is haemangiosarcoma. It typically presents as a mass of variable size, but its ultrasonographic appearance can be quite diverse. It may be solid or contain central area(s) of anechoic fluid accumulation. It may be isoechoic, hypoechoic or hyperechoic to the remainder of the spleen, or have a mixed echogenicity. It can also be ultrasonographically indistinguishable from benign mass lesions such as haematoma, infarct, abscess or haemangioma. Other malignant neoplasms that can have a similar appearance include other sarcomas (e.g. histiocytic sarcoma, fibrosarcoma, osteosarcoma, leiomyosarcoma, myxosarcoma, rhabdomyosarcoma, poorly differentiated sarcoma), lymphoma and metastatic disease (Figure 9.12). Both malignant and non-malignant lesions can bleed, so although the presence of concurrent haemoabdomen may raise the index of suspicion for a malignancy, it cannot be used to confirm the presence of haemangiosarcoma. Reduced total plasma protein and/or platelet count in such cases are most likely a consequence of severe haemorrhage and are not necessarily reliable biomarkers for predicting malignancy. The presence of schistocytes on a blood smear has been associated with haemangiosarcoma; however, they can be associated with non-malignant splenic lesions as well as other non-splenic diseases.

Contrast harmonic imaging has recently been used to evaluate splenic lesions in a number of studies, but experience so far is limited and more work needs to be done to fully assess its value. Ivancic *et al.* (2009) felt that it did not reliably differentiate haematoma from haemangiosarcoma, although there may be some value in differentiating metastatic nodules in the liver from benign hepatic nodular hyperplasia. Rossi *et al.* (2008) found that all malignant lesions became hypoperfused during the wash-out phase 30 seconds after injection, and this differed from all but one benign lesion. With a larger group of dogs, Ohlerth *et al.* (2008) found a greater overlap in the perfusion patterns of benign and malignant diseases, but extensive to moderate hypoechogenicity during all blood pool phases had a high association with malignancy.

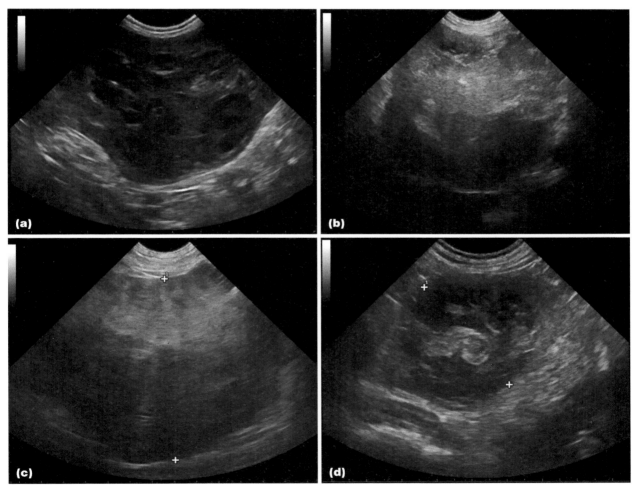

9.12 **(a)** Large hypoechoic mass in a canine spleen containing several anechoic areas representative of intralesional haemorrhage. The mass had a histopathological diagnosis of haemangiosarcoma. **(b)** Large mixed echogenic mass in a canine spleen containing a small amount of intralesional haemorrhage. The mass had a histopathological diagnosis of benign haemangioma. **(c)** Large mixed echogenic mass in a canine spleen with a histopathological diagnosis of benign nodular hyperplasia. **(d)** Large mixed echogenic mass in a canine spleen with a histopathological diagnosis of histiocytic sarcoma.

Although uncommon, solitary feline splenic masses (Figure 9.13) can have an appearance similar to that seen in dogs and have as wide a variety of differential diagnoses.

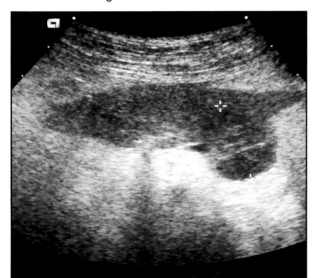

9.13 Ultrasonogram of a bulging nodule (between the callipers) that was isoechoic to the remainder of the cat's spleen. The mass had a cytological diagnosis of lymphoma.

Multiple lesions

Neoplasia of the spleen can manifest itself as hypoechoic or hyperechoic multiple nodules scattered throughout the parenchyma, and in this respect it can resemble nodular hyperplasia or extramedullary haemopoiesis. The more widespread and the greater the number of lesions, the higher the suspicion of malignant disease. However, tissue sampling may still be required to reach a diagnosis. The more common differential diagnoses for malignant multiple nodules include lymphoma (Figure 9.14a), histiocytic sarcoma, mast cell tumour, haemangiosarcoma and metastatic disease (Figure 9.14b).

Target lesions

Splenic target lesions are nodules or masses with a hypoechoic rim and a hyperechoic or isoechoic core, which resembles a bullseye target (Figure 9.15). They have been associated with malignancies in humans and it has been suggested that this may also be the case in dogs. However, they have a non-specific appearance, which requires tissue sampling to differentiate benign from malignant disease.

Nodular hyperplasia

Nodular hyperplasia is probably the most common cause of solitary or occasional nodules within the spleen of middle-aged or older dogs, and is an occasional finding in cats. The nodules are usually small (<3 cm in diameter), hypoechoic, hyperechoic or of mixed echogenicity, and may be within the parenchyma or bulging from a surface (Figure 9.16). In cases where they are isoechoic to the spleen, they may only be noticed as a surface bulge. Occasionally, nodular hyperplastic lesions can be quite numerous.

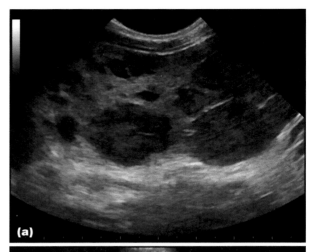

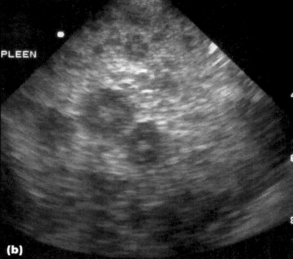

9.14 **(a)** Canine spleen containing numerous variably sized hypoechoic nodules scattered throughout the parenchyma. Cytological diagnosis was lymphoma. **(b)** Canine spleen containing numerous variably sized nodules scattered throughout the parenchyma, which range in appearance from hypoechoic to target-type nodules. Cytological diagnosis was metastatic carcinoma secondary to an anal sac tumour.

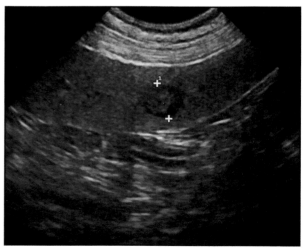

9.15 Small solitary canine splenic nodule with the appearance of a target lesion (between the callipers). Note the hyperechoic core and hypoechoic rim. Cytological diagnosis was nodular hyperplasia.

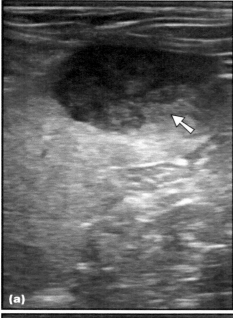

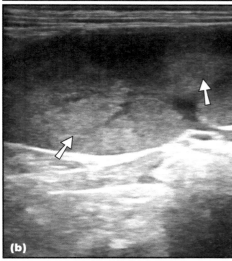

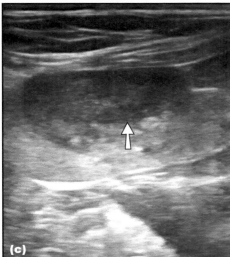

9.16 **(a)** Hypoechoic nodule (arrowed) in the spleen of an elderly dog. **(b)** Two hyperechoic nodules (arrowed) in the spleen of an elderly dog. **(c)** Mixed echogenic nodule (arrowed) in the spleen of an elderly dog. All of these lesions were diagnosed as nodular hyperplasia on fine-needle aspirate cytology.

Extramedullary haemopoiesis

Extramedullary haemopoiesis may result in generalized splenomegaly or manifest itself as solitary or multiple nodules within the spleen (Figure 9.17), and in this respect may be indistinguishable from nodular hyperplasia in appearance.

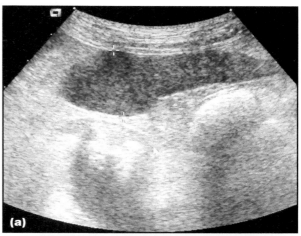

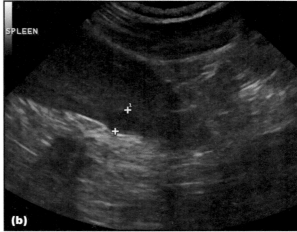

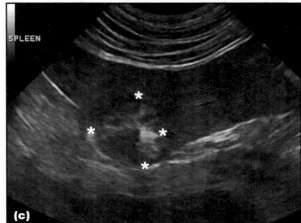

9.17 **(a)** Ultrasonogram of a 2 cm diameter mass in a cat with immune-mediated haemolytic anaemia. The mass is isoechoic to the remainder of the spleen. Fine-needle aspirate cytology diagnosed the mass as a focal region of extramedullary haemopoiesis. **(b)** Small hypoechoic nodule representing a focal area of extramedullary haemopoiesis. **(c)** Mixed echogenic splenic mass (*) diagnosed as a focal area of extramedullary haemopoiesis on fine-needle aspirate cytology.

Infarction

Splenic infarction may occur secondarily to hyperadrenocorticism, hypothyroidism, immune-mediated disease, protein-losing enteropathy, protein-losing nephropathy, bacterial endocarditis and neoplasia. The appearance of an infarct is variable and may change over time. They may extend over large areas, appear evenly hypoechoic and show no blood flow on Doppler assessment. Affected areas may contain hyperechoic flecks, giving a coarse lacy pattern ('starry sky' appearance) (Figure 9.18; see also **Splenic infarction (1)**, **(2)** and **(3)** clips on DVD). There may be haemorrhage within the lesion, resulting in a mass that resembles a neoplasm, haematoma or abscess. In time the affected area may reduce in size as it reorganizes, eventually resembling a hyperechoic scar associated with an overlying distortion of the splenic capsule.

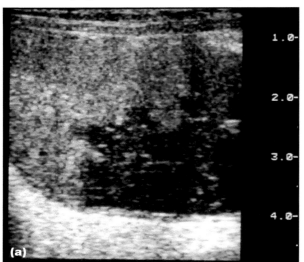

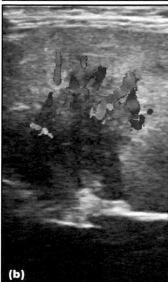

9.18
(a) Ultrasonogram of a canine spleen showing the demarcation line between the normal hyperechoic spleen (to the left of the image) and the hypoechoic infarcted spleen (to the right of the image). Hyperechoic flecks within the infarcted area give it a 'starry sky' appearance.
(b) Colour flow Doppler assessment shows flow in the normal hyperechoic splenic tissue, but no flow in the infarcted hypoechoic region of spleen.

Splenic torsion

Splenic torsion is most commonly associated with gastric dilatation and volvulus, but can occasionally occur as a primary problem, typically in large or giant-breed dogs, particularly German Shepherd Dogs and Great Danes. The clinical signs are usually vague and

non-specific, and may include abdominal pain or discomfort, weakness, tachycardia, hypotension, poor peripheral perfusion and collapse. The spleen is usually markedly enlarged, and may have a normal or reduced echogenicity. Free fluid may be present within the abdomen. Blood flow within the splenic vessels may be present or absent, depending upon the degree of torsion and the effect on its blood supply, and there may be areas of infarction with resultant coarse lacy parenchyma (Figure 9.19). Echogenic thrombi may be detected within the intrasplenic vessels and/or the splenic vein as it leaves the hilus. A hyperechoic invagination of mesenteric tissue around the hilar veins as they exit the spleen may be a further indication of torsion. However, this may be confused with myelolipidosis (described above), so care needs to be taken when interpreting this finding.

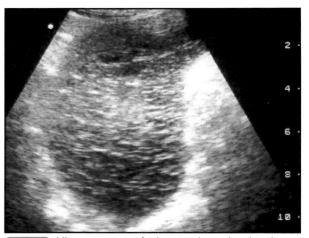

9.19 Ultrasonogram of a large spleen showing the 'starry sky' appearance of thrombosis. A laparotomy was performed and splenic torsion was confirmed as the underlying cause.

Splenic thrombosis

Splenic vein thrombosis (Figure 9.20) may occur without torsion or obvious infarction. Underlying diseases that may cause venous thrombosis include those listed for splenic infarction (see above).

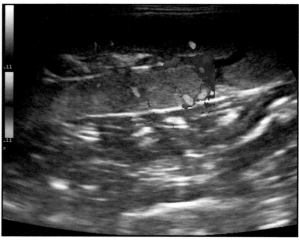

9.20 The splenic vein of this dog with hyperadrenocorticism was thrombosed. The colour flow Doppler shows recanalization of the vein with flow around and through the thrombus.

Particular considerations for sampling

It is not possible to differentiate neoplastic from non-neoplastic disease affecting the spleen using ultrasonographic appearance alone. The presence of lesions in other organs, abnormal intra-abdominal lymph nodes and/or peritoneal fluid may make neoplastic disease more likely, but without a definitive diagnosis, the clinician runs the risk of an incorrect diagnosis and subsequent inappropriate clinical decisions. In the United Kingdom where fungal diseases are rare, the presence of pulmonary nodules is the finding that gives the clinician the greatest confidence that a malignancy is likely. Ultimately, however, confirmation requires sampling.

When performing canine and feline splenic sampling for cytology, a non-aspiration technique is likely to give a superior sample when compared with an aspiration technique. Cell morphology is preserved, and there is higher cellularity because of reduced haemodilution. The technique is quick, minimally invasive and relatively simple to perform, and as long as the patient is adequately restrained to reduce the risk of splenic laceration, it is a relatively low risk procedure.

The limitations of cytological evaluation should also be understood. Errors in diagnosis can occur if:

- Inappropriate areas are sampled
- An insufficient number of samples are taken
- Samples are incorrectly presented or preserved
- The samples are evaluated by an inexperienced person
- Histopathology is required to differentiate between reactive and neoplastic conditions.

It is of limited value to attempt to reach a cytological diagnosis of a large splenic mass before splenectomy; once the spleen is removed, the entire mass should be sent for histopathological evaluation. In cases of splenic lymphoma, treatment with corticosteroids prior to sampling reduces the likelihood of a definitive diagnosis.

Sampling procedure
The author's preferred method for cytological sampling of the canine and feline spleen is given below.

Preparation
Preparation before sampling is very important as spleen samples clot very quickly in the needle.

- Place frosted slides on a bench nearby ready for the samples.
- Place several 5 ml syringes near the slides, and introduce 2–3 ml of air into each syringe ready for use after sampling.

Procedure
Spinal needles of a length suitable for the depth of sampling are used (22-gauge, 1.5 inches or 3.5 inches). The stilette is left inside the needle.

- Using ultrasound-guidance, place the needle tip at the margin of the region of interest.
- After a colleague gently removes the stilette, pass the needle through the region of interest once, and withdraw.
- Attach one of the pre-prepared 5 ml syringes and gently expunge the sample from the needle on to a slide.
- Make a smear and air-dry the sample.

This procedure is repeated several times for each area of interest. If the slides are to be sent away for evaluation, they should not be placed in the same package as anything in formalin, as exposure to formalin fumes inhibits routine staining, resulting in loss of cellular detail.

References and further reading

Cruz-Arambulo R, Wrigley R and Powers B (2004) Sonographic features of histiocytic neoplasms in the canine abdomen. *Veterinary Radiology and Ultrasound* **45**, 554–558

Cuccovillo A and Lamb CR (2002) Cellular features of sonographic target lesions of the liver and spleen in 21 dogs and a cat. *Veterinary Radiology and Ultrasound* **43**, 275–278

Fife WD, Samii VF, Drost WT, Mattoon JS and Hoshaw-Woodard S (2004) Comparison between malignant and non-malignant splenic masses in dogs using contrast-enhanced computed tomography. *Veterinary Radiology and Ultrasound* **45**, 289–297

Hanson JA, Papageorges M, Girard E et al. (2001) Ultrasonographic appearance of splenic disease in 101 cats. *Veterinary Radiology and Ultrasound* **42**, 441–446

Hammond TN and Pesillo-Crosby SA (2008) Prevalence of haemangiosarcoma in anemic dogs with a splenic mass and hemoperitoneum requiring a transfusion: 71 cases (2003–2005). *Journal of the American Veterinary Medical Association* **232**, 553–558

Ivancic M, Long F and Seiler GS (2009) Contrast harmonic ultrasonography of splenic masses and associated liver nodules in dogs. *Journal of the American Veterinary Medical Association* **234**, 88–94

LeBlanc CJ, Head LL and Fry MM (2009) Comparison of aspiration and non-aspiration techniques for obtaining cytological samples from the canine and feline spleen. *Veterinary Clinical Pathology* **38**, 242–246

Mai W (2006) The hilar perivenous hyperechoic triangle as a sign of acute splenic torsion in dogs. *Veterinary Radiology and Ultrasound* **47**, 487–491

O'Brien RT, Waller KR and Osgood TL (2004) Sonographic features of drug-induced splenic congestion. *Veterinary Radiology and Ultrasound* **45**, 225–227

Ohlerth S, Dennler M, Ruefli E, Hauser B, Poirier V, Siebeck N, Roos M and Kaser-Hotz B (2008) Contrast harmonic imaging characterisation of canine splenic lesions. *Journal of Veterinary Internal Medicine* **22**, 1095–1102

Ramirez S, Douglass JP and Robertson ID (2002) Ultrasonographic features of canine abdominal malignant histiocytosis. *Veterinary Radiology and Ultrasound* **43**, 167–170

Rossi F, Leone VF, Vignoli M, Laddaga E and Terragni R (2008) Use of contrast-enhanced ultrasound for characterization of focal splenic lesions. *Veterinary Radiology and Ultrasound* **49**, 154–164

Sato AF and Solano M (2004) Ultrasonographic findings in abdominal mast cell disease: a retrospective study of 19 patients. *Veterinary Radiology and Ultrasound* **45**, 51–57

Saunders HM, Neath PJ and Brockman DJ (1998) B-mode and Doppler ultrasound imaging of the spleen with canine splenic torsion: a retrospective evaluation. *Veterinary Radiology and Ultrasound* **39**, 349–353

Video extras

- Normal spleen in a cat
- Normal spleen in a dog
- Splenic infarction (1)
- Splenic infarction (2)
- Splenic infarction (3)

Access via QR code or bsavalibrary.com/ultrasound_9

10

Kidneys and proximal ureters

John P. Graham

Introduction

Ultrasonography is a versatile tool for evaluating the kidneys and ureters as it is quick, non-invasive and relatively sensitive. Changes in renal size, architecture and echogenicity can be assessed. However, it provides no data about renal function.

Indications

Common indications for renal ultrasonography include:

- Gross or microscopic haematuria
- Pyuria
- Proteinuria
- Suspected urolithiasis
- Bilateral or unilateral renomegaly/renal mass
- Acute renal failure
- Congenital renal dysplasia or familial nephropathy
- Polyuria/polydipsia
- Loss of retroperitoneal detail radiographically
- Chronic renal failure.

Suspected renal or ureteral disease is a common indication for abdominal ultrasonography. The kidneys should also be evaluated when scanning patients with clinical signs of lower urinary tract disease, as some conditions can affect multiple sites (e.g. urolithiasis) and lower urinary tract infections may ascend to cause pyelonephritis. Clinical tests of renal function are insensitive and only show changes once 70% or more of the functional nephrons have been destroyed. Ultrasonographic abnormalities are not always reflected in serum chemistry tests and urinalysis. Conversely, the ultrasonographic appearance of the kidneys may be normal even when significant renal compromise is present and the patient is azotaemic. Ultrasound examination is relatively unhelpful in assessing patients with chronic renal failure and azotaemia, as the findings are similar for almost all chronic renal diseases. Ultrasonography may be somewhat more helpful in investigating acute renal failure, determining its cause and in distinguishing acute from chronic renal failure.

Value of ultrasonography compared with radiography and computed tomography

Ultrasonography has largely supplanted survey and contrast radiography in evaluating the upper urinary tract. Radiographs are preferred for a global assessment of the urinary tract and for determining renal size and detecting mineralization. Ultrasonography is particularly helpful in patients with renal enlargement as it can distinguish between causes such as hydronephrosis, polycystic disease and renal masses.

Renal neoplasia may efface all normal architecture, so the ultrasonographic diagnosis may be based on being confident that the mass has not displaced a normal kidney. The pattern of organ displacement caused by a renal mass on survey radiographs usually points to the kidney as the probable organ of origin, and may help confirm the ultrasonographic diagnosis. Excretory urography can confirm the absence of a normal kidney. Ultrasonography is more sensitive than radiography for assessing local invasion by renal tumours, especially invasion or encasement of the vena cava and aorta. In cases where the mass is very large, this may be difficult and contrast-enhanced computed tomography (CT) is often more helpful.

With the exception of cysteine and urate calculi, uroliths can be seen on survey radiographs unless they are quite small. Ultrasonography is superior for detecting small renal calculi and sand-like material. It can also differentiate mineralization of the parenchyma from intraluminal mineralized structures. In addition, ultrasonography can be used to locate ureteral calculi, especially if ureteral dilatation is present. Tracing the ureter distally is difficult unless there is moderate or severe dilatation. Ultrasonography is best used in combination with radiography for evaluating ureteral calculi, especially if these are small or located distally.

In cases of abdominal trauma, excretory urography is the technique of choice to diagnose renal rupture, renal avulsion and ureteral rupture. Ultrasonography may show fluid within the retroperitoneal space, but cannot distinguish urine from haemorrhage and cannot confirm a ureteral laceration. In patients with little body fat or cachexia, ultrasonography is the preferred technique for assessing the kidneys.

Imaging technique

Patient preparation

The patient is prepared by clipping the hair coat and applying acoustic coupling gel.

Positioning

Dogs

The kidneys can be scanned with the patient in either dorsal or lateral recumbency. With the dog in dorsal recumbency, the left kidney is imaged through the left ventral abdominal wall, just caudal to the ribs. In most patients, minimal pressure is applied to the transducer to displace the small and large bowel. Both sagittal and transverse plane images should be obtained. For sagittal plane images, the transducer can be kept in one place and the beam fanned medially and laterally. For transverse plane images, the transducer must usually be moved cranially and caudally, sliding on the skin, as the kidney is relatively long. The descending colon may block this acoustic window. In this case, the transducer is moved laterally, pressure is applied, and the transducer is then swept medially to displace the colon towards the midline and reveal the kidney. In some patients, it may be easier to move the transducer medially, apply some pressure, and then attempt to displace the colon laterally. If this fails, the probe should be moved laterally and dorsally to the paralumbar fossa to locate an imaging window dorsal to the colon. Dorsal and transverse plane images should then be obtained.

The right kidney in dogs is more difficult to image because it is located further cranially and dorsally and deep to the ribs. Scanning the right kidney from the ventral abdomen requires pressure to be applied with the transducer to displace the pylorus, duodenum and ascending colon. The degree of force required depends upon the size of the dog, body condition, tension of the abdominal wall and filling of the gastrointestinal tract. From this approach, sagittal and transverse plane images should be obtained. If the patient is tense, obese, large or deep-chested or has abdominal pain, it may not be feasible to use a ventral abdominal window to scan the right kidney. In such patients, the transducer is moved either laterally and dorsally to scan through the last few intercostal spaces, or angled cranially and medially from caudal to the last rib whilst the patient is tilted to the left. Using this approach, dorsal and transverse plane images are obtained. The transducer will likely have to be moved back and forth between the intercostal spaces to avoid acoustic shadows from the ribs and to scan the entire kidney. This window has the advantage of placing the transducer closer to the kidney and requires little or no application of pressure, which is more comfortable for both patient and ultrasonographer.

When scanning a patient in lateral recumbency, the uppermost kidney is examined. The transducer is placed in the left paralumbar fossa to scan the left kidney. This has the advantage that the descending colon usually drops ventrally, away from the kidney.

However, the kidney also rotates medially and ventrally, and obtaining a true longitudinal image requires adjusting the image plane. When evaluating the right kidney, the transducer is placed in the last two or three intercostal spaces or immediately caudal to the last rib, and the kidney scanned in the same manner as described above.

Cats

In cats both kidneys are located caudal to the ribs, which makes the examination substantially easier. The imaging technique is the same as described for dogs, with the exception that an intercostal approach is almost never required to view the right kidney. If available, a linear transducer is preferred for the examination of cats as the image quality is superior.

Equipment

Linear transducers offer superior image quality and may be used to examine both kidneys in most cats. In dogs, it is usually not possible to view the right kidney with a linear transducer as the contact area of the probe is too large. For this reason curved array or sector transducers are more often used. The kidneys are superficial and for most patients high-frequency transducers (7–10 MHz) provide adequate penetration and good detail. In larger dogs, especially those with a deep-chested conformation, a lower frequency transducer may be needed, particularly for the right kidney.

Doppler ultrasonography

Colour Doppler ultrasonography of a kidney shows its rich vascular supply. Flow within the renal artery and vein and lobar vessels is clearly seen (Figure 10.1). Colour Doppler has been used to identify renal arteries in donor patients for renal transplants. Some cats have two major renal arteries, but this is only clinically significant when planning a nephrectomy or screening potential kidney donors.

Pulsed wave (PW) Doppler can be used to evaluate flow in the renal arcuate arteries. For this

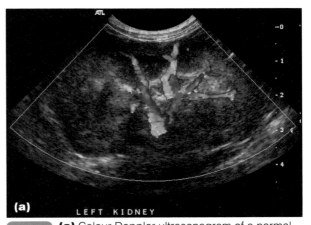

10.1 **(a)** Colour Doppler ultrasonogram of a normal left kidney showing the presence of multiple large vessels within the organ. The veins are larger than the arteries. Venous flow is shown as blue, indicating flow below the baseline or away from the transducer. Arterial flow is shown as red/orange, indicating flow towards the transducer. (continues) ▶

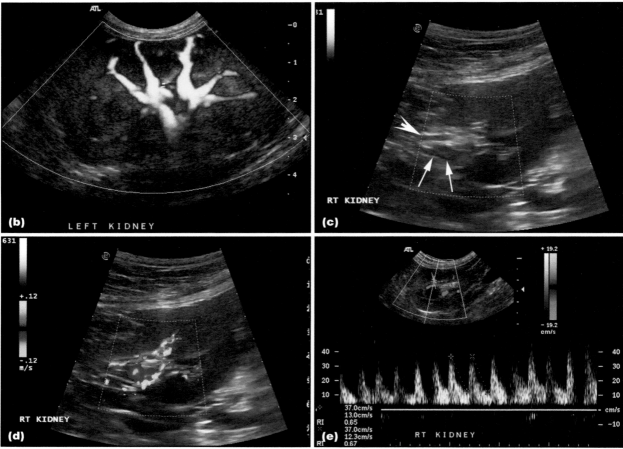

10.1 (continued) **(b)** Power Doppler ultrasonogram of a normal left kidney. Power Doppler is more sensitive to the presence of flow, but includes no information about flow direction or velocity. Transverse images of the hilus of the right kidney **(c)** without and **(d)** with colour flow Doppler. The greyscale image shows the renal artery (arrowhead) and renal vein (arrowed) at the renal hilus. The renal vein is much wider than the corresponding artery. The colour Doppler ultrasonogram shows flow within these vessels. **(e)** Doppler evaluation and RI in an arcuate artery. The arcuate artery was identified using colour flow Doppler, and a small (1–2 mm) PW Doppler sample volume was then placed over the artery. Normal flow within the arcuate arteries is characterized by rapid acceleration at the beginning of systole followed by gradual deceleration. Flow is present even during diastole. The RI in this patient is <0.70 and thus is normal.

technique, a colour Doppler box is placed on the kidney and an arcuate artery is identified at the corticomedullary junction. Using the colour Doppler image for guidance, a 1–2 mm PW Doppler sample volume is placed over the arcuate artery and a recording of flow made (Figure 10.1e). Several identical, sequential wave forms should be obtained. This is relatively easier in the left kidney as there is less motion from breathing; it can be quite difficult in the right kidney. The resistive index (RI) is calculated by the following formula:

$$RI = \frac{(\text{Peak systolic velocity} - \text{Minimum diastolic velocity})}{\text{Peak systolic velocity}}$$

Most ultrasound machines have software to calculate and display the RI on the monitor in realtime. Values in excess of 0.70 are considered abnormal. Increased RI values have been reported with obstruction of the ureter, in all acquired renal diseases, except chronic glomerular disease, and with rejection of renal transplants. Hypotensive animals will also exhibit an elevated RI. An increased RI is quite non-specific and is seldom used in clinical practice.

Pyelography

Ureteral obstruction can be confirmed with ultrasound-guided pyelography (Figure 10.2). The skin overlying the kidney is aseptically prepared and with ultrasound guidance a 22-gauge hypodermic needle is placed in the dilated renal pelvis. Urine is withdrawn and a similar volume of water-soluble iodinated contrast medium (at least 250 mgI/ml) is injected whilst observing filling of the pelvis. If leakage of contrast medium along the needle tract is seen, the injection is stopped. Lateral and ventro-dorsal radiographs are made at regular intervals for 20 minutes or until the contrast medium enters the bladder. The injection of contrast medium directly into the renal pelvis produces good filling, and evaluating the patency of the ureter is usually straightforward. The technique does not rely on the kidneys to concentrate the contrast medium and avoids the risk of contrast medium-induced renal failure or systemic hypotension. Leakage of contrast medium is usually confined to the subcapsular space or perirenal retroperitoneal space, and seldom hampers interpretation. Culture of the pelvic urine sample can confirm or exclude pyelonephritis.

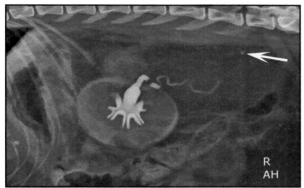

10.2 Lateral abdominal radiograph of an ultrasound-guided pyelogram in a cat. The contrast medium was injected into the renal pelvis following urine aspiration. Some contrast medium has accumulated between the renal cortex and capsule, creating a halo around the kidney. The renal pelvis and pelvic diverticula are moderately dilated and there is mild to moderate dilatation of the ureter. There is a small air bubble within the ureter just distal to the ureteropelvic junction. An obstructive calculus (arrowed) is present in the dorsal mid-abdomen. On subsequent radiographs there was no evidence of the contrast medium passing beyond the calculus.

Normal ultrasonographic appearance

The kidneys of dogs are paired elongated ovoid structures. There is a hilus at the medial aspect of the mid-body where the renal artery enters and the renal vein and ureter exit. The renal capsule is seen as a thin hyperechoic line when perpendicular to the ultrasound beam. When the beam strikes the capsule obliquely, the ultrasound waves are reflected away from the transducer and the capsule is not visible. The cortex has a very fine, uniform echotexture. The medulla is quite dark and appears almost anechoic by comparison (Figure 10.3a). The medulla is lobulated, divided by fine, radiating, echogenic lines. The arcuate vessels may be seen as small hyperechoic structures at the corticomedullary junction. The depth of the renal cortex and medulla are approximately the same. The renal pelvis, peripelvic fat (Figure 10.3b), proximal ureter, renal artery and vein appear as a hyperechoic structure at the medial aspect of the kidney. Pulsation of the renal artery may be seen on B-mode images, although the lumen is usually seen only in larger dogs. The renal vein is of larger calibre and is seen as an anechoic tubular structure (Figure 10.3c). The normal pelvic lumen and ureter are not seen as distinct structures.

When comparing echogenicity, the kidney must be scanned at the same depth and with the same machine settings as the reference organ. The right kidney is compared with the liver and the left with the spleen. The right kidney lies within the renal fossa of the caudate liver lobe, and in most dogs it is possible to obtain images of the right kidney in contact with the liver (Figure 10.4). The left kidney lies caudal to the last rib and is medial and caudal to the head of spleen, and the two are usually close together allowing comparison (Figure 10.5; see also **Normal kidney in a dog** clip on DVD). The cortex of the right

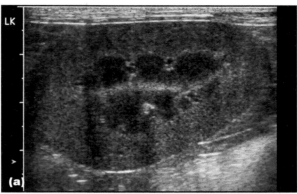

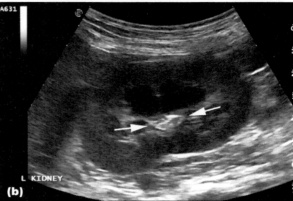

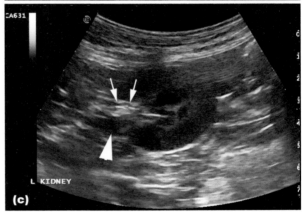

10.3 **(a)** Sagittal plane image of a normal left kidney in a dog. The cortex has a uniform granular echotexture and medium echogenicity. The medulla is hypoechoic in comparison to the cortex. There is good distinction between the cortex and medulla. **(b)** Dorsal plane image of a normal left kidney in a dog. The lateral cortex is in the near-field. Note the hyperechoic appearance of the renal pelvis and peripelvic fat at the renal hilus (arrowed). **(c)** Transverse plane image at the mid-body of a normal left kidney in a dog. The renal artery is seen as two parallel slightly irregular lines (arrowed). The renal vein is much larger and positioned slightly deeper (arrowhead). The papilla of the renal medulla is almost anechoic and protrudes slightly into the renal pelvis, which is hyperechoic and concave.

kidney is hypoechoic or isoechoic to the caudate lobe of the liver, and the cortex of the left kidney is hypoechoic to the spleen. In some normal patients, the cortex of the right kidney appears more echoic than the liver. These relationships are not absolute and can vary with different transducers, imaging frequencies and machine settings.

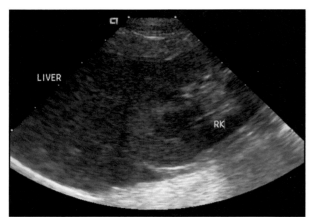

10.4 Sagittal plane image of a normal right kidney (RK) and the caudate lobe of the liver in a dog. The cranial two-thirds of the right kidney is seen. The cranial pole of the kidney sits in the renal fossa of the caudate lobe of the liver. The renal cortex is comparable in echogenicity and echotexture to the liver parenchyma.

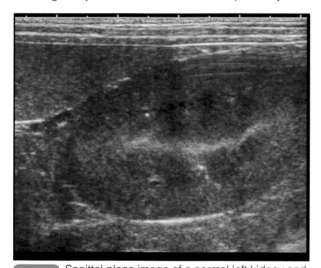

10.5 Sagittal plane image of a normal left kidney and spleen in a dog. The spleen is in the upper left corner of the image, in close contact with the cortex of the kidney. The splenic parenchyma is hyperechoic in comparison with the renal cortical parenchyma.

Feline kidneys are shorter and rounder than the kidneys of dogs (Figure 10.6; see also **Normal kidney in a cat** clip on DVD). The appearance of the medulla and renal hilus in a normal feline kidney is similar to that of a dog. Fat is deposited in renal tubular cells in cats with a moderate or large amount of body fat. This causes the cortex to appear much more echogenic than the medulla and enhances contrast between the two areas. In fat cats, a hyperechoic renal cortex should not be interpreted to indicate renal disease. The kidneys, liver and spleen are seldom in contact with each other in cats, which makes comparison more difficult. Normal feline kidneys measure 30–45 mm in length. The renal medulla is divided into segments by the diverticula and radiating lobar vessels. The renal pelvis is hyperechoic because of the presence of fat and fibrous tissue. The renal vein may be seen at the hilus with a high-frequency linear probe but the renal artery is usually too small to be seen.

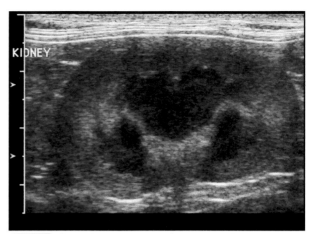

10.6 Dorsal plane image of a normal left kidney in a cat. The kidney is somewhat shorter and rounder than a normal canine kidney. The cortex is moderately echogenic, whilst the medulla is hypoechoic in comparison. The hyperechoic structure of the renal pelvis and hilar fat is seen at the medial aspect of the mid-body of the kidney.

Collecting system conditions

Hydronephrosis and hydroureter

Dilatation of the renal pelvis and ureter may be unilateral or bilateral and may be caused by lesions anywhere within the urinary tract. In normal patients, the renal pelvic lumen and ureteral lumen are too small to be seen with ultrasonography. Mild dilatation of the renal pelvis appears as a thin hypoechoic or anechoic line in the inner medulla in sagittal or dorsal (Figure 10.7a) plane images. Mild dilatation is easier to identify in transverse images, as it appears as a semilunar hypoechoic or anechoic area outlining the renal papilla (Figure 10.7b). Dilatation of 1–2 mm may be iatrogenic, caused by fluid administration, diuresis or even bladder distension. Dilatation of >2 mm should be considered abnormal and investigated (Figure 10.7c). Possible causes include chronic parenchymal renal disease, pyelonephritis and ureteral obstruction.

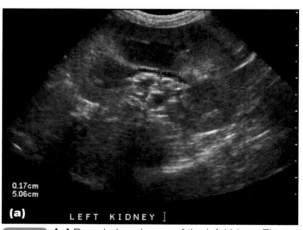

0.17cm
5.06cm

(a)   LEFT KIDNEY

10.7 **(a)** Dorsal plane image of the left kidney. The renal pelvis is mildly dilated, measuring slightly <2 mm in depth. There is increased cortical and medullary echogenicity with some loss of normal corticomedullary distinction. (continues) ▶

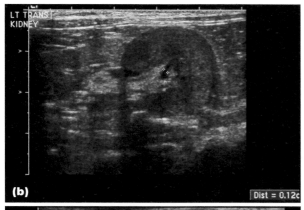

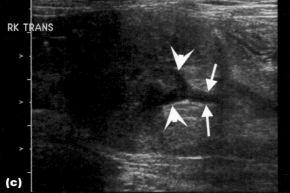

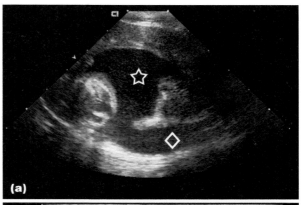

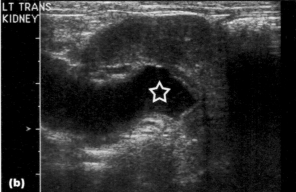

10.7 (continued) **(b)** Transverse plane image of the left kidney in a 17-year-old cat. The renal pelvis is mildly dilated, measuring slightly >1 mm in depth. It appears as a hypoechoic half moon-shaped structure, outlining the renal papilla at the renal hilus. The echogenicity of the cortex and medulla is comparable with little corticomedullary distinction. This is a non-specific indicator of chronic renal disease. **(c)** Transverse plane image of the right kidney in a cat. There is mild to moderate dilatation of the renal pelvis (arrowheads) and proximal ureter (arrowed). The urine within the pelvis and proximal ureter appears anechoic and outlines the renal papilla.

Uroliths are the most commonly encountered obstructive lesions. Complete ureteral obstruction by a urolith, iatrogenic ligation or other cause leads to progressive dilatation of the pelvis and ureter. Accumulation of urine and increased pressure within the pelvis causes the renal parenchyma to atrophy and the kidney to become grossly enlarged, which is termed hydronephrosis (see **Hydronephrosis** clip on DVD). In end-stage hydronephrosis, the normal architecture is completely effaced and the kidney becomes a thin-walled cavity filled with urine with no functional tissue left. Perirenal fluid accumulation may also be seen in acute obstructive renal failure. Partial obstruction may be caused by ureteral uroliths or by extrinsic compression by masses and tumours in the trigone area of the bladder. Partial obstruction is common with transitional cell carcinomas of the bladder and may affect one or both kidneys.

Left untreated, complete urethral obstruction causes severe urinary bladder distension and eventually bilateral renal pelvic and ureteral dilatation. Renal pelvic and ureteral dilatation is also common with ectopic ureters because of the partial obstruction of the distal ureter and ascending infection (Figure 10.8).

10.8 **(a)** Dorsal and **(b)** transverse plane images of the left kidney in a 1-year-old Golden Retriever. There is moderate to severe dilatation of the renal pelvis (☆) and similar dilatation of the ureter (◇). The urine within the collecting system is quite echogenic. There is atrophy of the medulla and increased cortical echogenicity. These abnormalities were the result of a partial obstruction caused by ureteral ectopia and chronic secondary pyelonephritis.

Uroliths

Uroliths can form anywhere in the upper urinary tract. In general, ultrasonography is more sensitive than radiography in detecting uroliths. Even in patients with signs of lower urinary tract disease, the kidney and ureters should be examined for evidence of uroliths. Uroliths which are large enough to block the entire ultrasound beam appear as a bright, echogenic interface with a distal acoustic shadow (Figure 10.9ab). If the uroliths are small, they may not be wide enough to block the ultrasound beam and there will not be an acoustic shadow. Renal parenchymal mineralization (nephrocalcinosis) may occur in chronic renal disease (e.g. interstitial nephritis) and can mimic small uroliths. Distinguishing small pelvic uroliths from nephrocalcinosis or mineralization of the renal pelvis may not be possible in all cases.

Smaller uroliths are usually located in the pelvic diverticula and are often multiple in number (see **Renal calculi** clip on DVD). Large uroliths may fill the renal pelvis and appear as a broad echogenic interface with an acoustic shadow in the centre of the medulla. The shape of the urolith may conform to the pelvis and diverticula, the so-called 'staghorn' (Figure 10.9c), or may be round or oblong. Dilatation of the renal pelvis may be present as a result of concurrent

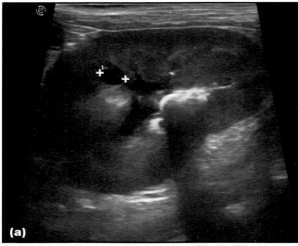

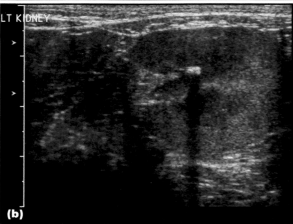

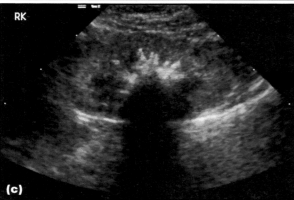

pyelonephritis, renal parenchymal atrophy or partial or complete ureteral obstruction. If the renal pelvis and proximal ureter are dilated, the ureter should be followed as far distally as possible to confirm or exclude the possibility of obstruction (Figure 10.10a). In some cases, multiple uroliths lodge at different points within the ureter (Figure 10.10b). If the dilatation abruptly ends at a ureteral urolith it should be considered to indicate that there is partial or complete obstruction. Following the ureter distally is quite challenging and may not be possible if the degree of dilatation is mild. Ingesta, gas and faeces in the gastrointestinal tract may obscure the lesion, especially in the distal half of the ureter. In such cases, ultrasonography should be supplemented with abdominal radiography. Diagnostic yield is improved if the patient is prepared as for a contrast study of the upper urinary tract.

Acute renal failure may be caused by ureteral obstruction as a result of calculus formation, especially in older cats. These patients have subclinical

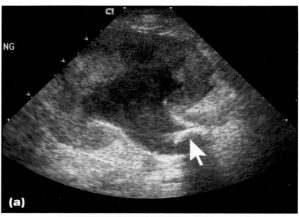

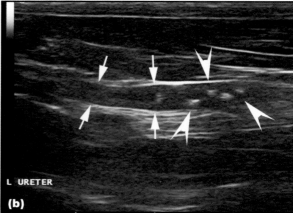

10.9 **(a)** Sagittal plane image of the left kidney in an elderly dog. There is a large calculus within the renal pelvis, seen as a curved hyperechoic interface with a distal acoustic shadow. A small calculus is present within one of the pelvic recesses, just above the large calculus. The renal pelvis is moderately dilated. A cyst (indicated by the cursors) is present at the corticomedullary junction of the kidney. There is increased cortical and medullary echogenicity with loss of corticomedullary distinction. **(b)** Transverse plane image of the left kidney in a cat. A small calculus is present within the renal pelvis, appearing as a hyperechoic structure with a well defined distal acoustic shadow. **(c)** Sagittal plane image of the right kidney in a 12-year-old Pomeranian. There is a large calculus within the renal pelvis. The calculus has an irregular shape and extends into the pelvic diverticula, giving a so-called 'staghorn' appearance. The calculus is quite large and generates a wide complete acoustic shadow.

10.10 **(a)** Dorsal plane image of the left kidney in a dog. There is moderate dilatation of the renal pelvis and proximal ureter with echogenic urine. The renal medulla is partly atrophied. A large calculus (arrowed) is present within the proximal ureter just distal to the ureteropelvic junction. There is no evidence of ureteral dilatation distal to the calculus, which indicates at least partial obstruction. **(b)** Sagittal plane image of the left ureter in the mid-abdomen. The ureter (arrowed) is mildly dilated and the ureteral wall appears mildly to moderately thickened. There are multiple small calculi within the ureter (arrowheads), which are too small to cause an acoustic shadow. There was similar dilatation of the ureter distal to these calculi, indicating that they are unlikely to be obstructive.

renal disease and the loss of renal function by unilateral ureteral obstruction is sufficiently great to cause clinical renal failure. This diagnosis should be suspected in patients with acute renal failure and mild or moderate renal pelvic and ureteral dilatation and pelvic calculi. The dilated ureter should be traced distally to locate the urolith, but it may be quite small and difficult to find. In patients where the ureteral dilatation ends abruptly at a urolith, acute obstructive renal failure is the presumptive diagnosis. The presence of fluid within the retroperitoneal space adjacent to the affected kidney is indicative of acute failure.

Ureteral rupture

With rupture of the ureter, ultrasonography shows anechoic or echogenic fluid within the loose fascia of the retroperitoneal space. However, ultrasonography cannot distinguish between urine and haemorrhage. In cases of ureteral rupture, both blood and urine may be present in the retroperitoneal space. Perirenal retroperitoneal fluid accumulation may also be caused by acute renal failure. Reported aetiologies include ethylene glycol poisoning in dogs, Easter Lily poisoning in cats and acute, complete ureteral obstruction. Ureteral rupture can only be definitively diagnosed by a contrast study, either using ultrasound-guided pyelography (as described above) or conventional excretory urography.

Diffuse parenchymal disease

Congenital

Young cats and dogs may present with chronic renal failure due to congenital or hereditary disease. This must be differentiated from acute renal failure caused by toxic agents such as ethylene glycol and aminoglycoside antibiotics. Familial nephropathies have been reported in numerous dog breeds. These patients present in renal failure quite young, often <1 year of age. The kidneys are small and diffusely hyperechoic with poor corticomedullary distinction, and the cortical surface and shape are irregular (Figure 10.11). There may be mild renal pelvic dilatation. In severely affected individuals the kidneys are

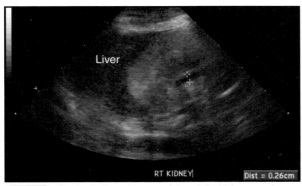

10.11 Sagittal plane image of the right kidney and caudate liver lobe in an 8-month-old Shih Tzu. The kidney is markedly hyperechoic in comparison with the caudate lobe of the liver. There is poor corticomedullary distinction and the cortical surface is irregular. Mild dilatation of the renal pelvis is also seen (indicated by the cursors). The final diagnosis was renal dysplasia.

sometimes difficult to identify. Rarely, the kidneys have normal echogenicity and internal architecture but are small. Similar abnormalities are seen in cases of renal dysplasia or hypoplasia. With unilateral hypoplasia there is often marked compensatory hypertrophy of the contralateral kidney.

Acute renal failure due to ingestion of or exposure to a toxin usually causes increased renal echogenicity with preserved size and architecture. In the case of ethylene glycol intoxication, the increased echogenicity is severe and the kidney may show acoustic shadowing.

Acquired

Acquired renal parenchymal diseases which are diagnosed in cats and dogs include:

* Chronic interstitial nephritis
* Glomerulonephritis
* Acute and chronic pyelonephritis
* Tubular necrosis
* Amyloidosis
* Nephrocalcinosis.

Chronic conditions

Chronic interstitial nephritis is a common cause of chronic renal insufficiency in both dogs and cats. The ultrasonographic changes identified in chronic renal parenchymal disease are non-specific. The most commonly observed abnormalities are alterations of renal echogenicity (Figure 10.12; see also **Chronic renal disease in a cat** clip on DVD). In some diseases, the cortex is more severely affected and appears hyperechoic with enhanced corticomedullary distinction. In chronic interstitial nephritis, there is usually increased echogenicity of both the cortex and medulla with reduced corticomedullary distinction. Small cyst-like lesions with anechoic contents may be seen within the cortex. The kidney may be reduced in

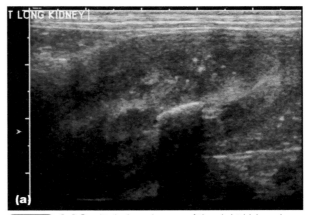

10.12 **(a)** Sagittal plane image of the right kidney in a 12-year-old Yorkshire Terrier. There is increased echogenicity of the cortex and medulla with near complete loss of normal corticomedullary distinction. Multiple small, pinpoint hyperechoic foci are seen within the medulla, consistent with nephrocalcinosis. These findings are non-specific and indicate chronic acquired renal disease. The patient was azotaemic and the final diagnosis was chronic interstitial nephritis. Note also the large calculus in the renal pelvis causing a well defined acoustic shadow. (continues) ▶

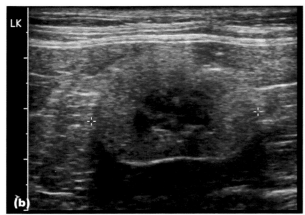

(continued) **(b)** Dorsal plane image of the left kidney in an elderly cat. The kidney is small measuring slightly less than the lower limit of the normal range (3.0–4.5 cm). The cortex is markedly hyperechoic and has an irregular contour. The medulla appears atrophied. These findings are consistent with chronic acquired renal disease such as chronic interstitial nephritis.

size and have an irregular cortical contour. In severe cases, there may be so-called 'end-stage' changes to the kidney, which appears as an amorphous, irregularly shaped, hyperechoic structure with little or no identifiable internal architecture. Determining that the abnormal structure is a kidney is based on its position and a thorough search which confirms that a normal kidney has not been overlooked.

Renal amyloidosis results in a marked increase in echogenicity of the cortex, which increases the normal corticomedullary distinction.

In some patients ultrasonographic abnormalities are seen without biochemical evidence of renal compromise because renal failure only occurs once 70% of the functional nephrons are destroyed (Figure 10.13). Conversely, some patients with azotaemia have no significant abnormalities on ultrasonography.

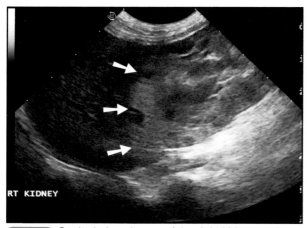

10.13 Sagittal plane image of the right kidney and caudate liver lobe of an 11-year-old Dachshund. The renal cortex is hyperechoic in comparison with the adjacent liver tissue. There are multiple small cysts (arrowed) within the cortex. The medulla is also increased in echogenicity with reduced corticomedullary distinction. These findings are consistent with chronic renal disease. However, this patient had no evidence of renal insufficiency and was diagnosed with a linear foreign body of the pylorus and descending duodenum.

A diagnosis of renal failure is typically based on serum chemistry and urinalysis findings. Some dogs with chronic severe renal failure may show characteristic ultrasonographic abnormalities. Chronic renal insufficiency leads to deranged calcium and phosphorus homeostasis and soft tissue mineralization. Uraemic gastropathy (Figure 10.14) causes mineralization of the mucosa seen as a prominent, thin, hyperechoic band close to the luminal surface. This finding indicates chronic severe renal insufficiency.

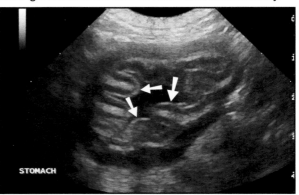

10.14 Sagittal plane image of the body of the stomach in a 10-year-old mixed-breed dog. A thin hyperechoic line (arrowed) is seen at the mucosal surface consistent with mineralization of the gastric mucosa, indicating uraemic gastropathy and chronic severe renal insufficiency.

Inflammation and infection

A number of infectious diseases may affect the kidney. The reported ultrasonographic changes in canine leptospirosis include increased renal cortical echogenicity, dilatation of the renal pelvis, renal enlargement, perirenal effusion and a hyperechoic band within the medulla. The latter finding is considered relatively characteristic of leptospirosis. The hyperechoic band extends from the renal pelvis to the mid-point of the medulla. A hyperechoic band in the outer medulla or at the corticomedullary junction has been reported with hypercalcaemia and in both normal cats and dogs.

Cryptococcus infection and granulomatous feline infectious peritonitis, caused by feline coronavirus infection, result in renal changes in cats. Abnormalities which may be seen include multiple small nodules or mass lesions within the cortex and medulla, and a band of hypoechoic tissue between the renal capsule and the cortex. There is often some distortion or blurring of the normal internal renal architecture. These findings are similar to those seen in renal lymphoma in cats.

Pyelonephritis may occur as a sequel to lower urinary tract infection. It is also a common concurrent condition with ureteral ectopia. The ultrasonographic findings in experimentally induced pyelonephritis in dogs include dilatation of the proximal ureter and renal pelvis, a hyperechoic line within the pelvis or ureter, and hyperechoic or hypoechoic foci within the renal cortex and medulla. In humans, acute pyelonephritis causes renal swelling, reduced echogenicity of the parenchyma and hyperechoic foci from haemorrhage. Acute pyelonephritis (Figure 10.15) should be

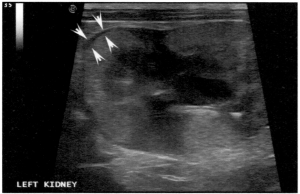

10.15 Dorsal plane image of the left kidney in a cat. The patient had been treated 1 week earlier for acute, complete urethral obstruction and presented with acute onset dullness, lethargy and abdominal pain. On physical examination the left kidney was palpably enlarged and appeared painful. Ultrasonography showed that the left kidney was larger than at the examination 1 week earlier. A thin hypoechoic rim is visible adjacent to the outer cortex (arrowheads), the cortex is hyperechoic, and a hypoechoic defect is seen within it in the near-field. There were large numbers of neutrophils in the urine and the patient had a marked leucocytosis. The diagnosis was acute pyelonephritis superimposed on chronic renal disease.

suspected if urine analysis confirms infection, and there is renal pelvic and ureteral dilatation and non-uniform altered parenchymal echogenicity. Chronic pyelonephritis causes abnormalities similar to chronic interstitial nephritis, with increased medullary and cortical echogenicity, pyelectasia, irregular cortical contours and reduced kidney size.

Metabolic conditions
Hypercalcaemic nephropathy in the dog has relatively characteristic ultrasonographic changes. Lymphoma is the most common cause of paraneoplastic hypercalcaemia in dogs. A hyperechoic band is present at the corticomedullary junction, sometimes referred to as the medullary rim sign. The increased echogenicity is a result of calcification of the Bowman's capsule and tubular epithelium within the cortex and medulla. The presence of these abnormalities and hypercalcaemia indicates a poor prognosis as there is extensive damage to the renal tubules. However, a hyperechoic medullary band has also been reported in patients with no clinical evidence of renal disease or hypercalcaemia (Figure 10.16); therefore, this finding should be evaluated in conjunction with a serum chemistry panel.

Toxic conditions
Ethylene glycol ingestion is a common cause of acute renal failure in the dog and cat as the substance is quite palatable and readily consumed. In acute cases, there is a severe increase in renal cortical echogenicity with enhanced corticomedullary distinction (Figure 10.17). This appearance is caused by renal tubular necrosis and deposition of calcium oxalate crystals within the renal tubules. There may be perirenal fluid accumulation as a result of the acute renal failure. The ultrasonographic changes develop within hours of

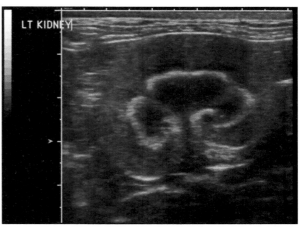

10.16 Dorsal plane image of the left kidney in a middle-aged cat. There is a thin, well defined hyperechoic line in the upper medulla close to the corticomedullary junction. This abnormality may be seen with hypercalcaemia, acute tubular necrosis and chronic renal disease. However, the patient had no evidence of renal insufficiency.

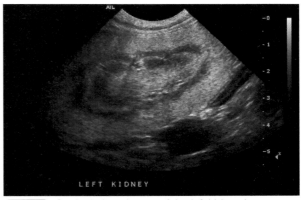

10.17 Sagittal plane image of the left kidney in a 1-year-old Australian Cattle Dog. The patient presented in acute renal failure. There is a marked increase in echogenicity of the renal cortex. An ill defined hyperechoic band is also present within the medulla. These abnormalities are the result of ethylene glycol poisoning.

ingestion of the toxin, so ultrasonography may be used to confirm a suspected diagnosis. In more chronic cases, there is increased renal and cortical echogenicity with loss of corticomedullary distinction. Similar abnormalities may be seen in cats with acute renal failure caused by eating the Easter Lily plant, and in dogs with acute renal failure as a result of consuming grapes.

Focal parenchymal disease

Cysts
Cysts within the cortex of the kidney are a common finding in chronic renal disease (see Figure 10.9a). They are usually small, well defined and have anechoic contents. These cysts do not disrupt or distort the normal outline of the kidney. Cysts can be distinguished from solid lesions by the presence of acoustic enhancement deep to the lesion. Single, large cysts are occasionally encountered in middle-aged and older patients (Figure 10.18).

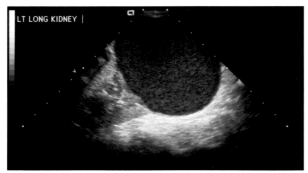

10.18 Sagittal plane image of the left kidney in a 12-year-old Schnauzer. The caudal half of the kidney has been replaced by a well defined, thin-walled cyst-like lesion with echogenic contents. The patient had no evidence of renal insufficiency. The lesion was presumed to be a benign renal cyst.

Polycystic kidney disease is a progressive condition, which may ultimately result in renal failure in affected animals. The condition is heritable in Persian and Himalayan cats, and Cairn Terriers. Ultrasonography was at one time used as a screening test to identify affected cats and remove them from the breeding population, but this has been supplanted by a recently developed genetic test. Affected cats have several cysts in each kidney, although the exact number and size vary considerably (Figure 10.19). These may be quite small in juvenile cats but are reliably detected by 10–12 months of age.

The cysts have thin walls, which blend with the kidney parenchyma, and originate in the cortex or at the corticomedullary junction. The cyst contents are usually anechoic and there is acoustic enhancement. Echogenic cyst contents may be found in some patients, but this finding is usually not significant. The cysts progressively enlarge, destroying normal parenchyma and ultimately causing gross renomegaly. In moderately and severely affected cats, progressive loss of normal renal tissue causes renal insufficiency. In severely affected, late-stage cases there is little or no recognizable normal renal architecture, as it has been replaced by numerous thin-walled cysts of varying size, with an appearance similar to a bunch of grapes.

Infarction

Renal infarcts are a common and usually incidental finding, especially in older cats. The lesions are cortical and result from occlusion of a branch of an arcuate artery by an embolus. In the acute phase the infarct appears hypoechoic and causes a slight bulge of the renal capsule. The lesion is wedge-shaped with the base at the renal capsule and apex at the corticomedullary junction (Figure 10.20a). Acute infarcts are more likely to be seen in patients with severe systemic illness and resultant hypercoagulability. In the chronic phase, the affected part of the renal cortex atrophies, resulting in a concave dimple at the capsule (Figure 10.20bc). Chronic infarcts usually have a hyperechoic appearance (see **Renal infarction (1)** and **(2)** clips on DVD). Multiple chronic infarcts may cause the kidney to appear small and have an irregular shape.

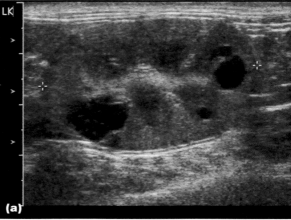

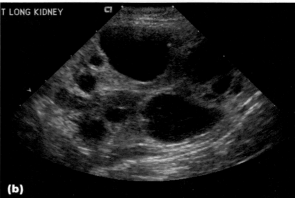

10.19 **(a)** Sagittal plane image of the left kidney in a Himalayan cat. There are several cysts within the renal cortex. The cyst at the lower left of the image contains some echogenic debris. The other cysts have anechoic contents, are well defined and the cyst walls blend with the renal cortex. These abnormalities are consistent with polycystic kidney disease. **(b)** Sagittal plane image of the left kidney in an 8-year-old Persian cat. There is gross enlargement of the kidney, which extends beyond the field-of-view. There are multiple, variably sized cysts within the kidney. These cysts have effaced all normal renal architecture. This patient had bilateral palpable renal enlargement and was azotaemic.

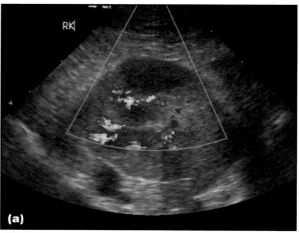

10.20 **(a)** Transverse plane image of the right kidney in a dog. There is a wedge-shaped hypoechoic lesion within the renal cortex in the near-field. The colour Doppler sample volume demonstrates absence of flow within this lesion consistent with an acute renal infarct. (continues) ▶

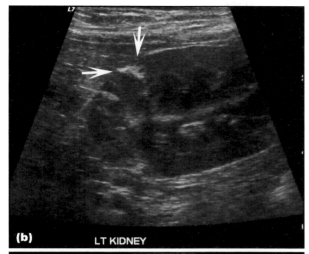

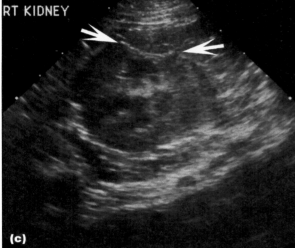

10.20 (continued) **(b)** Sagittal plane image of the left kidney in a dog. There are several well defined hyperechoic lesions within the renal cortex of the cranial pole of the kidney. These are wedge-shaped with the base at the cortical surface and apex at the corticomedullary junction. A shallow concave depression is seen in the cortical surface (arrowed), overlying the lesion in the near-field. The abnormalities are consistent with chronic renal infarcts. **(c)** Transverse plane image of the right kidney in a cat. There is a broad, well defined concave defect (arrowed) within the cortex in the near-field. This is consistent with local atrophy of the cortex as a result of a chronic infarct.

Neoplasia

Primary renal neoplasms include renal cell carcinoma, soft tissue sarcoma, transitional cell carcinoma and nephroblastoma. Synchronous bilateral primary renal tumours occur in about 4% of dogs. Renal cystadenocarcinoma with nodular dermatofibrosis is a syndrome of German Shepherd Dogs and has been shown to be hereditary. Renal lymphoma occurs rarely in dogs but is the most common renal neoplasm in cats.

Canine renal tumours are often quite large at the time of diagnosis. Many tumours completely efface the normal kidney and the diagnosis of a renal mass is based on the lesion position and the absence of a normal kidney (Figure 10.21a). In some cases,

scanning the mass reveals a vestige of normal kidney tissue, which makes confirmation of the diagnosis easier (Figure 10.21bc; see also **Renal lymphoma** clip on DVD). Adrenal carcinomas and phaeochromocytomas are locally aggressive and may invade and partly or completely efface the ipsilateral kidney. The ultrasonographic appearance of renal neoplasms is variable. The echogenicity is most often mixed or complex, and cystic or cavitated lesions are common. Definitive diagnosis requires fine-needle aspiration (FNA) or biopsy, but is more often obtained by surgical excision. The renal vessels, caudal vena cava and aorta should be examined for evidence of a tumour thrombus or encasement by the lesion, which may preclude surgical removal. Vascular invasion most likely indicates a malignant adrenal gland lesion such as adenocarcinoma or phaeochromocytoma. Transitional cell carcinomas which arise in the renal pelvis or proximal ureter may cause obstruction and dilatation of the renal pelvis, progressing to hydronephrosis. The mass is outlined by urine within the renal pelvis. Colour Doppler interrogation of the mass may be helpful in distinguishing it from a blood clot.

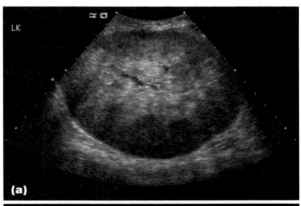

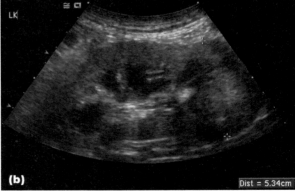

10.21 **(a)** Sagittal plane image of the left kidney in a 12-year-old Shetland Sheepdog. All normal renal architecture has been effaced by a mass. The mass lesion has a hypoechoic outer rim and an irregular hyperechoic centre with a few small cavitated areas. The mass was determined to be renal in origin based on the absence of a normal kidney and its location. The final diagnosis was renal carcinoma. **(b)** Dorsal plane image of the left kidney in a cross-breed German Shepherd Dog. There is a mixed echogenic mass slightly >5 cm in diameter at the caudal pole of the left kidney. The mass lesion has effaced the cortex in this area and expanded beyond the renal capsule. The histological diagnosis was haemangiosarcoma. (continues) ▶

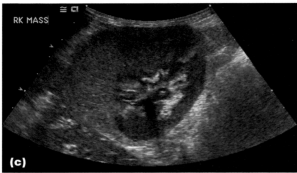

10.21 (continued) **(c)** Sagittal plane image of the right kidney in a dog. There is a well defined mass lesion of uniform echogenicity and echotexture originating from the cranial and ventral aspects of the right kidney. The mass lesion appears slightly hyperechoic in comparison with the normal renal cortex. The normal architecture of the renal medulla and pelvis have been partly preserved. This mass was diagnosed as lymphoma.

Lymphoma can affect one or both kidneys. There may be nodules or masses of the cortex and medulla. Some cats have diffuse infiltration of the kidney, which causes enlargement and partial or complete obliteration of the normal internal renal architecture. A hypoechoic subcapsular infiltrate or halo is a common appearance (Figure 10.22). This may also be caused by granulomatous feline infectious peritonitis (caused by feline coronavirus), *Cryptococcus* infection and acute pyelonephritis. Many cats with renal lymphoma also have lesions in the gastrointestinal tract.

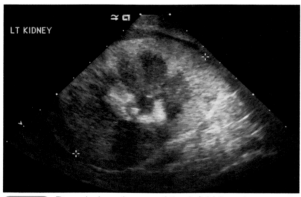

10.22 Dorsal plane image of the left kidney in a Domestic Shorthaired cat. There is gross enlargement of the kidney, which measures 7 cm in length. The medulla is expanded and the renal cortex is hyperechoic. In the near-field, an irregular hypoechoic rim can be seen between the renal capsule and cortex. This rim of hypoechoic tissue adjacent to the cortex is frequently seen in feline renal lymphoma. Lymphoma was confirmed by FNA.

Renal metastases are reported to be quite common at necropsy. However, in clinical practice these are identified relatively infrequently. Nodules and masses are most likely to be seen in the cortex. The size, number, echogenicity and echotexture are quite variable. In a patient with a proven malignancy, solid lesions in the renal cortex may represent acute infarcts or metastasis. Colour Doppler examination shows no blood flow within infarcts. Serial scans may be helpful in distinguishing infarcts as these lesions will usually become smaller over time, whereas metastases will usually grow. Definitive diagnosis requires FNA or biopsy.

Perirenal disease

Pseudocysts
Perirenal pseudocysts are found in older cats. The lesions cause severe, usually bilateral, renal enlargement. The pseudocyst appears as a large cyst-like structure with a thin, well defined wall and anechoic contents. The kidney is eccentrically placed within the pseudocyst (Figure 10.23). In most cases, the kidney is hyperechoic with reduced corticomedullary distinction as a result of disease (e.g. chronic interstitial nephritis). Pseudocysts can be drained quite easily with ultrasound guidance and this procedure makes the cat more comfortable. However, the fluid accumulates again, but this may take several months.

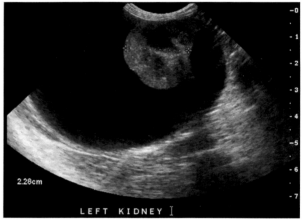

10.23 Sagittal plane image of the left kidney in a 15-year-old Domestic Shorthaired cat. The field-of-view is nearly completely filled by a large cyst-like lesion with anechoic contents. The left kidney is contained within the cyst and is seen in the near-field. The kidney is small (2.28 cm long; normal 3.0–4.5 cm), has increased cortical and medullary echogenicity and an irregular cortex. This is a perinephric pseudocyst.

Urinoma
A urinoma is an encapsulated extravasation of urine, also called a paraureteral pseudocyst. It has been reported in a dog as a sequel to ureteral trauma during ovariohysterectomy. The lesion formed a palpable mass and on ultrasonography appeared as a sharply marginated, anechoic mass with an irregular, hyperechoic wall caudal to the right kidney. There was dilatation of the ipsilateral renal pelvis and proximal ureter. Excretory urography showed no evidence of ureteral contrast medium distal to the urinoma. Transection of the ureter and an adjacent urinoma were found at surgery.

Particular considerations for sampling

Core biopsy samples and fine-needle aspirates may be obtained from the kidney. The indications for renal biopsy are limited as the treatment and prognosis for most forms of chronic renal disease are non-specific. For core biopsy, an 18-gauge needle device is preferred. When performing a renal biopsy, the most important consideration is to limit the path of the needle to the cortex to avoid laceration of the arcuate arteries, which will cause profuse haemorrhage and subsequent infarction. Cortical biopsy with an 18-gauge needle usually obtains samples with several glomeruli that are suitable for histopathological evaluation. General anaesthesia is preferred. Either kidney may be biopsied and the choice depends upon clinical indication and operator preference. In most patients, the left kidney is more accessible but more mobile. The right kidney is somewhat more difficult to access without interposed gastrointestinal structures and is subject to more respiratory motion.

The needle path and distance of travel must be carefully assessed when using automated biopsy devices. Devices which advance the obturator to transfix the target before the outer cutting sleeve is fired are preferred as there is far less risk of poor needle placement or overshooting the target. Overshooting the kidney can result in laceration of the aorta, caudal vena cava, renal artery or renal vein. There is a greater risk of iatrogenic injury of the right pancreas and major abdominal vessels when biopsying the right kidney. FNA is less hazardous and usually obtains a diagnosis for lesions such as renal neoplasia or metastasis. Gross haematuria is a common sequel to renal biopsy or FNA. In cats, ureteral obstruction associated with the resultant blood clots has been reported, and intravenous fluid administration during the biopsy procedure has been recommended to reduce this risk. Ultrasound guidance can also be used for pyelocentesis to confirm pyelonephritis.

References and further reading

Brinkman-Ferguson EL and Biller DS (2009) Ultrasound of the right lateral intercostal space. *Veterinary Clinics of North America: Small Animal Practice* **39**, 761–781

Bryan JN, Henry CJ, Turnquist SE, Tyler JW, Liptak JM *et al.* (2006) Primary renal neoplasia of dogs. *Journal of Veterinary Internal Medicine* **20**, 1155–1160

Chandler ML, Elwood C, Murphy KF, Gajanayake I and Syme HM (2007) Juvenile nephropathy in 37 boxer dogs. *Journal of Small Animal Practice* **48**, 690–694

d'Anjou MA (2008) Kidneys and ureters. In: *Atlas of Small Animal Ultrasonography*, ed. DG Penninck and MA d'Anjou, pp. 339–364. Blackwell, Ames

Feeney DA and Johnston GR (2007) Kidneys and ureters. In: *Textbook of Veterinary Diagnostic Radiology, 5th edn*, ed. DE Thrall, pp. 693–705. WB Saunders, Philadelphia

Holloway A and O'Brien R (2007) Perirenal effusion in dogs and cats with acute renal failure. *Veterinary Radiology and Ultrasound* **48**, 574–579

Ivancic M and Mai W (2008) Qualitative and quantitative comparison of renal versus hepatic ultrasonographic intensity in healthy dogs. *Veterinary Radiology and Ultrasound* **49**, 368–373

Mareschal A, d'Anjou MA, Moreau M, Alexander K and Beauregard G (2007) Ultrasonographic measurement of kidney-to-aorta ratio as a method of estimating renal size in dogs. *Veterinary Radiology and Ultrasound* **48**, 434–438

Nyland TG, Mattoon JS, Herrgesell ER and Wisner ER (2002) Urinary tract. In: *Small Animal Diagnostic Ultrasound, 2nd edn*, ed. TG Nyland and JS Mattoon, pp. 158–195. WB Saunders, Philadelphia

Valdes-Martinez A, Cianciolo R and Mai W (2007) Association between renal hypoechoic subcapsular thickening and lymphosarcoma in cats. *Veterinary Radiology and Ultrasound* **48**, 357–360

Wills SJ, Barrett EL, Barr FJ, Bradley KJ, Helps CR *et al.* (2009) Evaluation of the repeatability of ultrasound scanning for detection of feline polycystic kidney disease. *Journal of Feline Medicine and Surgery* **11**(12), 993–996

Zatelli A, D'Ippolito P and Zini E (2005) Comparison of glomerular number and specimen length obtained from 100 dogs via percutaneous echo-assisted renal biopsy using two different needles. *Veterinary Radiology and Ultrasound* **46**, 434–436

Video extras

- Chronic renal disease in a cat
- Hydronephrosis
- Normal kidney in a cat
- Normal kidney in a dog

- Renal calculi
- Renal infarction (1)
- Renal infarction (2)
- Renal lymphoma

Access via QR code or bsavalibrary.com/ultrasound_10

11

Stomach, small and large intestines

Lorrie Gaschen and Daniel Rodriguez

Indications

Abdominal ultrasonography has become in many instances a part of the minimum database in conjunction with abdominal radiography for the assessment of intestinal disease. Some of the most common indications for gastrointestinal ultrasonography include:

- Persistent or chronic vomiting
- Diarrhoea
- Abdominal pain
- Palpable abdominal mass
- Palpable thickening of the small intestinal loops
- Weight loss and anorexia
- Suspected ingestion of foreign bodies
- Staging of neoplasia
- Suspected hernias.

Value of ultrasonography compared with radiography and computed tomography

The greatest advantages of ultrasonography compared with computed tomography (CT) and conventional radiography are: the lack of any biological risks at commonly used frequencies (1–10 MHz); the fact that little patient preparation is needed; the ability to assess intestinal motility, wall thickness (Figure 11.1) and layering; and to be able to determine the type and origin of lesions. Abundant free and/or intraluminal gas can be problematic when assessing the gastrointestinal tract and other structures deep to the gas-filled viscus. Large volumes of faecal material can cause similar problems. Additional information can be gained from vascular assessment of the intestinal tract using Doppler ultrasonography. CT is an alternative to abdominal ultrasonography in situations where examination of the organs is difficult. This may occur in obese animals where good resolution is not possible as low frequency probes are required, or prior to surgery when there is pathology that is difficult to assess ultrasonographically.

Radiography of the abdomen is important in all patients with vomiting and diarrhoea, and the findings should be used to help interpret those of the ultrasound examination. Abdominal radiographs are standardized, rapidly performed and allow mechanical obstruction or radiopaque foreign material to be identified. Ultrasonography is a more targeted examination

Bodyweight (kg)	Jejunum (mm)	Duodenum (mm)
<10	4.1	5.1
10–20	4.1	5.0
21–30	4.4	5.3
31–40	4.4	6.0
>41	4.7	5.7

11.1 Intestinal wall measurements in relation to bodyweight.

and lacks the overview of the abdominal radiograph. If abdominal radiographs are unremarkable, ultrasonography is an excellent non-invasive method of further examining the gastrointestinal tract. In the hands of experienced operators, intestinal ultrasonography has largely replaced the use of barium contrast studies. Ultrasonography can be used to inspect the small intestines for wall layering, thickness, dilatation and peristalsis as well as for intraluminal, intramural and extraluminal causes of obstruction.

Abdominal radiography should also be the first diagnostic imaging examination performed in dogs and cats with constipation, haematochezia or painful defecation. Abnormalities of the colon such as obstruction, megacolon and obstipation can usually be recognized radiographically. Lateral and ventrodorsal radiographs that include the pelvic region can provide helpful information and rapid assessment of the size and content of the entire large intestine. Ultrasonography cannot provide the same information and is a more targeted examination of segments of the large intestine.

One major advantage of ultrasonography is its ability to assess the wall thickness and layering of the colon. Although not common, colonic torsion can occur causing severe dilatation and displacement of the colon from its normal location, and is best diagnosed radiographically. Mechanical obstruction of the descending colon and rectum due to previous pelvic trauma or space-occupying lesions can also be ruled out radiographically. Increased soft tissue opacities or displacement or compression of the colon within the pelvic canal, as well as a normal radiographic examination, are indications for ultrasonography of the colon in animals with appropriate clinical signs.

Stomach

Imaging technique

Patient preparation
Ventral abdominal clipping is necessary and the use of coupling acoustic gel helpful before starting the imaging procedure. Sedation may be necessary in some fractious patients. Withholding food for 12 hours (with access to water) prior to the examination is recommended to avoid excess gas within the stomach and prevent artefacts, although the effects of fasting may vary.

Positioning
Dorsal, left lateral and right lateral recumbency as well as a standing position can be used to examine the gastrointestinal tract. The purpose of multiple positions and acoustic windows is to displace luminal gas away from the area of interest. Left lateral recumbency improves visualization of the gastric fundus; right lateral recumbency of the pylorus; and the standing position enhances the ventral pylorus and body of the stomach. The transducer is commonly placed caudal to the costal arch, but in some deep-chested dogs (e.g. Dobermann, Greyhound, German Shepherd Dog) an intercostal approach is necessary. The stomach should be scanned from the fundus to the pylorus in both the transverse and sagittal planes.

Equipment
Medium to high frequency transducers are preferable (5–8 MHz) in medium to large sized patients, and high frequency transducers in small dogs and cats (7–10 MHz). Common ultrasound arrays include curvilinear, linear and sector (Figure 11.2). Small footprint curvilinear probes are ideal for the majority of the gastrointestinal tract, but high frequency linear probes often allow a higher resolution image of the intestinal walls of the jejunum and colon.

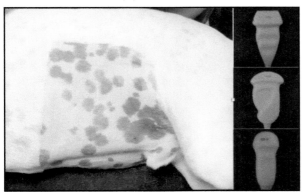

11.2 Transducer arrays and clipping area for abdominal ultrasonography. From top to bottom: multi-frequency linear; convex; and microconvex transducers.

Normal ultrasonographic appearance
The stomach and small intestines have a similar layered appearance ultrasonographically. The outermost layer corresponds to the serosal surface, followed by the muscularis, submucosal and mucosal layers, all of which can be seen ultrasonographically in a normal dog and cat. Hypoechoic layers correspond to the mucosa and muscularis; the remaining layers are hyperechoic. The normal stomach has a varied appearance, dependent mostly on the degree of intraluminal distension and intraluminal contents. The normal stomach may contain small amounts of fluid, gas or ingesta or a combination thereof. The rugal folds are prominent in the fundus of both dogs and cats, but as the stomach becomes distended the rugal folds become less apparent. One difference between the dog and cat is that the feline stomach resembles a 'wagon wheel' appearance in the transverse plane (Figure 11.3).

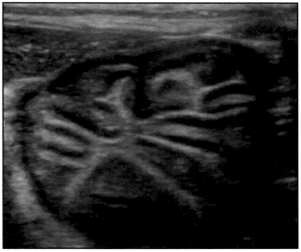

11.3 Short-axis view of a normal empty stomach of a cat showing the 'wagon wheel' appearance.

Measurements of the stomach wall should be made between the rugal folds on a transverse plane image. The inter-rugal fold thickness ranges between 3 and 5 mm in the dog, and is 2.2 mm in the cat. The rate of gastric peristalsis is variable and dependent on several factors. Intrinsic and extrinsic factors such as stress, caloric density of the meal, food particle size, tranquillizers and prokinetic drugs can all affect peristalsis. Normal gastric peristalsis in dogs accounts for five antral contractions per minute or one contraction every 12 seconds.

Functional abnormalities

Pylorospasm
Pylorospasm is impaired relaxation of the pyloric sphincter in the absence of a thickened pyloric muscular layer. This condition has been described in human infants and adults secondary to bile reflux from the duodenum, as an early functional manifestation of pyloric stenosis, and as an idiopathic condition. Ultrasonographically pylorospasm may be suspected if forceful contractions of the pylorus are observed without movement of ingesta into the duodenum and without evidence of abnormal muscular layer thickening. The normal ultrasonographic appearance of the pylorus is shown in Figure 11.4.

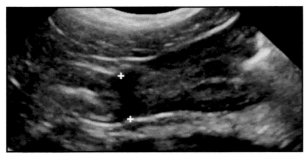

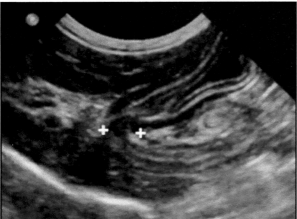

11.4 Long-axis view of the normal **(a)** canine and **(b)** feline pylorus.

Ileus

Paralytic ileus, also called adynamic ileus, is non-mechanical obstruction of the gastrointestinal tract due to reduced or absent peristalsis (Figure 11.5; see also **Functional ileus** clip on DVD). The aetiology is multifactorial and can be seen after surgery, and secondary to peritonitis, pancreatitis, neuromuscular intestinal disease and the administration of drugs such as atropine, opioids and vincristine. Paralytic ileus may also be seen in any condition in which serum potassium is reduced.

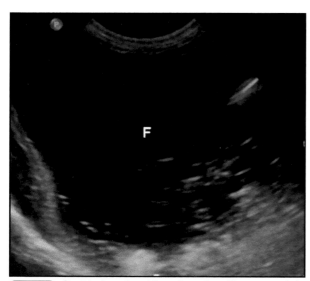

11.5 Gastric functional ileus in a dog. The stomach is severely dilated and fluid-filled (F) and does not show peristaltic activity.

Obstruction

Functional gastric outflow obstructions are difficult to document ultrasonographically. Measurement of the pyloric circumference may be made postprandially, but normal ranges have not been well established in dogs and cats. Pyloric wall thickness, especially the muscular layer, should be assessed to rule out mural infiltration or hypertrophy. Mechanical obstructive lesions can involve the antrum and pyloric canal and include foreign material, neoplasms and functional diseases. Common causes for gastric outflow obstruction are listed in Figure 11.6.

Cause	Comments
Functional obstruction	
Pylorospasm	Not described formally in veterinary patients; mostly anecdotal
Paralytic or adynamic ileus	Multifactorial; seen as a pseudo-obstructive pattern in parvovirus infection
Mechanical obstruction	
Foreign body	
Congenital or acquired (chronic) pyloric hypertrophy	Age or presentation may help differentiation; similar ultrasonographic findings for both diseases; in the acquired form the hypertrophy can affect the mucosa and muscularis
Neoplasia	Adenocarcinoma

11.6 Common causes of gastric outflow obstruction.

Foreign bodies

A strong and uniform acoustic shadowing artefact characterizes the ultrasonographic appearance of foreign bodies, although this appearance may vary depending upon the size and composition of the foreign material. The position of the gastric foreign body may change according to gravity, and placing the patient in right lateral recumbency on an echocardiography table may aid the examination of the dependent pylorus. Linear foreign bodies are common in both dogs and cats. They may be anchored around the tongue and extend in through the pylorus to the duodenum. The stomach, like the small intestine, can appear gathered up ultrasonographically if the linear foreign body is anchored at two ends. Gastric trichobezoars (hair balls) are also common in cats and the ultrasonographic appearance is usually of an irregular hyperechoic gas interface and strong uniform acoustic shadowing.

Diffuse lesions

Inflammation

Acute gastritis is rarely diagnosed with ultrasonography unless it is related to a foreign body. Chronic gastritis on the other hand may be seen ultrasonographically due to the insidious nature of the underlying cause, which may modify the normal ultrasonographic appearance of gastric walls. The hallmark finding is diffuse rather than focal wall thickening, with a hypoechoic or hyperechoic wall. Loss of layering can occur in severe cases (Figure 11.7; see also Gastric oedema clip on DVD). A fluid-filled stomach and enlarged rugal folds may also be seen.

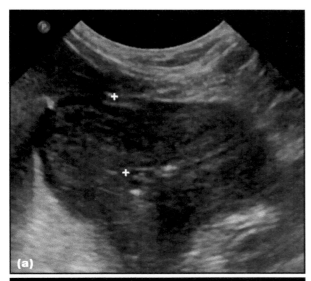

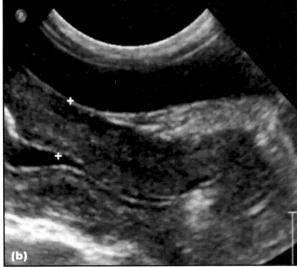

11.7 Severe gastritis in a dog with chronic vomiting. The wall (between the callipers) shows generalized thickening with loss of wall layering in both **(a)** long and **(b)** short-axis views.

Gastritis induced by uraemia may resemble non-specific gastritis ultrasonographically, but may also show a hyperechoic line at the mucosal/submucosal interface, likely representing mineralization. This type of mineralization generally does not cast an acoustic shadow. Differential diagnoses for this finding include gastric wall haemorrhage and oedema due to hypoalbuminaemia.

Eosinophilic and lymphocytic–plasmacytic gastritis may share ultrasonographic features (described above), and some overlap with diffuse neoplastic disease is possible.

Neoplasia
The most common diffuse gastric neoplastic disease in small animals is lymphoma, especially in cats. Other systemic infiltrative neoplasms such as mast cell tumours, especially the systemic form, affect the upper gastrointestinal tract including stomach, duodenum, liver, spleen and local lymph nodes. A predisposition in the Maltese Terrier has been observed in a retrospective study of 39 dogs with gastrointestinal mast cell disease (Ozaki, 2002). Diffuse complete loss of layering with wall thickening, hypoechoic walls and focal mass effect with regional lymphadenopathy are common ultrasonographic features of gastric lymphoma, especially in cats.

Ischaemia
Ischaemic gastropathy may be induced by uraemia, thrombosis, disseminated intravascular coagulation (DIC) and hypovolaemic shock. In humans, partial pancreatectomy and recent mesenteric angiography are two of the most common causes. The end result of an ischaemic event, if severe enough, is ulceration with necrosis.

Other
Pythiosis is caused by *Pythium insidiosum*, an aquatic pathogen belonging to the class Oomycetes in the Kingdom Stramenopila (Chromista). Endemic areas include the Gulf Coast states of North America as well as southeast Asia, eastern coastal Australia and South America. Ultrasonographic features include gastric transmural and occasionally circumferential wall thickening with some characteristics of malignancy, such as loss of layering and local lymphadenopathy. The duodenum and ileocolic junction may also be involved.

Focal lesions

Neoplasia
Benign and malignant neoplasia may create an obstruction at the pyloric outflow tract. Malignant neoplasia has been reported more frequently than benign, and occurs more commonly in males with the exception of adenomas, which are more frequent in females. Benign gastric polyps (also known as adenomatous hyperplasia) can be an incidental finding, but in some cases cause obstruction due to their large size or pedunculated or sessile shape. The ultrasonographic appearance of gastric polyps has been recently described and is summarized in Figure 11.8. Ultrasonographic features of malignant gastric neoplasia can include focal or diffuse loss of layering, usually with wall thickening (8–25 mm; median of 15 mm) and local lymphadenopathy. Some of the largest lesions may be ulcerated.

A high genetic predisposition for gastric carcinoma has been reported in Belgian Shepherd Dogs with an average age of occurrence at 8 years and a 2.5:1 dog to bitch ratio. Adenocarcinomas, carcinomas and lymphomas are commonly associated with local lymphadenopathy. Lymphoma can present as either a focal or diffuse, hypoechoic thickening with a

Appearance	Comments
Single mucosal antral lesion	Differential diagnoses include acquired pyloric hypertrophy, granulomatous gastritis and smooth muscle neoplasia (less common)
Hyperechoic to mixed echoic appearance	
No evidence of gastric layer disruption	A mild disruption of layers can be seen in larger polyps with adjacent wall oedema
No evidence of lymphadenopathy	

11.8 Ultrasonographic features of gastric polyps. Note: final diagnosis may require full-thickness biopsy.

loss of wall layering (Figure 11.9; see also **Gastric lymphoma** clip on DVD). A focal transmural thickening with *pseudolayering* of the affected segment has been reported as a common feature of carcinomas (see **Pseudolayering** clip on DVD). Histiocytic sarcomas rarely produce a solitary hypoechoic gastric mass. Leiomyosarcomas and leiomyomas (Figure 11.10) can be difficult to differentiate, especially in the early stages, due to the fact that both originate from the same layer and share echogenic features (hypoechoic lesions). Leiomyosarcomas tend to have a mixed echogenic pattern as they become larger in size. Biopsy of the lesion is always necessary to confirm the diagnosis. Figure 11.11 details the most common gastric tumours seen in dogs and cats.

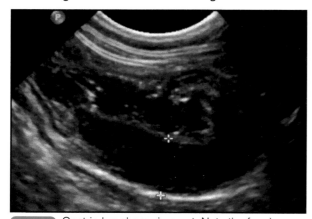

11.9 Gastric lymphoma in a cat. Note the focal thickened and hypoechoic wall with loss of wall layering (between the callipers).

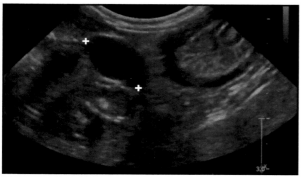

11.10 Focal leiomyoma (+–+) in a dog with hypoglycaemia.

Neoplasm	Location	Comments
Malignant		
Lymphoma	Commonly diffuse, can be local	Transmural hypoechoic loss of layering common
Adenocarcinoma	Lesser curvature and antrum of the stomach	Pseudolayering occurs
Histiocytic sarcoma		Rarely a solitary mass, liver and splenic involvement is more common
Leiomyosarcoma	Variable	Mixed pattern common
Benign		
Leiomyoma	Cardia	
Adenoma (polyp)	Pyloric antrum	

11.11 Common gastric neoplasms.

Hypertrophy

Normal pyloric muscular and complete wall thickness measurements have been reported to be <4 mm and <9 mm, respectively, in dogs. Congenital or acquired *pyloric hypertrophy* can be diagnosed if previous measurements are exceeded. Chronic acquired pyloric hypertrophy is a disease of small, middle-aged to older dogs; breeds reported to be frequently affected include Lhasa Apso, Shih Tzu and Pekingese. It has also been reported in Siamese cats in association with megaoesophagus.

Ultrasonographically, hypertrophic pyloric disease results in circumferential pyloric sphincter thickening involving the muscular layer and sometimes the mucosa (acquired form). Direct visualization with endoscopy and positive contrast gastrography may be necessary to confirm the diagnosis of obstructive/delayed emptying disease.

Ulcers

The ultrasonographic characteristics of a gastric ulcer include focal wall thickening, with or without loss of layering, and with or without an ulcer crater. The ulcer crater sometimes contains trapped gas, which appears as small hyperechoic foci that produce reverberation artefacts. The affected portion of the stomach wall may appear hypomotile or stiff. A small percentage of gastric ulcers are due to neoplasia and it has to be included in the differential diagnoses. If neoplasia is suspected fine-needle aspiration (FNA) or biopsy is recommended for a definitive diagnosis.

Duodenum

Imaging technique

Regardless of the recumbency used, the proximal duodenum is identified by scanning the right lateral abdomen as it lies just medial to the body wall. An intercostal approach is sometimes necessary to visualize the cranial duodenal flexure in deep-chested dogs. In dogs the duodenum is characterized by its right cranial abdominal location; its course is mostly superficial and its caudal flexure is usually cranial to the full urinary bladder (Figure 11.12). In cats the duodenum is more midline and can generally be identified by tracing the stomach from left to right. High frequency transducers are preferred (7.5–10 MHz) and small curvilinear arrays are recommended for an intercostal approach.

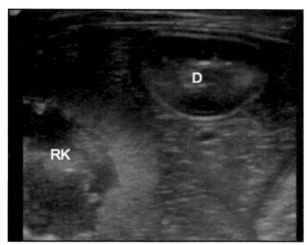

11.12 Normal anatomical location of the proximal duodenum viewed from a right dorsal acoustic window. Dorsal is towards the left of the image and the duodenum (D) is ventral to the short-axis of the right kidney (RK).

Normal ultrasonographic appearance

The normal duodenum (see **Normal duodenal contractions** clip on DVD) usually has a thicker wall than the small intestine with measurements that vary according to the patient's weight (see Figure 11.1). The duodenum, in common with the rest of the small bowel, has five ultrasonographically recognized layers: (from the lumen outward) mucosa, submucosa, muscularis, subserosa and serosa (Figure 11.13). The mucosa and muscularis are hypoechoic, the rest of the layers are hyperechoic. On occasion, hyperechoic indentations can be seen within the mucosal layer of the antimesenteric border of the duodenum; this has been histologically correlated with lymphatic tissue (Peyer's

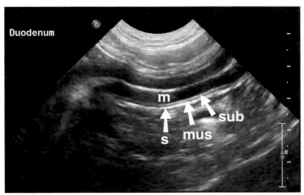

11.13 Duodenum in a dog showing normal wall layering. m = mucosa; mus = muscularis; s = serosa; sub = submucosa.

patches). The major duodenal papilla is usually recognizable in the cat, located close to the pylorus (see **Normal feline pylorus** clip on DVD), and appears as a small round nodule at the mesenteric border of the duodenal wall. The papilla can be more difficult to identify in dogs (see **Normal duodenal papilla** clip on DVD) if deep-chested.

Functional abnormalities

Paralytic ileus
The most common causes of paralytic ileus in small animals are pancreatitis and peritonitis, but it is important to remember that recent surgery and drugs, especially opioids and atropine, can also cause paralytic ileus. The duodenum appears mildly dilated, possibly rigid or corrugated, and the lumen is filled with fluid and gas.

Obstruction
Obstruction can occur either proximally in the descending duodenum (see **Inflammatory polyp** clip on DVD), or at the caudal flexure leading to dilatation of the duodenum and stomach. Proximal duodenal obstruction may not result in the degree of dilatation expected since most of the accumulated fluid can migrate to the stomach through a flaccid pyloric sphincter. Both intraluminal foreign material and mural infiltration with wall thickening or masses may lead to partial or complete obstruction.

Foreign bodies
Duodenal foreign bodies are not different from gastric foreign bodies in the sense that they share the same ultrasonographic characteristics. Linear foreign bodies occur frequently in cats; the affected segment of intestine may be thickened and bunched, and mildly fluid-filled intestinal loops can be seen in conjunction with plicated loops with an intraluminal echogenic structure. A systematic approach to the evaluation is important due to the fact that multiple foreign bodies can be located in the same patient. Chronic foreign bodies have the potential for intestinal perforation (see below).

Neoplasia
Neoplasia may lead to luminal occlusion and stenosis, especially if the growth pattern is concentric. Typically, a hypoechoic to mixed echoic mass with fluid-filled bowel proximal to the obstruction is seen, and efforts to examine the dilated segment as it enters the mass is recommended. The regional mesentery should be scanned for local lymphadenopathy and signs of perforation (free fluid or gas in the peritoneal cavity).

Adhesions
Adhesions may occur secondary to previous abdominal surgery. Trapped intestinal loops with strangulation may be seen with ultrasonography as an area of hyperechoic mesentery with adjacent hypomotile, fluid-filled intestinal loops and focal peritoneal fluid accumulation. Differential diagnoses for the same changes are as for intestinal perforation and infarction.

Diffuse lesions

Inflammation
Inflammatory bowel disease (IBD) can affect the duodenum as well as the rest of the small intestinal tract. There is an overlap of ultrasonographic changes associated with diffuse neoplasia and IBD (Figure 11.14). Commonly, IBD produces a focal to diffuse thickening of the intestinal layers with intact layers and with or without mild lymphadenopathy. In severe cases of IBD a partially disrupted intestinal layer may be seen. In cats, a thickened muscularis has been reported with IBD and in these cases an overlap with lymphoma is present as well. Full-thickness biopsy is warranted to further characterize the most severe cases.

Parameter	Enteritis	Neoplasia
Motility	No significant difference	Same
Distribution	72% diffuse 28% focal	2% diffuse 98% focal
Layering	88% normal or reduced 11% not present	1% normal or reduced 99% not present
Wall thickness (cm)	0.2–2.9	0.5–7.9
Lymph node size (thickness; cm)	0.6–2.6	0.3–9.0

11.14 Ultrasonographic differences between enteritis and neoplasia in the duodenum.

Neoplasia
Diffuse thickening of the duodenal walls with loss of layering and local lymphadenopathy would be expected as ultrasonographic signs of infiltrative diffuse neoplasia. Differential diagnoses include lymphoma, mast cell tumour and IBD since some overlap in their ultrasonographic appearance exists. Mast cell tumours in cats tend to be more focal, but this is not invariably so.

Lymphangiectasia
Lymphangiectasia can be congenital or secondary to intestinal disease such as IBD or neoplasia. Ultrasonographic changes seen in patients with lymphangiectasia are non-specific and may include hyperechoic mucosal striations (Figure 11.15), intestinal wall thickening, a small amount of free anechoic fluid, hypermotility, corrugated small intestines (not only the duodenum) and in some cases lymphadenopathy. Hyperechoic mucosal speckling (Figure 11.16) may also be seen with lymphangiectasia, but can be a normal variation. In dogs with clinical signs, mucosal biopsy is necessary.

Focal lesions

Neoplasia
Lymphoma is common in cats and in dogs and can involve the duodenum. It can lead to either a focal or a diffuse duodenal lesion. There are six different

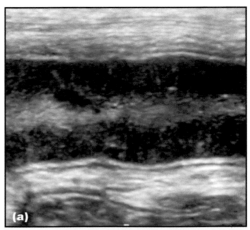
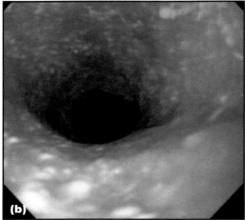

11.15 Intestinal lymphangiectasia in a Yorkshire Terrier. **(a)** Long-axis ultrasonogram of the proximal duodenum and **(b)** the corresponding endoscopic view. There are hyperechoic striations in the mucosa, which are arranged parallel to one another and perpendicular to the long axis. The endoscopic image shows multifocal pinpoint white raised structures representing the dilated lacteals.

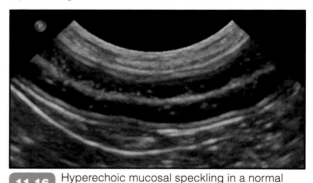

11.16 Hyperechoic mucosal speckling in a normal dog. Small pinpoint hyperechoic foci are present throughout the mucosa and can be seen as a normal variation.

ultrasonographic patterns described for intestinal lymphoma in cats and all except the diffuse mucosal infiltration are transmural.

Ultrasonographically, focal wall thickening with a hypoechoic to mixed echoic appearance, loss of layering and local lymphadenopathy are common findings for intestinal lymphoma. Less commonly, leiomyomas, adenocarcinomas, leiomyosarcomas and mast cell tumours can be focal in distribution, especially in the cat. On occasion, the layer of origin, size of the mass at presentation and pattern observed may guide the differential diagnosis. Large (>3 cm) eccentric, mural masses originating from the muscularis layer have been described as ultrasonographic features of leiomyosarcomas. Be-nign neoplasms such as leiomyomas can be found incidentally in the intestinal tract, most commonly in the stomach, but also in the small intestines including the duodenum. The ultrasonographic appearance is usually homogeneous and hypoechoic or hyperechoic (Figure 11.17). Leiomyomas can be a cause of intestinal intussusception in dogs.

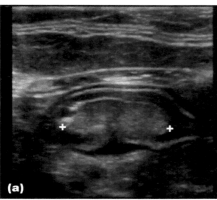
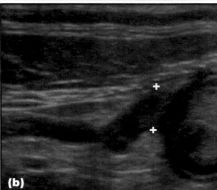

11.17 Duodenal polyp in a cat with hyperbilirubinaemia. **(a)** Ultrasonogram showing the long-axis of the polyp (+–+), which is well marginated, ovoid and homogeneously hyperechoic. **(b)** Ultrasonogram showing dilatation and likely partial obstruction of the common bile duct (+–+).

Ulcers
Duodenal ulcers are common in patients undergoing long-term anti-inflammatory therapy, either non-steroidal or steroidal, and to a lesser degree in patients with chronic severe uraemia. Ulceration with duodenal tumours is also possible, especially in larger fast-growing masses in which the tumour outgrows its vascular supply. They appear similar to those in the stomach with focal wall thickening and loss of layering. An irregularly shaped crater at the mucosal surface with trapped hyperechoic gas bubbles may also be detected.

Gastrointestinal perforation
Perforation of the gastrointestinal tract is multifactorial. The common causes are:

- Gastric dilatation and volvulus; intestinal volvulus
- Surgical dehiscence; percutaneous gastrostomy site leakage
- Gastric and duodenal ulcers
- Neoplasia
- Penetrating or blunt trauma
- Foreign body
- Intussusception.

The ultrasonographic appearance of gastrointestinal perforation includes:

- Regional hyperechoic mesentery
- Peritoneal effusion
- Fluid-filled stomach and/or intestines
- Gastric or intestinal wall thickening with loss of layering
- Regional lymphadenopathy
- Intestinal corrugation.

Jejunum
Imaging technique
Patient preparation
Withholding food for 12 hours (with access to water) as for general abdominal ultrasonography is adequate preparation of the patient for examination of the small intestines.

Positioning
The patient can be positioned in dorsal, right lateral or left lateral recumbency. More than one position may be required to examine the bowel segment of interest due to the presence of gas or overlying faecal material. For example, examination of the intestines from the dependent aspect of the abdomen allows better visualization of the wall layering, since gas rises to the non-dependent portion of the abdomen. Each jejunal segment should be traced from proximal to distal as far as possible. Due to the twisting and turning nature of the intestines, it is generally not possible to trace the jejunum completely. The wall thickness, layering, mucosal echogenicity, luminal diameter and content should be assessed. Attention to the echogenicity of the surrounding mesentery, regional lymph nodes and presence of free fluid is important in every examination.

Doppler ultrasonography
Colour Doppler ultrasonography can be helpful in assessing the vascularity of masses or for determining whether blood flow is present in the mesenteric arteries and veins when strangulated bowel or an intussusception is detected.

Normal ultrasonographic appearance
The jejunum can be differentiated from the duodenum, ileum and colon based on its location, wall layering and communication with adjacent intestinal segments. Jejunal segments in the right lateral abdomen can be confused with the duodenum. However, as they are traced cranially they do not travel towards

the pylorus as does the duodenum. Furthermore, the jejunal wall is not as thick as that of the duodenum. The ileum is identified by its communication with the colocaecal junction and its more prominent submucosal layer compared with the jejunum. Contractions can be observed in two-dimensional (2D) real-time imaging, and approximately 1–3 per minute is considered normal for the small intestine. Recently, investigators have tried to correlate intestinal wall thickness with bodyweight in healthy dogs. In that study, the authors (Delaney *et al.*, 2003) suggested normal values for the jejunal wall thickness of ≤4.1 mm for dogs up to 20 kg, ≤4.4 mm for dogs between 20 and 39.9 kg, and ≤4.7 mm for dogs 40 kg or over. The wall layering is the same as that of the duodenum (see Figure 11.13). Normal luminal content depends on the stage of fasting and dietary composition. A completely empty and contracted lumen is expected in healthy animals, but a small amount of gas or fluid can be present. It is important that the luminal content appears similarly throughout the entire jejunum.

Functional abnormalities

Chronic diarrhoea due to small intestinal disease is common in dogs and cats. Survey radiographs are often non-specific, and gastrointestinal contrast studies are often unrewarding for detecting wall infiltration in the majority of cases. For detecting intestinal wall infiltrates, ultrasonography is superior to both survey and contrast radiography. Abdominal ultrasonography allows for assessment of wall thickness, layering, localization of lesions, peristalsis and involvement of the regional lymph nodes and mesentery.

As seen with abdominal radiography, functional ileus appears ultrasonographically as mild generalized dilatation of the jejunum, usually with fluid and some gas content (Figure 11.18). The intestinal diameter is fairly uniform from one segment to the next. Little if any peristaltic activity is observed and the fluid content tends to have a to-and-fro movement, often random or synchronized with abdominal wall movement and respiration. Causes include enteritis, peritoneal inflammation, abdominal pain, anticholinergic

drugs, malabsorption, partial obstruction, vascular compromise and postoperative abdomen. Wall layering may be affected with some causes of functional ileus such as IBD. In puppies with parvovirus enteritis, mild generalized dilatation and increased fluid content is observed together with decreased thickness (1 mm) of the mucosal layer compared with normal puppies (Stander *et al.*, 2010).

Obstruction

Scanning the jejunal segments for non-uniformity of intestinal diameter is an important part of the ultrasound examination in vomiting animals. Signs of mechanical obstruction on ultrasonography are similar to those seen on radiography. There is often a mixed population of intestinal diameters present, with those proximal to the obstruction being moderately to severely dilated whilst those distal are empty or only mildly dilated. The abnormal segments should be examined for wall thickening, loss of wall layering and for hyperechoic content that creates acoustic shadows.

Foreign bodies

Intestinal foreign bodies may be detected using ultrasonography, regardless of whether or not they are evident radiographically. Radiolucent foreign bodies such as wood, clothing (Figure 11.19), plastic and rubber can be detected since solid material generally appears as a hyperechoic interface, which casts an acoustic shadow from the intestinal lumen. Balls have a round or curvilinear surface, peach pits (see **Jejunal foreign body** clip on DVD) are irregular, and bones generally have a smooth regular surface. The intestinal segment just proximal to the obstruction is markedly dilated and often fluid-filled. Foreign bodies tend to remain fixed in the same position and a repeat examination a short time later shows that they have not moved. Care should be taken not to misinterpret a gas–liquid interface in dilated bowel segments as an obstruction. These interfaces appear as linear, hyperechoic intraluminal structures with acoustic shadowing. However, the bowel often has a similar diameter proximally and distally to the artefact; this is usually not the case with intraluminal foreign bodies causing obstruction.

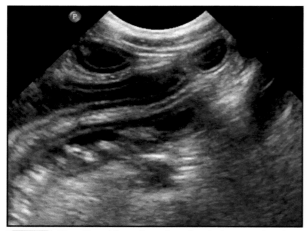

11.18 Functional ileus in a dog due to haemorrhagic gastroenteritis. Note the normal wall layering and mild distension of the jejunal segments, which are fluid-filled. A uniform population of mildly distended small intestines is common with functional ileus.

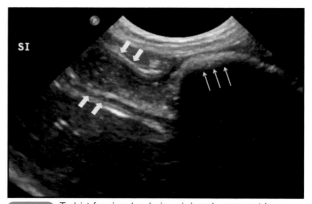

11.19 T-shirt foreign body in a jejunal segment in a dog. There is a smooth hyperechoic structure with clean distal shadowing (arrowed) within the lumen of one jejunal segment. The fluid distending the lumen proximal to it is echogenic (between thicker arrows).

Linear foreign bodies can sometimes be identified in plicated segments of small bowel. Plication appears as small intestinal segments gathered up with the linear foreign material binding them together. The surrounding mesentery should be examined for increased echogenicity and free fluid, which could be indicative of rupture. The presence of pneumoperitoneum together with abdominal effusion on a radiograph should alert the clinician that bowel perforation has occurred.

Neoplasia

Localized mural infiltrations due to inflammation or neoplasia can slowly narrow the intestinal lumen causing complete or, more commonly, partial obstruction. Some degree of intestinal dilatation is often present and solid foreign material such as small stones or dehydrated ingesta can collect proximal to the stricture. Ultrasonographically, neoplastic infiltrates produce intestinal wall thickening often with a loss of wall layering.

Lymphoma is the most common intestinal tumour in cats (see **Jejunal lymphoma** clip on DVD) and also occurs frequently in dogs (Figure 11.20a). It commonly leads to either a symmetrical or asymmetrical, transmural, circumferential thickening. The wall layers are difficult to identify and the entire wall appears hypoechoic to anechoic. The infiltration of the intestinal wall may be solitary, diffuse or multifocal, and the regional lymph nodes may be enlarged (Figure 11.20b). Intestinal carcinoma often produces a solitary intestinal mass, as can polyps, leiomyomas and leiomyosarcomas. Carcinomas tend to be annular, irregular infiltrations that invade the lumen and cause obstruction. Regional lymphadenopathy can also commonly be identified. As the ultrasonographic appearance of the bowel wall alone is not sufficient for a definitive diagnosis, full-thickness biopsy, ultrasound-guided percutaneous biopsy or FNA of the bowel wall is required for a definitive diagnosis of tumour type and to rule out non-neoplastic causes.

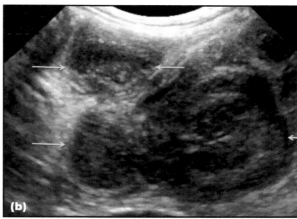

11.20 (continued) Intestinal lymphoma in a dog. **(b)** There is also regional lymphadenopathy due to the lymphoma. The jejunal lymph nodes (arrowed) are severely enlarged, rounded, hypoechoic and display a heterogeneous echotexture.

Non-neoplastic focal masses

Hypertrophy, fungal infections, abscesses, haematomas and foreign body granulomas may cause focal intestinal masses with complete or partial obstruction. Jejunal smooth muscle hypertrophy has been described in the cat and can cause focal wall thickening, but the wall layering is maintained. Fungal granulomas can occur in endemic areas and are often due to pithiosis or histoplasmosis (Figure 11.21). They often lead to either masses or diffuse wall infiltration with loss of wall layering and regional lymphadenopathy, which cannot be differentiated from neoplasia and require histology for a definitive diagnosis.

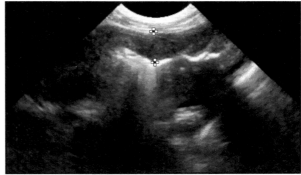

11.21 Histoplasmosis in a dog. There is focal jejunal wall thickening with loss of wall layering (between the callipers). The wall appears hypoechoic in the affected region. Histopathology confirmed the presence of histoplasmosis. Differential diagnoses include lymphoma, mast cell tumour, foreign body granuloma and other types of fungal and neoplastic disease.

Torsion, intussusception and ischaemia

Volvulus or mesenteric thromboembolism is usually recognized radiographically; patients present in shock or with an acute abdomen and cannot usually undergo abdominal ultrasonography due to the severe gas distension of the jejunum. Generalized, severely dilated and air-filled jejunal segments in combination with the clinical signs are usually diagnostic. Other complicated forms of ileus include thromboembolism and intussusception. Intestinal intussusception can

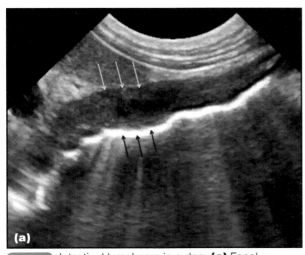

11.20 Intestinal lymphoma in a dog. **(a)** Focal hypoechoic thickening of the wall is present with a loss of wall layering (arrowed). (continues) ▶

usually be quickly diagnosed with ultrasonography. Multilayered, concentric rings of bowel can be identified (Figure 11.22). The outer bowel segment is often thickened, oedematous and hypoechoic. More normal appearing inner segments can be identified. Hyperechoic tissue representing invaginated mesenteric fat may also be detected. In older animals, careful examination of the affected bowel for nodular infiltrations of the bowel wall and regional lymphadenomegaly is important since underlying neoplastic disease may be responsible for the intussusception. Doppler ultrasonography can be used to determine whether the mesenteric vessels within the intussusception (central bowel segments) show flow or not.

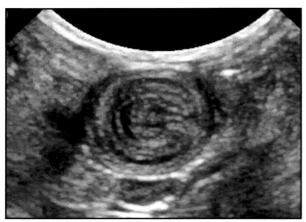

11.22 Intestinal intussusception in a puppy. Concentrically layered intestinal walls are evident in this cross-section of a jejunal intussusception.

Small intestinal corrugation can be seen in dogs and cats with pancreatitis, peritonitis (Figure 11.23), enteritis (including lymphocytic–plasmacytic enteritis), neoplasia, thrombosis, infarction and protein-losing enteropathy (Moon *et al.*, 2003). Corrugation and plication may initially appear similar; however, with corrugation the wall has an undulating appearance and with plication the wall appears gathered up in association with a linear foreign body.

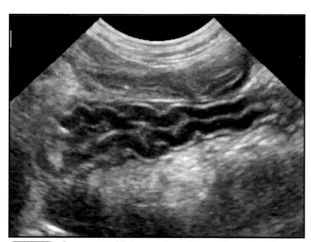

11.23 Corrugated jejunum in a dog with peritonitis. The jejunal segment has an undulating course that is fairly regular. Note the lack of plication associated with linear foreign bodies.

Strangulation, entrapment and adhesions

Intestinal entrapment and strangulation can lead to ischaemia and luminal obstruction and can occur within adhesions or rents in the mesentery or omentum (Swift, 2009). Fortunately, these are rare in cats and dogs. They have been reported secondary to adhesion formation following surgery, omental tears or rupture of the duodenocolic ligament. Abdominal herniation of intestines can also lead to entrapment and ischaemia. Clinical signs include vomiting, lethargy, pain, collapse and haematochezia. Ultrasonographically, the entrapped portion of jejunum is often surrounded by hyperechoic mesentery, and peritoneal effusion is present. The entrapped intestine may have a thickened or corrugated wall or altered layering or appear amotile.

Diffuse lesions

A number of gastrointestinal diseases lead to diffuse infiltration of the small intestinal wall (see **Hypereosinophilic syndrome** clip on DVD). Ultrasonography is important for localizing lesions within the gastrointestinal tract and allowing further characterization of the degree of infiltration inferred from wall thickness and the appearance of wall layering. The mucosa, submucosa and muscularis are most commonly affected.

Inflammatory diseases of the small intestines are common in dogs and cats, but do not always result in gross changes that can be detected with ultrasonography. IBD in cats and dogs must be confirmed histopathologically, either with mucosal or full-thickness biopsy samples. The abnormalities are generally diffuse, but the disease can also present focally or segmentally. Inflammatory disease generally leads to mild to moderate transmural thickening of the intestinal wall with preserved wall layering. Decreased intestinal motility due to wall thickening can also be seen with diffuse or segmental inflammatory disease. The relative thickness of the layers may also change whilst maintaining a normal total wall thickness. Although wall layering is generally preserved, in some instances it can be indistinct or completely lost. A 2D ultrasonography score has been established for canine chronic enteropathies. The number of intestinal wall abnormalities has been shown to correlate with the canine IBD clinical activity index (CIBDAI) at initial presentation when the disease is clinically active. However, improvement in the CIBDAI does not correlate with improvement of the ultrasonography score upon follow-up examinations. Therefore, intestinal ultrasonography is considered a poor method for monitoring intestinal wall abnormalities in dogs diagnosed with IBD.

In cats, the muscular layer is often selectively thickened (Figure 11.24). This finding in cats has also been attributed to lymphoma (Zwingenburger *et al.*, 2010). Lymphoma is the most common neoplastic cause of diffuse infiltration and wall thickening, which can appear similar to inflammatory disease.

The mucosa may also exhibit alterations in echogenicity, varying in severity from diffuse pinpoint hyperechogenic foci to generalized hyperechogenicity (Figure 11.25). Severe mucosal thickening with

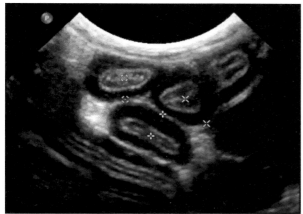

11.24 Muscularis thickening in a cat with lymphoma. The muscular layer is markedly thickened in all jejunal segments. When diffuse, the main differential diagnosis is inflammatory bowel disease. Intestinal biopsy is required to differentiate neoplasia from inflammation.

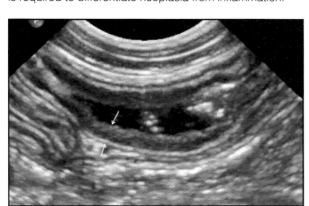

11.25 Inflammatory bowel disease in a dog. Mild generalized thickening of the mucosa is present with mild luminal distension. The mucosa has an increased echogenicity (arrowed) but the wall layering is preserved. Intestinal biopsy is necessary to rule out neoplasia.

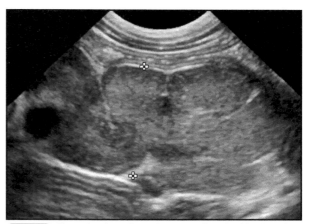

11.26 Reactive lymph nodes associated with chronic inflammatory bowel disease (between the callipers). The lymph nodes are increased in size and somewhat irregular in shape. The echogenicity is close to normal, being moderately echogenic, but with a heterogeneous architecture.

increased echogenicity may be seen in animals with protein-losing enteropathy and lymphangiectasia. In dogs with lymphangiectasia, hyperechoic striations arranged perpendicularly to the long axis of the intestine can be detected (see Figure 11.15); these represent dilated lacteals. Free peritoneal fluid is also often present in these patients. In addition, the small intestine generally shows some dilatation with fluid and gas, and may have decreased motility or a rigid appearance, representing a functional ileus.

Jejunal lymph nodes may appear rounded, heterogeneous, and possibly show target lesions in patients with both inflammatory (Figure 11.26) and neoplastic disease. However, lymph nodes tend to be more severely enlarged, rounded and hypoechoic when neoplasia is present.

Perforation

Complicated forms of jejunal disease include bowel perforation with peritonitis and free air in the abdominal cavity (Figure 11.27). The presence of pneumoperitoneum together with abdominal effusion on a radiograph should alert the clinician that bowel perforation may be the cause. Ultrasonography may be

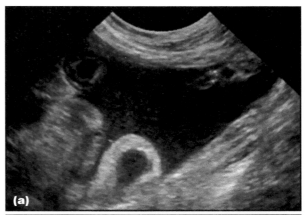

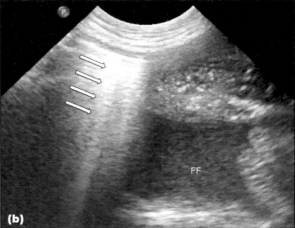

11.27 **(a)** Peri-intestinal focal free fluid and hyperechoic mesentery associated with an intestinal perforation due to a long-standing linear foreign body. **(b)** Free peritoneal air. There is a hazy hyperechoic reverberation artefact (arrowed) at the non-dependent margin of the peritoneum. This represents free air following an intestinal perforation. Care is required not to confuse with gas-filled bowel loops adjacent to the non-dependent aspect of the abdomen. If in doubt, radiographs should be performed to assess for free air. FF = free fluid.

used to identify the site or sites of perforation and help to elucidate the cause.

Masses due to granulomatous or neoplastic infiltration can perforate the intestinal wall due to necrosis. Perforations may also be caused by administration of non-steroidal anti-inflammatory medications, which cause ulcers. Ulceration of the small intestine can appear ultrasonographically similar to malignant disease. Both benign and malignant ulcerations can appear as focal wall thickening with a focal accumulation of hyperechoic air bubbles at the mucosal surface. Foreign bodies may also perforate the small intestine; these are commonly wooden sticks or screws. A foreign body may also cause indirect wall perforation due to necrosis following long-standing mechanical obstruction. The surrounding mesentery at the perforation site appears hyperechoic and variable amounts of free fluid are present in the abdomen, depending on the size and duration of the perforation. Regional lymph nodes may be enlarged when neoplastic disease is present. Full-thickness biopsy of the affected intestinal segments should be performed to rule out neoplastic disease.

Large intestine

Imaging technique

Patient preparation
No additional patient preparation is required for the initial examination of the colon. If an excessive amount of faeces is present, a cleansing enema may be required to examine not only the colon but also the remainder of the abdomen ultrasonographically. If a mechanical obstruction is present, it may not be possible to evacuate the colon. However, ultrasonography can still be useful for differentiating intramural from extramural lesions as the cause of the obstruction.

Positioning
The descending colon can be scanned from the pelvic inlet along the left abdominal wall where it lies very superficially. Placing the transducer transversely at the level of the urinary bladder shows the colon to be located dorsally. Tracing the colon cranially, it can be observed to turn towards the right just caudal to the stomach. From a right-sided acoustic window, the ascending colon and caecum can be identified. Using the descending duodenum as a landmark, the ascending colon can be searched for medial to it. The ileum can then be identified as it enters the colon at the ileocolic junction by sweeping the probe back and forth in the mid-abdomen on the right side. The ileum appears to end bluntly in a large intestinal segment. In cats, there may be no faeces or air in the caecum and therefore fewer reverberation artefacts.

Normal ultrasonographic appearance
The ileum, ileocaecal junction, caecum, and ascending, transverse and descending colon can be identified. When distended, the wall of the colon should have the appearance of having three to five layers and a thickness of 1–2 mm (Figure 11.28). The colon

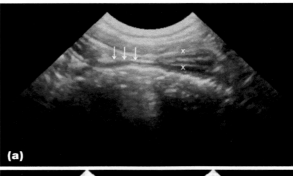

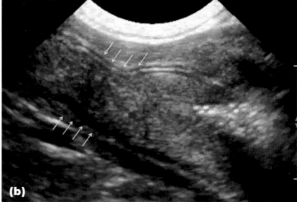

11.28 Normal colon. **(a)** The colon wall (arrowed) is thin with alternating hyperechoic and hypoechoic layers that are equal in diameter. Only the near wall is visible when the colon is filled with gas or faeces. Note the jejunal segment (between the callipers) adjacent to the colon whose thick mucosa helps to differentiate the two types of bowel. **(b)** Normal fluid-filled colon. Due to the lack of solid faeces, both the near and far wall can be identified (arrowed).

is often observed as a bright hyperechoic linear structure causing reverberation artefacts due to the presence of gas and faecal matter. The empty colon appears contracted and many stacked layers can be appreciated. This should not be misinterpreted as colonic wall thickening. Due to the presence of air and faeces, only the near wall (close to the transducer) can be examined from one acoustic window. Left, right and ventral acoustic windows are likely necessary to examine the wall more completely.

The colon can be differentiated from small intestine by its thickness and wall layering. The colonic layers are thin and equal in thickness compared with the greater thickness of the jejunal mucosa. The ileum can be identified medial to the duodenum and appears as a short segment with small bowel layering but with a prominent hyperechoic submucosa in both dogs and cats. Its identity can also be differentiated from the jejunum by its entrance site at the ileocaecocolic junction (Figure 11.29). Unlike the stomach and jejunum, peristaltic activity is not evident in the normal colon. The bony pelvis also limits examination of the colon, but the rectum as well as the perirectal and perineal regions can be examined via a perineal approach. If the region of interest within the pelvic canal cannot be assessed due to overlying bone, radiographic contrast studies, CT or magnetic resonance imaging (MRI) may be required to fully assess the extent of disease affecting the colon and rectum.

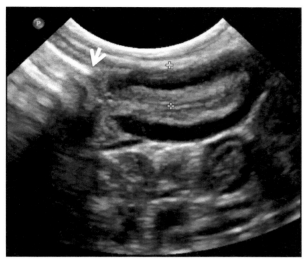

11.29 Ileum showing the ileocaecocolic junction in a cat with inflammatory bowel disease. The short ileum enters the colon (arrowed). The muscular layer is thickened. A plasmacytic–lymphocytic–eosinophilic inflammatory infiltration was present.

Diffuse lesions

Ultrasonographically, the colon can be evaluated for wall thickening and loss of layering as well as regional lymphadenopathy. Neoplastic, inflammatory and infectious diseases can cause severe diffuse colon wall thickening. Colitis due to diffuse, mild to moderate lymphocytic–plasmacytic infiltration often shows no radiographic or ultrasonographic changes, and colonoscopy is the diagnostic method of choice when clinical suspicion of colitis exists. Severe or chronic disease may result in diffuse, moderate thickening of the wall (Figure 11.30a). The colon lumen may also be fluid-filled in patients with colitis (Figure 11.30b). However, ultrasonography is an important screening examination when haematochezia is present in order to rule out a colonic wall mass. Lesions that can be missed are those that are located in the pelvic canal, which lacks a good acoustic window. Severe diffuse thickening of the colon wall may occur in ulcerative colitis, fungal infections and diffuse neoplastic processes such as lymphoma.

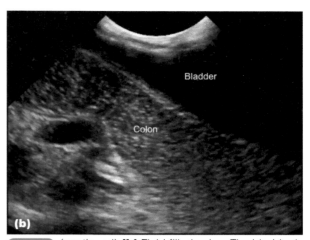

11.30 (continued) **(b)** Fluid-filled colon. The bladder is a good landmark for confirming that a fluid-filled bowel segment is colonic by its dorsal location to the bladder.

Focal lesions

Focal infiltration of the colon by neoplastic masses may be recognized radiographically if the lesions are large enough; however, they are not always evident. Ultrasonographically, focal infiltrations or intramural masses of the colonic wall may be detected with high frequency transducers and are usually associated with either neoplasms (Figure 11.31) or granulomas. Both MRI and CT are alternative methods for examining the pelvic region or determining the involvement of the colon and surrounding tissues, especially when space-occupying lesions are present in that region or radiation therapy may be required.

Neoplastic masses usually appear large and irregularly shaped with a loss of wall layering (see **Colonic carcinoma** clip on DVD). Masses are usually heterogeneous with a mixture of echogenicities. Dystrophic mineralization may also be present in colonic wall masses, and may occur in both neoplastic and granulomatous diseases. Mineralization appears as multifocal hyperechoic structures with distal acoustic shadowing. The sublumbar lymph nodes are often enlarged and can be rounded and hypoechoic when colonic neoplasia is present. However, fungal infection

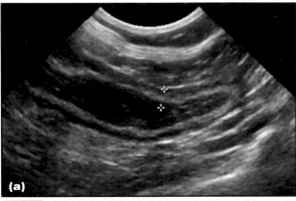

11.30 **(a)** Mildly, diffusely thickened colon wall in a cat with chronic, severe colitis diagnosed by mucosal biopsy. The wall layering is less distinct than normal, the wall thickness is 3.5 mm (normal is 1 mm) and it appears hyperechoic. The lumen is fluid-filled. (continues) ▶

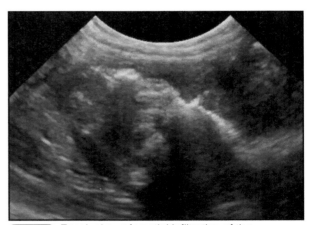

11.31 Focal, circumferential infiltration of the descending colon wall in a cat. The thickened portion has a heterogeneous, hypoechoic appearance with loss of wall layering. Biopsy confirmed a carcinoma.

can also lead to lymphadenopathy. In addition, lymphoma has a hypoechoic appearance with wall thickening and loss of layering, which can also be diffuse. Mast cell infiltration and leiomyosarcomas can have a similar appearance. Adenocarcinomas generally cause a circumferential and focal thickening of the colon with stricture. Adenocarcinoma is the most common colonic neoplasm in cats, followed by malignant lymphosarcoma. Leiomyosarcoma can also be found in the large intestine.

Focal masses can also be caused by pyogranulomatous colitis, resulting from histoplasmosis in dogs from endemic regions. Therefore, obtaining cytological or histological confirmation is critical for a definitive diagnosis. FNA with a 22–25-gauge needle for cytology can be performed on the thickened colon wall or mass if an appropriate acoustic window can be obtained. This is usually easier to perform in the caudal abdomen where the colon is more fixed in position. Tissue core biopsy can be performed on colonic wall masses if large enough: a rule of thumb is a minimum size of 2.5 cm in diameter. This will also depend on the penetration depth of the biopsy needle, which must be verified prior to performing the biopsy.

Intussusception

Ultrasonography can be very helpful for diagnosis of large intestinal intussusception and caecal inversion, and is usually preferred to contrast studies by experienced ultrasonographers. Lesions appear similar to small intestinal intussusceptions and have a multi-layered wall appearance in the region of the ascending or transverse colon on both longitudinal and transverse views. They occur most commonly at the ileocolic junction and can be ileocolic, caecocolic (caecal inversion), ileocaecal and colocolic. Small intestinal dilatation can occur secondarily with obstruction.

Perforation

Colonic perforation can occur secondary to neoplasia or surgical dehiscence. Other causes are non-steroidal anti-inflammatory medications, steroids, pelvic fractures and foreign bodies. Ulceration of the colonic mucosa is difficult to detect with either contrast radiography or ultrasonography. However, secondary signs of perforation include a perilesional zone of hyperechoic mesentery, free fluid and possibly free air. These findings in a patient with an acute abdomen should raise suspicion of perforation. If the rectal area is affected, these abnormalities may be present in the retroperitoneal space. Perforations affecting the ascending, transverse and descending colon result in peritoneal free fluid or gas.

References and further reading

Biller DS, Partington BP, Miyabayashi T and Leveille R (1994) Ultrasonographic appearance of chronic hypertrophic pyloric gastropathy in the dog. *Veterinary Radiology and Ultrasound* **35**, 30–33

Boysen SR, Tidwell AS and Penninck DG (2003) Sonographic findings in dogs and cats with intestinal perforation: a retrospective study (1995–2001). *Veterinary Radiology and Ultrasound* **44**, 556–564

Choi M, Seo M, Jung J, Lee K, Yoon J, Chang D and Park RD (2002) Evaluation of canine gastric motility with ultrasonography. *Journal of Veterinary Medical Science* **64**, 17–21

Cohen HL, Zinn HL, Haller JO et al. (1998) Ultrasonography of pylorospasm: findings may simulate hypertrophic pyloric stenosis. *Journal of Ultrasound in Medicine* **17**, 705–711

Delaney F, O'Brien RT and Waller K (2003) Ultrasound evaluation of small bowel thickness compared to weight in normal dogs. *Veterinary Radiology and Ultrasound* **44**, 577–580

Gaschen L, Kircher P, Stüssi A, Allenspach K, Gaschen F et al. (2008) Comparison of ultrasonographic findings to clinical activity index (CIBDAI) and diagnosis in dogs with chronic enteropathies. *Veterinary Radiology and Ultrasound* **49**, 56–64

Graham JP, Newell SM, Roberts GD and Lester NV (2000) Ultrasonographic features of canine gastrointestinal pithiosis. *Veterinary Radiology and Ultrasound* **41**, 273–277

Grooters AM, Miyabayashi T, Biller DS et al. (1994) Sonographic appearance of uremic gastropathy in four dogs. *Veterinary Radiology and Ultrasound* **35**, 35–40

Kondo S, Katoh H, Hirano S et al. (2004) Ischemic gastropathy after distal pancreatectomy with celiac axis resection. *Surgery Today* **34**, 337–340

Louvet A and Denis B (2004) Ultrasonographic diagnosis – small bowel lymphangiectasia in a dog. *Veterinary Radiology and Ultrasound* **45**, 565–567

Matthews AR, Penninck DG and Webster CR (2008) Postoperative ultrasonographic appearance of uncomplicated enterotomy or enterectomy sites in dogs. *Veterinary Radiology and Ultrasound* **49**, 477–483

Moon ML, Biller DS and Armbrust LJ (2003) Ultrasonographic appearance and etiology of corrugated small intestine. *Veterinary Radiology and Ultrasound* **44**, 199–203

Newell SM, Graham JP, Roberts GD, Ginn PE and Harrison JM (1999) Sonography of the normal feline gastrointestinal tract. *Veterinary Radiology and Ultrasound* **40**, 40–43

Ozaki K, Yamagami T, Nomura K and Narama I (2002) Mast cell tumours of the gastrointestinal tract in 39 dogs. *Veterinary Pathology* **39**, 557–564

Paoloni MC, Penninck DG and Moore AS (2002) Ultrasonographic and clinicopathologic findings in 21 dogs with intestinal adenocarcinoma. *Veterinary Radiology and Ultrasound* **43**, 562–567

Patsikas MN, Jakovljevic S, Moustardas N, Papazoglou LG, Kazakos GM and Dessiris AK (2003) Ultrasonographic signs of intestinal intussusception associated with acute enteritis or gastroenteritis in 19 young dogs. *Journal of the American Animal Hospital Association* **39**, 57–66

Patsikas MN, Papazoglou LG, Jakovljevic S and Dessiris AK (2005) Color Doppler ultrasonography in prediction of the reducibility of intussuscepted bowel in 15 young dogs. *Veterinary Radiology and Ultrasound* **46**, 313–316

Pearson H, Gaskell CJ, Gibbs C et al. (1974). Pyloric and oesophageal dysfunction in the cat. *Journal of Small Animal Practice* **15**, 487–501

Penninck DG (1998) Characterization of gastrointestinal tumors. *Veterinary Clinics of North America: Small Animal Practice* **28**, 777–797

Penninck DG, Matz M and Tidwell AS (1997) Ultrasonographic detection of gastric ulceration. *Veterinary Radiology and Ultrasound* **38**, 308–312

Penninck DG, Nyland TG, Kerry LY et al. (1990) Ultrasonographic evaluation of the gastrointestinal diseases in small animals. *Veterinary Radiology and Ultrasound* **31**, 134–141

Rivers BJ, Walter PA, Johnston GR, Feeney DA and Hardy RM (1997) Canine gastric neoplasia: utility of ultrasonography in diagnosis. *Journal of the American Animal Hospital Association* **33**, 144–155

Stander N, Wagner WM, Goddard A and Kirberger RM (2010) Ultrasonographic appearance of canine parvoviral enteritis in puppies. *Veterinary Radiology and Ultrasound* **51**, 69–74

Swift I (2009) Ultrasonographic features of intestinal entrapment in dogs. *Veterinary Radiology and Ultrasound* **50**, 205–207

Tidwell AS and Penninck DG (1992) Ultrasonography of gastrointestinal foreign bodies. *Veterinary Radiology and Ultrasound* **33**, 160–169

Valdes-Martinez A and Waguespack RW (2006). What is your diagnosis? Cecocolic intussusception. *Journal of the American Veterinary Medical Association* **228**, 847–848

Watson PJ (1997) Gastroduodenal intussusception in a young dog. *Journal of Small Animal Practice* **38**, 163–167

Yam PS, Johnson VS, Martineau HM, Dickie A and Sullivan M (2002) Multicentric lymphoma with intestinal involvement in a dog. *Veterinary Radiology and Ultrasound* **43**, 138–143

Zwingenberger AL, Marks SL, Baker TW and Moore PF (2010) Ultrasonographic evaluation of the muscularis propria in cats with diffuse small intestinal lymphoma or inflammatory bowel disease. *Journal of Veterinary Internal Medicine* **24**, 289–292

Video extras

- Colonic carcinoma
- Functional ileus
- Gastric lymphoma
- Gastric oedema
- Hypereosinophilic syndrome

- Inflammatory polyp
- Jejunal foreign body
- Jejunal lymphoma
- Normal duodenal contractions
- Normal duodenal papilla
- Normal feline pylorus
- Pseudolayering

Access via QR code or bsavalibrary.com/ultrasound_11

12

Pancreas

Silke Hecht and Matt Baron

Indications

As clinical signs of pancreatic disease are variable and often non-specific, evaluation of the pancreas should form part of every complete abdominal ultrasonographic examination. Specific indications include:

- Anorexia
- Weight loss
- Vomiting
- Diarrhoea
- Abdominal pain
- Palpable abdominal mass
- Therapy-resistant diabetes mellitus
- Hypoglycaemia
- Icterus.

Pancreatic disease may result in complications affecting other organs (e.g. extrahepatic biliary obstruction) or may be associated with concurrent disorders such as inflammatory bowel disease (IBD) or cholangiohepatitis. Therefore, ultrasonographic evaluation of the entire peritoneal cavity is warranted if pancreatic disease is of concern.

Value of ultrasonography compared with radiography and computed tomography

Radiography

Radiography is often the first diagnostic imaging modality employed in working up abdominal disorders in small animals. Unfortunately, radiographs are of little value in the diagnosis of pancreatic disease. The normal pancreas is not observed in dogs on abdominal radiographs, and is only occasionally visible in cats, if they are obese. Furthermore, the utility of abdominal radiographs in diagnosing pancreatic diseases is limited; in dogs, their sensitivity for the diagnosis of severe pancreatitis is as low as 24% (Hess *et al.*, 1998). The accuracy of abdominal radiography for the diagnosis of feline pancreatitis has not been quantified to the authors' knowledge, but is considered low. Whilst the sensitivity of abdominal radiography for the detection of pancreatic tumours in dogs has also been shown to be low (19%) (Lamb *et al.*, 1995), radiographic abnormalities were observed in 100% of cats with pancreatic malignancies and pancreatic nodular hyperplasia according to one study (Hecht *et al.*, 2007). However, in no case were the radiographic

abnormalities observed necessarily specific to the pancreas, and pancreatic nodular hyperplasia could not be distinguished from pancreatic malignancy based on radiographic findings.

Ultrasonography

Abdominal ultrasonography allows visualization of the normal pancreas in the majority of dogs and cats, and has proven useful in the diagnosis of various pancreatic disorders. In dogs, abdominal ultrasonography was found to have a sensitivity of 68% for the detection of severe pancreatitis (Hess *et al.*, 1998), and a sensitivity of 75% was reported for the diagnosis of pancreatic neoplasia (Lamb *et al.*, 1995). Ultrasonography is of limited value in the detection of endocrine pancreatic tumours, likely due to their small size (Robben *et al.*, 2005). It may be inferred from one retrospective study that abdominal ultrasonography is not as helpful in the diagnosis of pancreatitis in cats as it is in dogs: most reports indicate a sensitivity of 11–35% (Gerhardt *et al.*, 2001; Saunders *et al.*, 2002), although one study reports a sensitivity of 80% (Forman *et al.*, 2004). Abdominal ultrasonography fares well at identifying and characterizing lesions in cats with pancreatic neoplasia and nodular hyperplasia: in a retrospective study, ultrasonography revealed pancreatic abnormalities in 16 of 17 cats with pancreatic malignancy and 5 of 5 cats with nodular hyperplasia (Hecht *et al.*, 2007). There was considerable overlap in ultrasonographic findings between the two diseases, although a solitary mass of >2 cm appeared to be specific for malignancy.

Computed tomography

Contrast-enhanced computed tomography (CT) is considered the modality of choice for the diagnosis of acute pancreatitis and other pancreatic disorders in human medicine. Disadvantages of CT in veterinary medicine in comparison with radiography and ultrasonography include cost and the need for general anaesthesia. Initial case studies describing the use of CT in the diagnosis of canine pancreatitis yielded promising results (Jaeger *et al.*, 2003). Studies investigating the use of contrast-enhanced CT in the diagnosis of feline pancreatitis indicated that this modality was largely unhelpful, with a sensitivity as low as 20% (Gerhardt *et al.*, 2001; Forman *et al.*, 2004). Recent reports investigating the use of CT for diagnosing pancreatic neoplasms such as insulinoma in dogs (Robben *et al.*, 2005) yielded promising results.

Imaging technique

Patient preparation
Patient preparation (sedation if necessary, clipping and application of ultrasonographic coupling gel) is performed in a routine manner.

Positioning
In most patients the pancreas can be examined using a routine ventral abdominal approach with the patient positioned in dorsal recumbency. However, especially in deep-chested dogs and animals with severe abdominal pain, a right intercostal approach with the patient in left lateral recumbency may be chosen to facilitate evaluation of the body and right lobe of the pancreas.

Equipment
Choice of transducer is dictated by availability and personal preference, and both linear and curvilinear transducers may be used. Due to the small size of the pancreas, the examination should be performed using the highest frequency possible. In small dogs and cats, an 8–15 MHz transducer is typically used. In large dogs, a lower frequency transducer (5–8 MHz) may be needed to increase penetration depth.

Normal ultrasonographic appearance

As the pancreas is a fairly inconspicuous organ, it is important to be familiar with anatomical landmarks to aid in identification (Figure 12.1). The pancreas in both the dog and cat is a slightly ill defined organ,

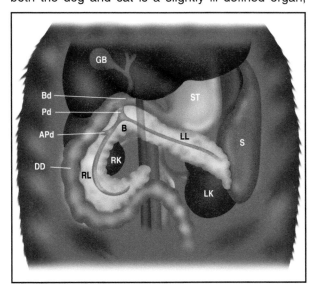

12.1 Pancreas and associated anatomical landmarks. The left lobe of the pancreas (LL) can be found caudal to the stomach (ST) and is intimately associated with the splenic vein. The body of the pancreas (B) is located ventral to the portal vein. The right lobe of the pancreas (RL) follows the descending duodenum (DD). APd = accessory pancreatic duct; Bd = common bile duct; GB = gallbladder; LK = left kidney; Pd = pancreatic duct; RK = right kidney; S = spleen. (Reproduced from the *BSAVA Manual of Canine and Feline Abdominal Imaging*)

normally isoechoic to the surrounding mesentery, isoechoic to slightly hyperechoic to the adjacent liver, and hypoechoic to the spleen.

It is important to remember that the pancreas can appear ultrasonographically normal even when diseased, especially in cats. This is particularly true in many cases of pancreatitis and certain neoplastic disorders (e.g. insulinoma). Therefore, a normal ultrasonographic examination should not solely be relied upon to rule out pancreatic pathology.

Dogs
Pancreatic size in the dog is variable and has been reported to range from 1–3 cm in width and up to 1 cm in thickness. The right lobe of the pancreas is often the more readily observable lobe. It can be found by identifying the descending duodenum in transverse section, and then looking for a triangular portion of tissue lying medially, dorsally or sometimes laterally to it. The cranial pancreaticoduodenal vein is often readily observable within this triangularly shaped tissue, and may aid in identification of the pancreas (Figure 12.2; see also **Normal pancreas (dog)** clip on DVD). The vein runs parallel to the long axis of the right lobe of the pancreas and the descending duodenum. The body and left lobe of the pancreas are more difficult to identify and are located ventral to the portal vein and between the stomach and transverse colon, respectively.

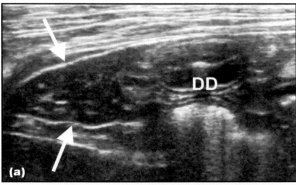
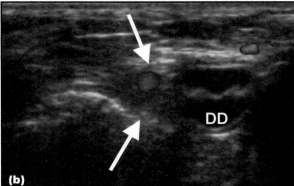

12.2 Ultrasonograms of the normal canine pancreas. **(a)** Transverse view. The right pancreatic lobe (between arrows) manifests as a triangular structure of intermediate echogenicity, immediately adjacent to the descending duodenum (DD). **(b)** The centrally located round anechoic structure represents the pancreaticoduodenal vein, which exhibits a flow signal on colour Doppler examination.

Cats

In cats, the pancreas measures approximately 0.5–1.0 cm in thickness. The left lobe and the pancreatic body are the most readily identifiable parts. With the transducer oriented parallel to the long axis of the patient, just to the left of the midline, the left lobe of the pancreas should be observed between the stomach cranially and the transverse colon caudally. Turning the transducer transversely, the pancreatic body is located ventral to the portal vein, at approximately the level where the splenic vein enters the portal vein (Figure 12.3; see also **Normal pancreas (cat)** clip on DVD). The remainder of the splenic vein may be traced just caudal to the left lobe of the pancreas, running parallel to the lobe. The pancreatic duct is usually visible in cats as a tubular, anechoic, approximately 1–2 mm structure in the centre of the pancreas, and is often crucial in the identification of the organ. The right pancreatic lobe is often difficult to observe in the cat. When seen, it is usually located dorsomedially to the descending duodenum.

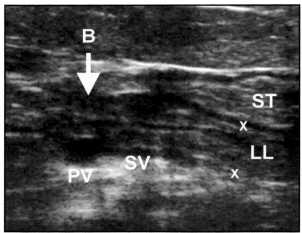

12.3 Ultrasonogram of the normal pancreas in a cat. The transducer is positioned in transverse orientation to the patient, allowing visualization of the long axis of the pancreatic body (B) and left lobe (LL; between the cursors). Note the associated anatomical landmarks: portal vein (PV); splenic vein (SV); and stomach (ST). The pancreas is of intermediate echogenicity and is readily identified by the centrally located tubular anechoic pancreatic duct.

Diffuse disease

Inflammation

Acute pancreatitis

Acute pancreatitis is a common pancreatic pathology in the dog, and less so in the cat. Classic ultrasonographic features of acute pancreatitis in both species include an enlarged pancreas, hypoechoic pancreatic parenchyma, surrounding hyperechoic mesentery, focal peritoneal fluid accumulation, corrugated duodenum, and focal mild intestinal dilatation with decreased intestinal motility (indicative of focal ileus) (Figure 12.4; see also **Acute pancreatitis in a dog** clip on DVD).

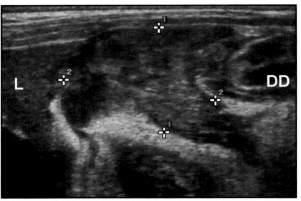

12.4 Acute pancreatitis in a 5-year-old Miniature Schnauzer presented with a 3-day history of vomiting and abdominal pain. Transverse image of the right cranial abdomen showing enlargement and hypoechogenicity of the right lobe of the pancreas (between the cursors) and adjacent strongly hyperechoic fat. Abdominal effusion was also noted in this patient (not shown). DD = duodenum; L = liver.

Observation of all of these 'classic' findings is not necessary to make a diagnosis of pancreatitis, and in many cases not all are present. Common bile duct dilatation may be seen if pancreatic inflammation causes (partial) obstruction due to external compression of the distal duct. Dilatation of the pancreatic duct in association with pancreatitis has been reported. Pancreatic cysts, pseudocysts, necrosis and abscesses can be seen in association with acute pancreatitis in dogs and cats. Although ultrasonography is highly specific for acute pancreatitis in the dog, it has only moderate sensitivity. Therefore, an ultrasonographically normal pancreas does not rule out pancreatitis. In cats, the sensitivity of ultrasonography in the diagnosis of acute pancreatitis is poor, indicating that in most cases the pancreas appears ultrasonographically normal.

Chronic pancreatitis

Chronic pancreatitis affects both dogs and cats, and is more common than acute pancreatitis in cats. Ultrasonographically, chronic pancreatitis can have a variable appearance, and often the abnormalities observed are more subtle and subjective than in acute pancreatitis. Ultrasonographic findings of chronic pancreatitis include a hypoechoic irregular pancreas, hyperechoic pancreatic parenchyma believed to represent pancreatic fibrosis, and hyperechoic mineralized foci with distal acoustic shadowing within and/or surrounding the pancreatic parenchyma, resulting from dystrophic mineralization of chronically inflamed pancreatic and peripancreatic tissue (Figure 12.5; see also **Chronic pancreatitis in a cat** clip on DVD). Displacement of the stomach and/or duodenum may be seen if adhesions develop secondary to chronic inflammation in the pancreatic region. In cats, chronic pancreatitis has been associated with hepatic lipidosis, IBD and cholangiohepatitis, and therefore concurrent ultrasonographic changes in the liver and small intestine may be encountered.

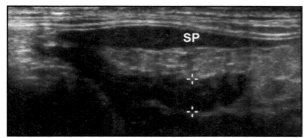

12.5 Chronic pancreatitis in an 8-year-old cat presented with anorexia. The pancreas is hypoechoic, nodular, irregular and more conspicuous than usual. The ultrasonogram of the left cranial abdomen shows the extremity of the left lobe of the pancreas (between the cursors) at the level of the spleen (SP).

Neoplasia

Pancreatic tumours most commonly manifest as focal pancreatic or peripancreatic nodules or masses (see below). Diffuse infiltration of the pancreas can be seen with various tumour types, including adenocarcinoma and lymphoma (Figure 12.6), which may result in diffuse thickening, abnormal echogenicity and/or nodular contour of the pancreas. Diffuse pancreatic neoplasia may mimic other diffuse pancreatic diseases, especially pancreatitis.

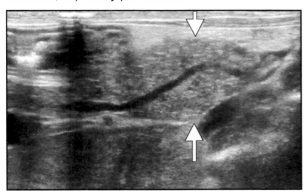

12.6 Pancreatic lymphoma in a 16-year-old cat. The pancreas (left lobe shown between the arrows) is diffusely enlarged (1.5 cm thickness), hyperechoic and heterogeneous. Fine-needle aspiration of the pancreas was performed and yielded a diagnosis of lymphoma.

Oedema

Pancreatic oedema has been associated with hypoalbuminaemia, portal hypertension and experimentally induced pancreatitis. Ultrasonographically, it appears as thickening of the pancreas with multiple hypoechoic striations dissecting between the pancreatic parenchyma, producing a characteristic 'tiger stripe' appearance (Figure 12.7).

Focal lesions

It must be emphasized that it is often difficult to distinguish different types of focal pancreatic lesions via ultrasonography alone. Although colour Doppler examination may be helpful in select cases, tissue sampling such as ultrasound-guided fine-needle aspiration (FNA) is commonly needed to establish a diagnosis.

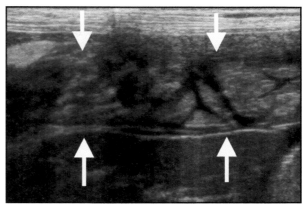

12.7 Pancreatic oedema in a 6-year-old Cocker Spaniel with chronic hepatopathy and portal hypertension. Longitudinal image of the right lobe of the pancreas (arrowed) showing generalized thickening and a classic 'tiger stripe' appearance.

Neoplasia

Pancreatic neoplasms are rare in dogs and cats. Adenocarcinoma is the most common exocrine tumour affecting the pancreas. Other tumour types include adenoma, squamous cell carcinoma, lymphoma, lymphangiosarcoma and spindle cell sarcoma. Insulinoma is the most common endocrine tumour of the pancreas. A pancreatic neoplasm most commonly manifests as a pancreatic or peripancreatic nodule or mass lesion of variable size and echogenicity (Figures 12.8 and 12.9; see also **Insulinoma** clip on DVD).

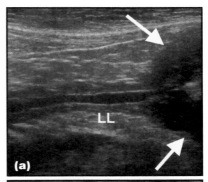

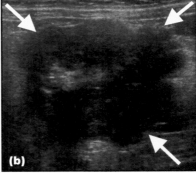

12.8 Exocrine pancreatic tumour (adenocarcinoma) in a 16-year-old Scottish Fold presented for lethargy and anorexia. Transverse ultrasonograms of **(a)** the mid and **(b)** the left cranial abdomen showing a solid, irregularly marginated, mixed echogenic mass (arrowed), approximately 4 cm in diameter, originating from the extremity of the left lobe of the pancreas (LL). (Courtesy of Dr G. Henry, University of Tennessee)

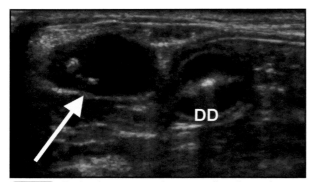

12.9 Endocrine pancreatic tumour (insulinoma) in a 16-year-old West Highland White Terrier presented with a history of trembling, seizures and hypoglycaemia. Transverse image of the right cranial abdomen demonstrating a hypoechoic nodule, approximately 8 mm in diameter, with a few hyperechoic shadowing foci associated with the right lobe of the pancreas (arrowed). DD = descending duodenum.

Other common ultrasonographic features include multifocal pancreatic nodules, pancreatic enlargement, abdominal effusion and extrahepatic biliary obstruction. Potential pitfalls for the imaging diagnosis of pancreatic neoplasms include:

- Variations of the normal ultrasonographic appearance of the pancreas
- Abnormal lymph nodes in close proximity to the pancreas
- Masses arising from neighbouring structures
- A similar ultrasonographic appearance of malignant and benign pancreatic lesions such as abscesses and nodular hyperplasia.

Ultrasonography is fairly sensitive in the diagnosis of exocrine pancreatic tumours; however, identification of endocrine pancreatic tumours is often limited by their small size. Metastases are a common feature of malignant pancreatic neoplasms. Lymphatic drainage of the pancreas is provided by the splenic, hepatic, pancreaticoduodenal and jejunal lymph nodes. As all of these lymph nodes are also involved in drainage of other abdominal structures, the aetiology of lymphadenomegaly may be difficult to determine. Hepatic metastases may manifest as nodules of variable echogenicity. Metastatic spread to the mesentery (carcinomatosis) manifests as numerous hypoechoic nodules emanating from the connecting peritoneum, commonly associated with abdominal effusion.

Nodular hyperplasia

Pancreatic nodular hyperplasia is a common incidental finding in old dogs and cats. Ultrasonographically, nodular hyperplasia in cats manifests as multiple, <1 cm diameter, mostly isoechoic or hypoechoic nodules associated with the pancreas and pancreatic enlargement (Figure 12.10). Ultrasonographic findings in dogs have, to the authors' knowledge, not been reported, but would be expected to have a similar appearance. Hyperplastic nodules may mimic other focal pancreatic lesions (such as pancreatic neoplasms) and cytology or histopathology is required to establish a definitive diagnosis.

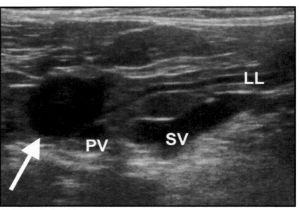

12.10 Incidental finding of pancreatic nodular hyperplasia in a 15-year-old cat with a history of numerous non-pancreatic diseases, including chronic renal failure, hyperthyroidism and hypertrophic cardiomyopathy. The pancreas contained numerous hypoechoic nodules. The largest nodule (arrowed) measured approximately 1 cm in diameter and was associated with the body of the pancreas. LL = left lobe of the pancreas; PV = portal vein; SV = splenic vein.

Cysts and pseudocysts

Congenital pancreatic cysts are of uncertain significance and are occasionally seen as incidental findings in dogs or cats. They have also been documented in association with feline polycystic renal and liver disease. Pancreatic cysts and pseudocysts may occur as sequelae of acute or chronic pancreatitis. Pseudocysts appear to be more common than true cysts, although this differentiation cannot be made based on ultrasonography. Both cysts and pseudocysts appear as variably sized, anechoic, spherical to lobulated structures with thin walls and distal acoustic enhancement (Figure 12.11). Large lesions may displace or indent adjacent viscera.

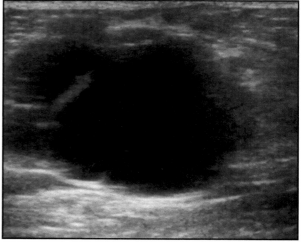

12.11 Pancreatic cyst in an 11-year-old cat with a history of diabetes mellitus and chronic pancreatitis. Ultrasonographic examination revealed a thin-walled structure, approximately 3 cm in diameter, containing anechoic fluid in the right cranial abdomen adjacent to the descending duodenum. Exploratory laparotomy revealed a cystic lesion associated with the right lobe of the pancreas, which was drained and omentalized. An endothelial lining found on histological examination was consistent with a true cyst.

Abscesses

Pancreatic abscesses, like pancreatic cysts and pseudocysts, may be sequelae of pancreatitis but may also develop secondary to systemic sepsis. They are more common in dogs than in cats. Ultrasonographically, they can have a variable appearance. The walls of an abscess are commonly thick, irregular and highly echogenic (Figure 12.12). The central portion may be anechoic, hypoechoic to the surrounding tissue, or even isoechoic to the abscess wall, creating the impression of a solid mass. Swirling debris may be observed in the central portion of the abscess upon mild agitation. Hyperechoic bubbles with associated reverberation artefacts may be seen if the abscess contains gas, potentially from gas-producing bacteria.

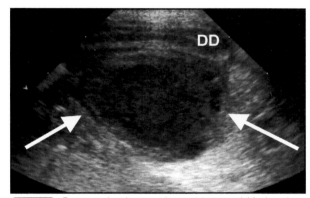

12.12 Pancreatic abscess in an 11-year-old Labrador Retriever presented with a 1-month history of vomiting. Sagittal ultrasonogram of the right cranial abdomen showing a thick-walled mass lesion (arrowed), approximately 3 cm in diameter, containing echogenic fluid adjacent to the descending duodenum (DD). FNA cytology yielded a diagnosis of septic suppurative inflammation.

Other diseases

Pancreatolithiasis

Mineralized calculi within the pancreatic duct have been described in cats and are believed to occur most commonly as sequelae to chronic pancreatitis. Ultrasonographic findings include a hyperechoic structure with distal acoustic shadowing within the pancreatic duct, and pancreatic duct dilatation upstream from the calculus.

Exocrine pancreatic insufficiency

Exocrine pancreatic insufficiency (EPI) is characterized by a lack of adequate amounts of digestive enzymes necessary for sufficient breakdown of nutrients from the intestinal tract. In dogs, this disease is most commonly due to pancreatic acinar atrophy. Ultrasonographic findings in dogs with EPI have, to the authors' knowledge, not been described in the literature. Feline EPI is uncommon, and the underlying cause is often unable to be determined. On ultrasonographic examination the pancreas may appear normal, may be diffusely hyperechoic, or may have a heterogeneous echogenicity and contain nodules.

Pancreatic bladder and pseudobladder

Pancreatic (pseudo)bladder is a rare abnormal focal expansion of the pancreatic ductal system. These lesions can have a similar appearance as pancreatic cysts and pseudocysts. A single case report exists in the veterinary literature describing a cat with a pancreatic pseudobladder that developed secondary to pancreatolithiasis (Bailiff *et al.*, 2004).

Particular considerations for sampling

FNA or biopsy of diffuse or focal pancreatic lesions can be performed safely following the usual precautions. Pancreatic cysts and pseudocysts can be differentiated from cystic lesions arising from other abdominal viscera by fluid sampling and enzyme analysis, as fluid aspirated from lesions of pancreatic origin should have a high lipase activity. In addition to obtaining diagnostic samples, ultrasound guidance can be used to monitor therapeutic drainage of fluid-filled pancreatic lesions.

References and further reading

Akol KG, Washabau RJ, Saunders HM *et al.* (1993) Acute pancreatitis in cats with hepatic lipidosis. *Journal of Veterinary Internal Medicine* **7**, 205–209

Bailiff NL, Norris CR, Seguin B *et al.* (2004) Pancreatolithiasis and pancreatic pseudobladder associated with pancreatitis in a cat. *Journal of the American Animal Hospital Association* **40**, 69–74

Baron ML, Hecht S, Matthews AR *et al.* (2010) Ultrasonographic observation of secretin-induced pancreatic duct dilation in healthy cats. *Veterinary Radiology and Ultrasound* **51**, 86–89

Bennett PF, Hahn KA, Toal RL *et al.* (2001) Ultrasonographic and cytopathological diagnosis of exocrine pancreatic carcinoma in the dog and cat. *Journal of the American Animal Hospital Association* **37**, 466–473

Etue SM, Penninck DG, Labato MA *et al.* (2001) Ultrasonography of the normal feline pancreas and associated anatomic landmarks: a prospective study of 20 cats. *Veterinary Radiology and Ultrasound* **42**, 330–336

Ferreri JA, Hardam E, Kimmel SE *et al.* (2003) Clinical differentiation of acute necrotizing from chronic non-suppurative pancreatitis in cats: 63 cases (1996–2001). *Journal of the American Veterinary Medical Association* **223**, 469–474

Forman MA, Marks SL, De Cock HE *et al.* (2004) Evaluation of serum feline pancreatic lipase immunoreactivity and helical computed tomography *versus* conventional testing for the diagnosis of feline pancreatitis. *Journal of Veterinary Internal Medicine* **18**, 807–815

Gerhardt A, Steiner JM, Williams DA *et al.* (2001) Comparison of the sensitivity of different diagnostic tests for pancreatitis in cats. *Journal of Veterinary Internal Medicine* **15**, 329–333

Hecht S and Henry GA (2007) Sonographic evaluation of the normal and abnormal pancreas. *Clinical Techniques in Small Animal Practice* **22**, 115–121

Hecht S, Penninck DG and Keating JH (2007) Imaging findings in pancreatic neoplasia and nodular hyperplasia in 19 cats. *Veterinary Radiology and Ultrasound* **48**, 45–50

Hecht S, Penninck DG, Mahony OM *et al.* (2006) Relationship of pancreatic duct dilation to age and clinical findings in cats. *Veterinary Radiology and Ultrasound* **47**, 287–294

Hess RS, Saunders HM, Van Winkle TJ *et al.* (1998) Clinical, clinicopathologic, radiographic and ultrasonographic abnormalities in dogs with fatal acute pancreatitis: 70 cases (1986–1995). *Journal of the American Veterinary Medical Association* **213**, 665–670

Jaeger JQ, Mattoon JS, Bateman SW *et al.* (2003) Combined use of ultrasonography and contrast enhanced computed tomography to evaluate acute necrotizing pancreatitis in two dogs. *Veterinary Radiology and Ultrasound* **44**, 72–79

Lamb CR (1999) Pancreatic edema in dogs with hypoalbuminemia or portal hypertension. *Journal of Veterinary Internal Medicine* **13**, 498–500

Lamb CR, Simpson KW, Boswood A *et al.* (1995) Ultrasonography of pancreatic neoplasia in the dog: a retrospective review of 16 cases. *Veterinary Record* **37**, 65–68

Larson MM, Panciera DL, Ward DL et al. (2005) Age-related changes in the ultrasound appearance of the normal feline pancreas. *Veterinary Radiology and Ultrasound* **46**, 238–242

Nyland TG, Mattoon JS, Herrgesell EJ et al. (2002) Pancreas. In: *Small Animal Diagnostic Ultrasound, 2nd edn*, ed. TG Nyland and JS Mattoon, pp. 144–157. WB Saunders, Philadelphia

Nyland TG, Mulvany MH and Strombeck DR (1983) Ultrasonic features of experimentally induced, acute pancreatitis in the dog. *Veterinary Radiology* **24**, 260–266

Penninck DG (2008) Pancreas. In: *Atlas of Small Animal Ultrasonography*, ed. DG Penninck and MA d'Anjou, pp. 319–337. Blackwell Publishing, Ames

Rademacher N, Ohlerth S, Scharf G et al. (2008) Contrast-enhanced power and color Doppler ultrasonography of the pancreas in healthy and diseased cats. *Journal of Veterinary Internal Medicine* **22**, 1310–1316

Robben JH, Pollak YW, Kirpensteijn J et al. (2005) Comparison of ultrasonography, computed tomography, and single-photon emission computed tomography for the detection and localization of canine insulinoma. *Journal of Veterinary Internal Medicine* **19**, 15–22

Saunders HM, VanWinkle TJ, Drobatz K et al. (2002) Ultrasonographic findings in cats with clinical, gross pathologic, and histologic evidence of acute pancreatic necrosis: 20 cases (1994–2001). *Journal of the American Veterinary Medical Association* **221**, 1724–1730

Skrodzki M, Kattinger P and Trautvetter E (1992) Polyzystische Veränderungen in Leber, Niere, Pankreas und Bronchialdrüsen bei einer Perserkatze. *Kleintierpraxis* **37**, 599–605

Smith SA and Biller DS (1998) Resolution of a pancreatic pseudocyst in a dog following percutaneous ultrasonographic-guided drainage. *Journal of the American Animal Hospital Association* **34**, 515–522

Thompson KA, Parnell NK, Hohenhaus AE et al. (2009) Feline exocrine pancreatic insufficiency: 16 cases (1992–2007). *Journal of Feline Medicine and Surgery* **11**, 935–940

VanEnkevort BA, O'Brien RT and Young KM (1999) Pancreatic pseudocysts in 4 dogs and 2 cats: ultrasonographic and clinicopathologic findings. *Journal of Veterinary Internal Medicine* **13**, 309–313

Wall M, Biller DS, Schoning P et al. (2001) Pancreatitis in a cat demonstrating pancreatic duct dilatation ultrasonographically. *Journal of the American Animal Hospital Association* **37**, 49–53

Video extras

- **Acute pancreatitis in a dog**
- **Chronic pancreatitis in a cat**
- **Insulinoma**
- **Normal pancreas (cat)**
- **Normal pancreas (dog)**

Access via QR code or bsavalibrary.com/ultrasound_12

13

Adrenal glands

Livia Benigni

Indications

Common indications for ultrasonography of the adrenal glands include:

- To differentiate between primary and secondary hyperadrenocorticism
- To investigate a retroperitoneal or dorsal abdominal mass
- To investigate hypertension or other clinical signs which may be related to phaeochromocytomas
- To search for metastasis in known cases of extra-adrenal primary malignancy.

Value of ultrasonography compared with radiography and computed tomography

Radiography

Compared with ultrasonography, radiography is a less sensitive imaging modality for the evaluation of the adrenal glands. The normal adrenal glands are not usually visible radiographically, although incidental mineralization in older cats is not uncommon and is easily recognized. Adrenal masses must be of relatively large dimensions in order to be identified on a radiograph. However, in cases where a specific diagnosis of adrenal disease has not yet been made, an abdominal radiograph can be useful to provide an overview of the abdomen. In cases of hyperadrenocorticism, for example, associated hepatomegaly and calcinosis cutis may be seen on the abdominal radiograph.

Ultrasonography

Ultrasonography is preferred when assessing the size, shape and internal structure of the adrenal glands. It is also useful to check for abdominal metastasis and/or vascular invasion in cases of adrenal neoplasia, and to assess the liver in cases of hyperadrenocorticism. Typically, the liver of patients suffering from hyperadrenocorticism appears hyperechoic and diffusely enlarged on ultrasound examination.

Computed tomography

Computed tomography (CT) can also be used to assess the size, shape and internal structure of the adrenal glands, but is less widely available than ultrasonography in veterinary practice. CT requires a heavily sedated or anaesthetized patient, whereas ultrasonography can be performed in conscious or lightly sedated patients. A further advantage of ultrasonography over CT is that if multiple follow-up examinations are needed, these can be repeated without being too costly for the owner (e.g. follow-up of a clinically silent adrenal mass). CT is very valuable for the investigation of adrenal masses which show local invasion. Compared with ultrasonography, CT is considered easier to interpret and more reliable in the determination of the margins and the extent of the lesion. On post-contrast CT images the demarcation between affected and non-affected soft tissue may be further enhanced by the different distribution of the contrast media in the two areas. CT may also help in differentiating benign from malignant masses based on their characteristic attenuation and enhancement. CT angiography is used to evaluate whether there is vascular invasion. CT is considered by many to be the imaging modality of choice when planning surgical removal of some adrenal masses. In cases of adrenal malignancy, another advantage of CT over ultrasonography is the possibility of assessing the thorax for the presence of pulmonary metastasis.

Imaging technique

The adrenal glands are usually evaluated using a 5–7.5 MHz transducer in dogs and a 7.5–10 MHz transducer in cats.

Positioning

The patient can be scanned in either dorsal or lateral recumbency.

Dogs

With the patient in right lateral recumbency, the left adrenal gland can usually be visualized by positioning the transducer on the dorsal aspect of the left lateral abdominal wall, ventral to the lumbar musculature, and just caudal to the last rib, at the level of the left kidney (Figure 13.1a). In some deep-chested breeds (e.g. Pointer, Greyhound) the left adrenal gland is visualized from an intercostal window (12th intercostal space). At the level of the left kidney, the aorta should be identified as the closer of the two large vessels running in a craniocaudal direction (the other being the caudal vena cava). The left renal artery can be used as a second landmark. The renal artery is directed caudally at the exit from the aorta, but after a short path it hooks cranially to reach the renal hilus. The adrenal gland is found between the aorta and the left kidney and cranial to the hook made by the left renal artery (Figure 13.1b). The transducer is aligned to the long axis of the aorta and from this position, by slowly fanning the plane of the ultrasound beam dorsally and ventrally, the ultrasonographer should be able to identify the left adrenal gland. It should be noted that the position of the probe on the skin is maintained whilst undertaking the fanning movement. Owing to the variable position of the left kidney, the aorta and the left renal artery are more reliable landmarks to locate the left adrenal gland than the kidney itself.

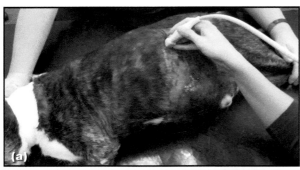

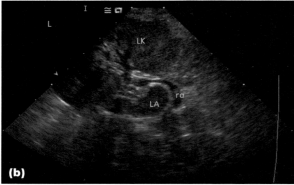

13.1 **(a)** The position of the transducer for imaging the left adrenal gland with the dog in right lateral recumbency. **(b)** Ultrasonogram obtained from the left window with the dog in right lateral recumbency showing the landmarks used to locate an enlarged left adrenal gland (LA). The left adrenal gland is found cranial to the left renal artery (ra) and medial to the left kidney (LK). Note the enlarged caudal pole of the adrenal gland.

With the patient in left lateral recumbency, the right adrenal gland can be visualized either with the probe placed on the abdominal wall just caudal to the 13th rib (transabdominal approach, excellent for small-breed dogs) (Figure 13.2) or with an intercostal approach (often necessary in very deep-chested dogs). The landmarks for locating the right adrenal gland are the caudal vena cava and right kidney. If the transabdominal window is used, the probe is positioned just ventral to the lumbar muscles and caudal to the edge of the last rib. The ultrasound beam is then oriented parallel to the length of the caudal vena cava and pointed cranially to visualize the caudal vena cava at the level of the cranial pole of the right kidney. From this position, the ultrasound probe is

slowly fanned laterally and medially. By doing so the right adrenal gland is generally visualized parallel to the caudal vena cava at the level of the cranial pole of the right kidney. In some dogs, when using this approach, it may be difficult to differentiate between the right adrenal gland and caudal vena cava as they lie very close together. In such cases changing the angulation of the probe slightly may help; otherwise an alternative approach can be attempted.

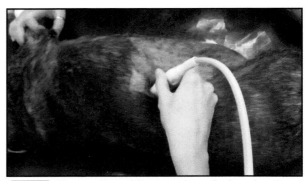

13.2 The position of the transducer for imaging the right adrenal gland with the dog in left lateral recumbency.

From an intercostal approach (11th or 12th intercostal space) the right adrenal gland can be located using a transverse or a dorsal plane to the patient. If the right adrenal gland is imaged in a transverse plane it is located by following the caudal vena cava and is seen lying lateral to the caudal vena cava at the level of the cranial pole of the right kidney. If a dorsal plane is used then the right adrenal gland is seen medially to the cranial pole of the right kidney, between the right kidney and the caudal vena cava. When scanning with the patient in dorsal recumbency, the same anatomical landmarks are used to locate the adrenal glands.

Cats

The feline adrenal glands are imaged using similar techniques to those described above for dogs. The only major difference is that in cats the adrenal glands are positioned more cranially along the main abdominal vessels with respect to the position of the kidneys. They are often visualized immediately cranial to the cranial pole of the respective kidney.

Normal ultrasonographic appearance

The adrenal glands are relatively small elongated structures located in the retroperitoneal space along the main abdominal vessels at the level of the corresponding kidney. The right adrenal gland is often adjacent to the caudal vena cava, whereas the left adrenal gland is often separated from the aorta by some fat, making it easier to identify. Being fairly uniformly hypoechoic, the adrenal glands can be easily confused with portions of the regional vessels (renal artery and veins). Occasionally, a hypoechoic outer and hyperechoic inner region may be recognized. If the internal structure of the adrenal gland is visible, then it is easier to identify them with certainty; colour flow Doppler techniques may help in this respect by showing the blood flow within the regional vessels. Two small vessels, the phrenicoabdominal artery and vein, pass dorsally and ventrally, respectively, to each adrenal gland. On the left the vein is frequently visualized with good quality ultrasound equipment.

Dogs

In dogs the size and shape of the adrenal glands may vary with bodyweight and breed. The left adrenal gland of small-breed dogs has a typical bilobed appearance (Figure 13.3a), often described as peanut-shaped; in large-breed dogs the shape becomes more elongated (Figure 13.3b; see also **Normal left adrenal gland in a dog** clip on DVD). In a transverse plane both the left and right adrenal glands appear oval or round to triangular. When visualized in a long-itudinal plane from a transabdominal window, the right adrenal gland often appears 'L'-shaped (also described as pistol- or arrow-shaped) (Figure 13.4a). When visualized in a longitudinal plane from an intercostal approach it appears more elongated (Figure 13.4b; see also **Normal right adrenal gland in a dog** clip on DVD).

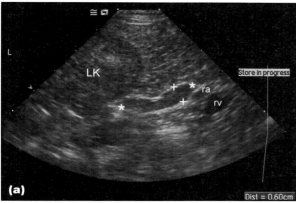

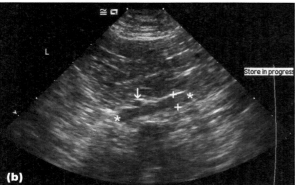

13.3 **(a)** Ultrasonogram of the normal left adrenal gland in a Cocker Spaniel. The thickness of the caudal pole is measured between the callipers and the length of the gland is indicated between the asterisks. **(b)** Ultrasonogram of the left adrenal gland in an Irish Setter. The thickness of the caudal pole is measured between the callipers and the length of the gland is indicated between the asterisks. Note the elongated appearance of the gland and the adjacent phrenicoabdominal vein seen in cross-section (arrowed). LK = left kidney; ra = renal artery; rv = renal vein.

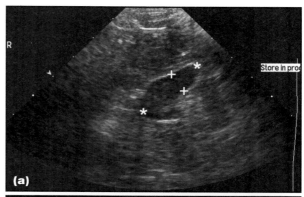

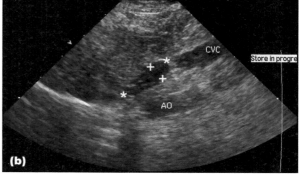

13.4 **(a)** Right adrenal gland viewed from a transabdominal window. Note the 'L' (or pistol) shape of the gland. The thickness of the caudal pole is 7.5 mm and is measured between the callipers. The length of the adrenal gland is denoted by the asterisks. **(b)** Right adrenal gland viewed from an intercostal approach. Note that the gland looks more elongated when imaged using this window. The thickness of the caudal pole is measured between the callipers and the length of the adrenal gland is denoted by the asterisks. AO = aorta; CVC = caudal vena cava.

A wide range of normal adrenal gland size has been reported in dogs. Subjective assessment of the size and shape of the adrenal glands is used by the experienced ultrasonographer to raise suspicion for enlargement. As a general rule it has been suggested that 7.4 mm be used as the upper normal limit of adrenal gland diameter. When measuring the adrenal glands, it must be borne in mind that some healthy dogs have normal adrenal glands measuring >7.4 mm in diameter and many dogs with hyperadrenocorticism have normal-sized adrenal glands. Therefore, the ultrasonographic findings need to be interpreted in light of the clinical signs and the blood analysis results. A finding of normal adrenal glands on ultrasonography is not sufficient to rule out hyperadrenocorticism.

Cats

In cats the adrenal glands are more oval than in the dog and are generally uniformly hypoechoic (see **Normal right adrenal gland in a cat** clip on DVD). It is rarer to see a corticomedullary distinction (Figure 13.5) within the adrenal glands in cats than in dogs. The short diameter of the adrenal glands in healthy cats and in cats that have non-adrenal dependent illness has been reported to range between 2.8 and 5.5 mm. Mineralization of the adrenal glands is a common incidental finding in cats (Figure 13.6); in

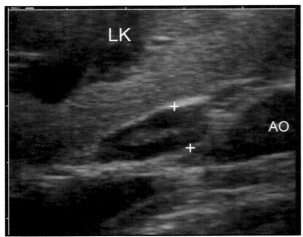

13.5 Ultrasonogram of the normal left adrenal gland in a cat. The thickness of the caudal pole is 3.9 mm and is measured between the callipers. Adrenal glands in cats are generally uniformly hypoechoic, but in this case a corticomedullary distinction is seen. AO = aorta; LK = left kidney.

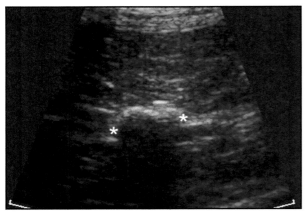

13.6 Ultrasonogram of the mineralized left adrenal gland in a cat (between the asterisks). Note the hyperechoic, hyper-reflective appearance of the adrenal gland, causing an acoustic shadow. (Courtesy of P. Mantis)

these cases the adrenal glands appear hyperechoic and, if the mineralization is substantial, a distal acoustic shadow is present. The size of the adrenal glands remains unchanged.

Hyperplasia

Approximately 80% of dogs with hyperadrenocorticism have pituitary-dependent hyperadrenocorticism (PDH). Ultrasonography may reveal bilateral adrenomegaly (Figure 13.7) in a large proportion of dogs and cats with PDH. The adrenal glands appear symmetrically enlarged and rounded, reflecting generalized cortical hyperplasia secondary to pituitary disease. However, bilateral adrenal gland enlargement may occasionally be found in patients with chronic, non-endocrine disease. The findings of normal or asymmetrically enlarged adrenal glands does not exclude the possibility of PDH. Nodular hyperplasia is responsible for asymmetrical enlargement of the adrenal

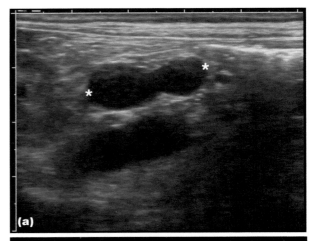

(a)

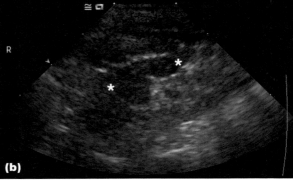

(b)

13.7 Ultrasonograms of the bilaterally enlarged **(a)** left and **(b)** right adrenal glands in a dog suffering from PDH. Note that the shape of the glands is bilaterally preserved; however, both glands appear 'plumped'. Asterisks indicate the long axis of the gland.

glands and is found in a small proportion of PDH cases. A large hyperplastic nodule looks similar to an adrenocortical adenoma; therefore, ultrasonography is not always helpful in differentiating between PDH and adrenal-dependent hyperadrenocorticism.

Bilateral enlargement of the adrenal glands can be found in dogs with PDH treated with trilostane (3β-hydroxysteroid dehydrogenase inhibitor). It has been suggested that the changes observed on ultrasonography reflect hypertrophy of the adrenal cortex due to increased adrenocorticotropic hormone (ACTH) stimulation.

Reduced cortisol production and diminished negative feedback on ACTH production explain the effect of trilostane on the adrenal glands. After trilostane treatment a change in the echogenicity of the adrenal gland may be noticed. In some cases the difference in echogenicity between the central and outer layers may become more marked, and in other cases the adrenal gland may become more heterogeneous in echogenicity. It is hypothesized that haemorrhage and/or hyperplasia may be responsible for the change in the echogenicity of the adrenal glands observed following trilostane treatment (Figure 13.8).

It is important therefore to perform ultrasonography before commencing treatment with trilostane, in order to differentiate between changes in the adrenal gland due to disease, and those which may be as a consequence of therapy.

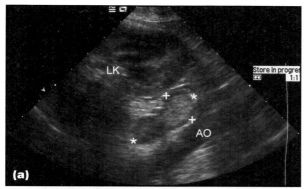

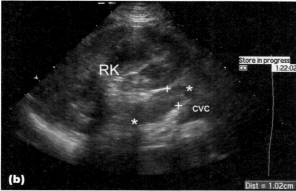

13.8 Ultrasonograms of the bilaterally enlarged **(a)** left and **(b)** right adrenal glands in a dog treated with trilostane. The asterisks denote the long axis of the gland and the callipers indicate the caudal pole. Note the hyperechoic appearance of the caudal pole of the left adrenal gland in (a) which, in the case of trilostane treatment, may be related to intraparenchymal haemorrhage and/or hyperplasia. AO = aorta; CVC = caudal vena cava; LK = left kidney; RK = right kidney.

Neoplasia

The finding of an adrenal nodule or mass on ultrasonographic examination does not necessarily indicate neoplasia. Furthermore, most of the adrenal neoplasms encountered are not malignant. There is a surprisingly high incidence of clinically silent adrenal lesions in older dogs; often they represent adrenal nodular hyperplasia (Figure 13. 9), with only a small proportion found to be neoplastic. Further investigations that may be indicated include function tests (e.g. ACTH stimulation test) and repeat imaging in 1–3 months. Further ultrasonographic monitoring of the nodule or mass can be performed at 3–6 monthly intervals. In many cases the final diagnosis is only reached at necropsy.

In dogs showing signs of hyperadrenocorticism, the finding of an adrenal nodule leads to the differential diagnoses of cortical adenoma, cortical adenocarcinoma and hyperplastic nodule. The ultrasonographic appearance of these lesions is non-specific. Nodules or masses >2 cm and/or showing mineralization are considered less likely to represent nodular hyperplasia and more likely to be either benign or malignant neoplasia. Therefore, in such cases the findings are suggestive of adrenal-dependant hyperadrenocorticism. If the mass is ≥4 cm then a malignant rather than a benign neoplastic lesion should be suspected (Figure 13.10).

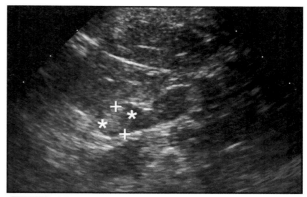

13.9 Ultrasonogram of a hyperechoic nodule (between the asterisks) found incidentally within the cranial pole of the left adrenal gland (between the callipers). The differential diagnoses include myelolipoma, hyperplastic nodule and neoplastic nodule (primary or metastatic). In cases of incidentally found nodules, follow-up ultrasonography of the adrenal gland is suggested.

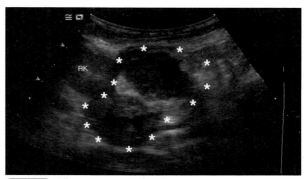

13.10 Ultrasonogram of a large heterogeneous mass found in the region of the right adrenal gland (periphery of the mass is highlighted by the asterisks). The final diagnosis was adrenal adenocarcinoma. RK = right kidney.

When an adrenal nodule or mass is found, there are a number of further possible differential diagnoses, including:

- Myelolipoma
- Phaeochromocytoma
- Metastatic tumour (see **Metastatic nodule** clip on DVD)
- Haematoma
- Granuloma
- Cyst.

Myelolipomas are benign, endocrinologically inactive tumours, occasionally found in the adrenal glands of dogs. They appear as hyperechoic adrenal nodules on ultrasonography. Their fatty component can be recognized on CT images and because of this, CT may be useful in differentiating myelolipomas from other lesions.

Phaeochromocytomas are relatively rare catecholamine-secreting tumours arising from the chromaffin cells of the adrenal medulla. The presenting signs are often non-specific (e.g. weakness/lethargy, tachyarrhythmia, polyuria/polydipsia, pale or injected mucous membranes, collapse, vomiting, tachypnoea, panting/dyspnoea, anorexia/inappetence and fever) and result either from the direct presence and space-occupying nature of the tumour, or are secondary to the excretion of excessive amounts of catecholamines. Feline phaeochromocytomas are extremely rare.

Metastases to the adrenal glands are common. In dogs the tumours found to most commonly metastasize to the adrenal glands are pulmonary, mammary, prostatic, gastric and pancreatic carcinomas, squamous cell and transitional cell carcinomas, melanomas, histiocytic sarcomas and haemangiosarcomas. In cats those tumours which commonly metastasize to the adrenal glands are renal and colonic carcinoma, haemangiosarcoma and melanoma.

Ultrasonography is useful in the investigation of hyperaldosteronism. Primary hyperaldosteronism results from either an adrenal tumour or adrenal hyperplasia affecting the mineralocorticoid-producing zona glomerulosa of the adrenal cortex. Persistent hypokalaemia is associated with the disease. Aldosterone-secreting tumours are rare in both dogs and cats. Aldosterone-producing tumours in cats have been reported to be frequently hypoechoic, rounded and variable in size (0.9–3 cm).

Occasionally bilateral adrenal nodules or masses can be found (Figure 13.11). As previously mentioned, it is not possible to differentiate with ultrasonography an endocrinologically active from an inactive mass/nodule. Therefore, in cases where bilateral adrenal masses/nodules are found with signs of hyperadrenocorticism, ultrasonography may not be particularly helpful in suggesting which of the lesions is responsible for the disease. It is important to combine ultrasonographic with clinical and laboratory findings, and to consider follow-up imaging studies before undertaking an unnecessary complicated surgical procedure.

In some cases an adrenal mass may invade adjacent organs (e.g. kidney; see **Left adrenal gland tumour** clip on DVD) and disrupt the normal regional anatomy. Finding signs of local invasion is a strong indicator of malignancy (adenocarcinoma or phaeochromocytoma; Figure 13.12). Large adrenal masses may bleed, leading to an ultrasonographic finding of retroperitoneal fluid.

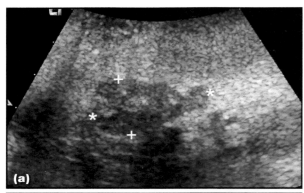

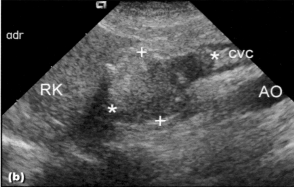

13.11 Ultrasonograms of adrenal masses/nodules in (a) the left and (b) the right adrenal glands in a dog. The asterisks denote the long axis of the gland and the callipers indicate the cranial pole. **(a)** The cranial pole of the left adrenal gland is deformed by a fairly isoechoic nodule. **(b)** The cranial pole of the right adrenal gland is deformed by a hyperechoic nodule. The dog was asymptomatic and it was not possible to confirm a diagnosis. A repeat ultrasound examination was performed 1–3 months later to monitor the size of the lesions. AO = aorta; CVC = caudal vena cava; RK = right kidney.

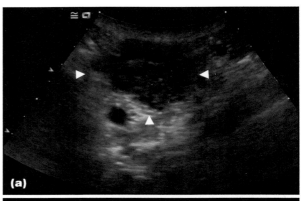

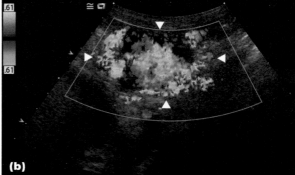

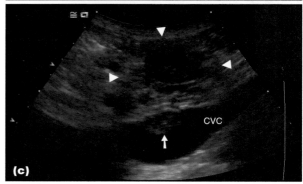

13.12 **(a)** Ultrasonogram of an irregularly marginated mass (arrowheads) in the region of the right adrenal gland. **(b)** Doppler ultrasonography confirmed that the mass (arrowheads) was highly vascularized. **(c)** Ultrasonogram showing the mass (arrowheads) invading the caudal vena cava (CVC) (arrowed). The final diagnosis was phaeochromocytoma.

Vascular invasion

A common complication observed ultrasonographically with adrenal gland malignancies is neoplastic invasion of the caudal vena cava (Figure 13.13; see also **Phaeochromocytoma** clip on DVD). This is more frequently observed with neoplasia of the right adrenal gland, but aggressive tumours of both the left and right adrenal glands can reach the caudal vena cava by invading the local vasculature (renal veins, adrenal gland veins and phrenicoabdominal vessels) and extending into the caudal vena cava. The presence of static echogenic material within the caudal vena cava adjacent to an adrenal mass is suggestive of a tumour thrombus. Colour or power Doppler may help confirm the presence of a mass. However, it is difficult to determine ultrasonographically how much of the mass observed is neoplastic tissue and how much is thrombus. A negative finding of local vascular invasion on ultrasonography is not sufficient to exclude this possibility. In cases of large masses adjacent to the caudal vena cava and main vasculature, vascular invasion should be suspected, and further investigation by CT angiography should be considered.

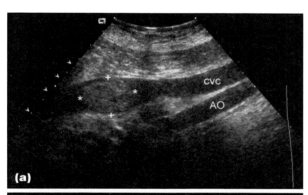

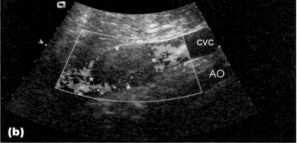

13.13 **(a)** Ultrasonogram of a hyperechoic thrombus (between the asterisks) causing widening of the lumen of the caudal vena cava (at the level of the callipers). **(b)** Colour Doppler ultrasonogram showing absence of flow at the level of the thrombus (between the asterisks). AO = aorta; CVC = caudal vena cava.

Atrophy

In patients with suspected hypoadrenocorticism, the finding of small adrenal glands (Figure 13.14) or failure to find the adrenal glands is supportive of the clinical diagnosis. In dogs, the adrenal glands are considered small when the left adrenal gland is <3 mm and the right adrenal gland is <3.4 mm in thickness. Due to the large variation in adrenal gland size in dogs, and the difficulty in finding the adrenal glands

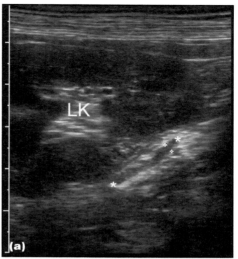

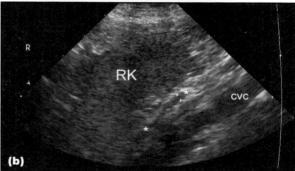

13.14 Ultrasonograms of the bilaterally small **(a)** left and **(b)** right adrenal glands in a case of hypoadrenocorticism. The callipers are used to measure the thickness of the caudal pole: left adrenal gland = 2.1 mm; right adrenal gland = 2.3 mm. The asterisks indicate the long axis of the gland. CVC = caudal vena cava; LK = left kidney; RK = right kidney.

in some patients, the ultrasonographic findings alone cannot be used to make a diagnosis of hypoadrenocorticism. In cats, a subjective assessment is used to judge whether the adrenal glands are small.

Mitotane therapy induces ultrasonographically recognizable bilateral reduction in size of the adrenal glands (compared with the size before treatment). Measurement of the adrenal glands during therapy cannot be used to differentiate adequate and inadquate control of adrenal cortical secretion. Small adrenal glands can be found in patients receiving long-term corticosteroid treatment; an associated hyperechoic and uniformly enlarged liver is generally found in these patients.

Particular considerations for sampling

Sampling of the adrenal gland is not commonly undertaken. Fine-needle aspirates are often unrewarding in the differentiation of hyperplasia and benign and malignant adrenocortical tumours. In the case of phaeochromocytoma, tissue core biopsy and fine-needle aspiration can both be extremely dangerous, as they may cause paroxysmal hypertension and/or uncontrollable haemorrhage.

References and further reading

Ash RA, Harvey AM and Tasker S (2005) Primary hyperaldosteronism in the cat: a series of 13 cases. *Journal of Feline Medicine and Surgery* **7**(3), 173–182

Barthez PY, Marks SL, Woo J *et al.* (1997) Pheochromocytoma in dogs: 61 cases (1984–1995). *Journal of Veterinary Internal Medicine* **11**(5), 272–278

Barthez PY, Nyland TG and Feldman EC (1998) Ultrasonography of the adrenal glands in the dog, cat and ferret. *Veterinary Clinics of North America: Small Animal Practice* **28**(4), 869–885

Besso JG, Penninck DG and Gliatto JM (1997) Retrospective ultrasonographic evaluation of adrenal lesions in 26 dogs. *Veterinary Radiology and Ultrasound* **38**(6), 448–455

Chiaramonte D and Greco DS (2007) Feline adrenal disorders. *Clinical Techniques in Small Animal Practice* **22**(1), 26–31

Douglass JP, Berry CR and James S (1997) Ultrasonographic adrenal gland measurements in dogs without evidence of adrenal disease. *Veterinary Radiology and Ultrasound* **38**(2), 124–130

Feldman EC and Nelson RW (2004) Canine hyperadrenocorticism. In: *Canine and Feline Endocrinology and Reproduction 3rd edn*, ed. EC Feldman and RW Nelson, pp. 283–288. WB Saunders, Missouri

Graham J (2008) Adrenal glands. In: *Atlas of Small Animal Ultrasonography*, ed. D. Penninck and M d'Anjou, pp. 385–396. Blackwell Publishing, Iowa.

Kintzer PP and Peterson ME (1997) Primary and secondary canine hypoadrenocorticism. *Veterinary Clinics of North America: Small Animal Practice* **27**(2), 349–357

Labelle P and De Cock HE (2005) Metastatic tumors to the adrenal glands in domestic animals. *Veterinary Pathology* **42**(1), 52–58

Mantis P, Lamb CR, Witt AL et al. (2003) Changes in ultrasonographic appearance of the adrenal glands in dogs with pituitary-dependent hyperadrenocorticism treated with trilostane. *Veterinary Radiology and Ultrasound* **44**(6), 682–685

Myers NC III (1997) Adrenal incidentalomas: diagnostic workup of the incidentally discovered adrenal mass. *Veterinary Clinics of North America: Small Animal Practice* **27**(2), 381–399

Rosenstein DS (2000) Diagnostic imaging in canine pheochromocytoma. *Veterinary Radiology and Ultrasound* **41**(6), 499–506

Schultz RM, Wisner ER, Johnson EG and MacLeod JS (2009) Contrast-enhanced computed tomography as a preoperative indicator of vascular invasion from adrenal masses in dogs. *Veterinary Radiology and Ultrasound* **50**, 625–629

Tidwell AS, Penninck DG and Besso JG (1997) Imaging of adrenal gland disorders. *Veterinary Clinics of North America: Small Animal Practice* **27**(2), 237–254

Video extras

- Left adrenal gland tumour
- Metastatic nodule
- Normal left adrenal gland in a dog
- Normal right adrenal gland in a cat
- Normal right adrenal gland in a dog
- Phaeochromocytoma

Access via QR code or bsavalibrary.com/ultrasound_13

14

Bladder and urethra

Esther Barrett

Indications

Common indications for ultrasonography of the bladder in the dog and cat include:

- Dysuria/haematuria/stranguria
- Acute, chronic or recurrent urinary tract infections
- Abnormalities identified on urinalysis
- Urinary incontinence
- Evaluation of suspected ectopic ureters
- Assessment of bladder integrity following trauma
- Palpable caudal abdominal mass
- Evaluation of perineal or inguinal rupture/hernia
- As part of an abdominal ultrasound examination
- As a crude assessment of urine output
- To obtain a urine sample by cystocentesis.

Value of ultrasonography compared with radiography and computed tomography

Ultrasonography and radiography are generally considered to be complementary imaging techniques in the evaluation of the bladder and urethra. Computed tomography (CT), although still not widely available, has the advantage of providing cross-sectional images which can then be reformatted into any plane, providing superior visualization of structures which may otherwise be obscured by the pelvic canal. Figures 14.1 and 14.2 compare the technical considerations and diagnostic usefulness of each technique.

Factor	Plain radiography	Contrast radiography	Ultrasonography	Computed tomography
Availability	Widely available	Widely available	Reasonably widely available	Limited
Cost	Low	Low to medium	Low	High
Safety	Ionizing radiation	Ionizing radiation: personnel are required to be in closer proximity for contrast procedures. Possible adverse reaction to positive contrast media. Small risk of air embolism with negative contrast studies	Safe	High-dose ionizing radiation. Possible adverse reaction to positive contrast media. Small risk of air embolism with negative contrast studies
Invasiveness	Sedation/general anaesthesia usually needed for restraint	General anaesthesia needed. Positive/negative contrast media instilled into the bladder/urethra. Urethral catheterization required	Non-invasive. May need sedation for fractious patients	General anaesthesia usually required. Intravenous contrast media routinely used. Positive/negative contrast media may be instilled into the bladder/urethra
Operator dependence	Accurate positioning required	Accurate positioning required. Ability to catheterize bladder ± place Foley catheter in distal urethra also needed	Results obtained depend on the quality of the ultrasound machine and experience of the operator	Straightforward procedure, but experience with CT needed to facilitate accurate positioning, acquisition, reconstruction and interpretation of images
Artefacts	Avoidable with good technique. Beware of nipples, dirt on the hair coat and small skin masses mimicking radiopaque calculi	Avoidable with good technique. Beware of air bubbles lying within the luminal contrast medium puddle mimicking radiolucent calculi	Several important artefacts need to be recognized: side and grating lobe artefacts and slice thickness artefacts can give the false impression of material present within the bladder lumen. Acoustic enhancement is recognized deep to the bladder. Acoustic shadowing is useful in the identification of calculi	Partial volume averaging makes detailed assessment of the curved surface of the bladder lumen difficult

14.1 Technical considerations for the different imaging modalities available to examine the bladder and urethra.

Consideration	Plain radiography	Contrast radiography	Ultrasonography	Computed tomography
General comments	Allows the identification of bladder shape and size and the detection of radiopaque calculi. The ureters are not usually seen	Retrograde contrast studies provide more information about the bladder lumen and the location of the urethra. Ureters will only be seen following an intravenous urogram (IVU)	Good for evaluation of the bladder, but the inability to image through bone limits its usefulness for assessment of the pelvic urethra. Ureteral terminations can usually be identified with experience and patience	Intravenous ± retrograde contrast studies facilitate good visualization of the ureters, bladder and urethra, but detailed assessment of the mucosal surface is inferior to double contrast radiography/ultrasonography due to partial volume averaging
Intraluminal calculi	Larger radiopaque calculi are usually recognized. Small and radiolucent calculi are not seen. Evaluate the whole urethra from the bladder neck to the external orifice when looking for urethral calculi. Calculi within the pelvic urethra may be difficult to identify	Bladder contrast studies (positive/negative/ double contrast) should detect both radiopaque and radiolucent calculi. Beware of 'drowning' calculi in too much contrast material. A positive contrast urethrogram should highlight urethral calculi as filling defects	Sensitive in the identification of calculi, which should collect in the most dependent aspect of the bladder. Most calculi will cast an acoustic shadow, even if radiolucent. Ballotte the bladder/turn the animal and use gravity to disturb the calculi and assess their individual size. It is not possible to accurately assess the pelvic urethra for calculi	Limited reports on detection of bladder calculi, but unlikely to be more sensitive than ultrasonography. Good for evaluation of the urethra due to the lack of superimposition in the images
Bladder wall	Plain radiographs are insensitive in the detection of wall lesions/masses. The wall and any soft tissue lesions silhouette with the urine and are seen as a single soft tissue opacity	A double contrast cystogram provides excellent luminal mucosal detail, and reasonable filling of the bladder should allow an accurate assessment of wall thickness. All bladder contrast studies should allow identification of mural masses	Ultrasonography has the potential for excellent visualization of the different layers making up the bladder wall, but it is important to use a high frequency (ideally ≥10 MHz) transducer with good near-field imaging. If the bladder is empty, the wall may appear artefactually thickened. Mural masses should be readily identified	Partial volume averaging makes assessment of the bladder wall less accurate. CT is sensitive in the identification of mural masses and in determining their exact location and extent
Bladder and/or urethral rupture	Not possible to diagnose from plain radiographs, but a loss of contrast in the caudal abdomen due to the presence of free fluid may be recognized	A positive contrast cystogram is considered the gold standard for the diagnosis of bladder rupture. A positive contrast urethrogram is sensitive in the detection of urethral rupture	Free abdominal fluid should be readily identified, but the defect within the bladder wall is rarely recognized	Although free abdominal fluid can be recognized, the wall defect is unlikely to be identified without the use of intraluminal contrast medium
Ectopic ureters	Ureters will not be recognized unless severely dilated	An IVU allows visualization of the ureters and is reasonably sensitive in the detection of abnormally terminating ureters. However, due to ureteral peristalsis, the termination is not always seen, which can make a definitive diagnosis of ectopia difficult. If available, fluoroscopy may be useful	With experience and patience, the termination of the ureters on to the bladder neck can be recognized in most cases, allowing ectopic ureters to be ruled out. Where a normal termination is not seen, it may be possible to identify termination of a (usually dilated) ureter in an abnormal location (most commonly the urethra)	CT allows superior identification of the ureters, and is very accurate in the identification of abnormal termination
Obtaining samples	No imaging guidance available	No imaging guidance available	Ultrasound-guided cystocentesis is a very commonly used and useful procedure. Where bladder masses are identified, the preferred method is to pass a urinary catheter via the urethra, using ultrasonography to guide the catheter to the mass	Although CT-guided biopsy is theoretically possible, this is not a recommended technique for the evaluation of bladder lesions
Evaluation of possible metastatic disease	Local lymphadenopathy will be recognized only if moderate to severe. Inflated right and left lateral thoracic radiographs allow evaluation of the lungs for pulmonary metastases	As for plain radiography	Very sensitive in the detection of local lymphadenopathy, and can be used to guide fine-needle aspiration to obtain samples for cytological assessment. Ultrasonography cannot be used to visualize the air-filled lung	Very sensitive in the detection of local lymphadenopathy. CT-guided biopsy is possible, but technically more challenging than ultrasound-guided sampling. CT is the gold standard for the identification of pulmonary metastases

14.2 Diagnostic usefulness of the different imaging modalities available to examine the bladder and urethra.

Imaging technique

Patient preparation

To facilitate accurate ultrasonographic evaluation of the bladder, the patient needs to be calm, relaxed and comfortable. Depending on patient temperament, this may require sedation. As with any ultrasound examination, the skin should be properly clipped and cleaned to maximize the transmission of ultrasound waves into the patient. For optimal imaging, the bladder needs to be moderately full; if the bladder is empty, ideally the examination should be postponed, giving the bladder a chance to fill. Alternatively, intravenous furosemide can be given to accelerate bladder filling, or the bladder can be distended with sterile saline, infused via a urinary catheter.

Protocol

The bladder should be examined from several different angles and in at least longitudinal and transverse planes. Ballotting the bladder and repositioning the patient during the examination is useful in disturbing any sediment or calculi.

A medium to high frequency transducer (≥7.5 MHz) should be used for imaging the bladder. A convex or linear transducer is ideal, but sector probes can also be used. As the bladder is fluid-filled, there will be less attenuation of the ultrasound beam in comparison with the adjacent soft tissue structures, and it may be necessary to reduce the overall gain and adjust the time–gain compensation to optimize the image.

To facilitate accurate evaluation of the bladder wall, the focal zone should be aligned with the wall and the transducer positioned so that the beam is perpendicular to the area of interest. With a high frequency (≥10 MHz) linear transducer, the large near-field of view may allow detailed evaluation of the bladder wall closest to the transducer. However, it is often more accurate to image the far wall of the bladder, especially when using a transducer with a lower frequency or more limited near-field of view, making sure that the wall lies within the focal zone. Slow systematic evaluation of the wall should minimize the chance of missing a focal mural lesion.

The bladder neck should be followed caudally as far as possible in both longitudinal and transverse planes; in most animals this facilitates examination of the cranial urethra before it is shadowed by the bony confines of the pelvis. A transducer with a small contact area (such as a microconvex probe) may be useful in angling the ultrasound beam further caudally into the pelvis. Ultrasonographic evaluation of the feline and the canine (bitch) urethra is generally limited to this cranial section. However, in the male dog it is possible to examine a large part of the membranous and penile urethra as it passes through the perineal area and penis. A high frequency (≥10 MHz) linear transducer is ideal: the urethra is fairly superficial at this point and is examined through the overlying perineal and penile skin, which should be appropriately clipped and prepared. Passing a urinary catheter may be helpful in identifying the course of the urethra.

Normal ultrasonographic appearance

The normal canine and feline bladder should be approximately pear-shaped, with a rounded cranial apex tapering to the bladder neck. When full, the bladder should lie within the caudoventral abdomen; the empty bladder tends to move caudally towards, and in the dog sometimes partly into, the pelvic inlet. The feline bladder tends to have a longer bladder neck and usually remains cranial to the pelvis. Although normal urine should be anechoic, swirling sediment is a common and often clinically insignificant finding. In particular, fat droplets, seen as hyperechoic speckles, are a frequent and incidental component of feline urine.

Using a high frequency probe, it should be possible to identify three layers within the bladder wall (Figure 14.3):

- An inner (luminal) hyperechoic layer, which corresponds to the submucosa
- A middle hypoechoic layer, which comprise three layers of smooth muscle
- An outer hyperechoic serosal layer.

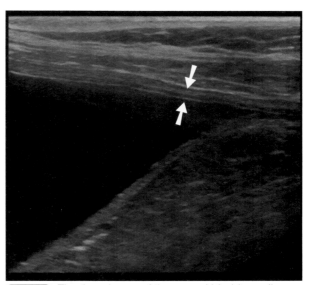

14.3 The three layers of the normal bladder wall (between the arrows) are clearly seen using a high frequency linear probe in this Domestic Shorthaired cat. (Sagittal plane; cranial is to the left of the image.)

A further hypoechoic mucosal layer may occasionally be recognized on the inside of the submucosa. Normal bladder wall thickness in the dog varies with bladder distension and bodyweight, with one study demonstrating the mean wall thickness to decrease from 2.3 mm in minimally distended bladders to 1.4 mm in moderately distended bladders (Geisse *et al.*, 1997). Normal bladder wall thickness in the cat varies from 1.3–1.7 mm (Finn-Bodner, 1995). There should be a smooth internal surface and fairly uniform wall thickness throughout the bladder, with the exception of the ureteral papillae which are recognized as small focal wall thickenings on the dorsolateral aspect of the bladder trigone. With a high frequency probe, intermittent jets of urine may be seen entering the bladder as small 'clouds' of echoes mixing with the anechoic urine. If available, colour Doppler can be used to enhance the signal from these moving jets of urine, displaying them as small bursts of colour (Figure 14.4; see also **Ureteric jet** clip on DVD). There is no obvious delineation between the bladder and the urethra at the bladder neck, although the layers within the urethral wall become less obvious as it passes into the pelvis, and the lumen of the distal urethra is usually not seen unless it is abnormally dilated.

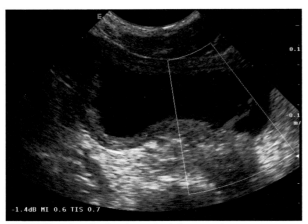

14.4 A jet of urine from the left ureter is seen as a burst of colour on colour Doppler. (Transverse plane; right is to the left of the image.) (Courtesy of the University of Bristol)

Important artefacts

Artefacts frequently recognized during ultrasonographic evaluation of the urinary bladder include:

- Acoustic enhancement – seen beyond the fluid-filled bladder
- Acoustic shadowing – seen deep to the bladder calculi
- Edge shadowing – seen due to the differential refraction of the ultrasound beam at the curved fluid:soft tissue interfaces of the bladder margins.

Side lobes, grating lobes and slice thickness artefacts are further important artefacts resulting in the apparent presence of additional intraluminal echoes. Side lobes and grating lobes result from secondary ultrasound beams, arising from the transducer and travelling into the patient in a different direction to the primary beam. Side lobes are generated by all transducers, whilst grating lobes are unique to linear transducers. As these secondary beams follow a different path into the patient, they are reflected by different structures to those encountered along the path of the primary beam. The ultrasound machine cannot differentiate between echoes returning from the primary and secondary beams, and displays all the information as if it was generated by interfaces along the path of the primary beam. This results in multiple faint images generated by each secondary ultrasound beam being superimposed on the primary image. In most situations, these faint secondary images are lost

in the stronger echoes from the primary beam; however, when imaging the bladder, the lack of echoes from the fluid-filled lumen provides an ideal background against which these additional echoes can be recognized. The typical appearance of secondary lobe artefacts is as faint curvilinear echoes within the bladder lumen. Due to the weak nature of these echoes, they disappear if the power or gain settings are turned down. Reducing the number of focal zones and placing the focal zone deeper within the bladder may also help to eliminate these artefacts (Figure 14.5).

Slice thickness artefacts are a consequence of the third dimension (thickness) of the ultrasound beam, which is not separately represented on two-dimensional (2D) images. This creates a problem at fluid: soft tissue interfaces, where both structures lie within the finite width of the same ultrasound beam. The strength of the returning echoes represents the 'average echogenicity' of the fluid and adjacent soft tissue, resulting in artefactual echoes being displayed at the periphery of the bladder lumen and giving the appearance of 'pseudosludge'. These artefactual echoes can be differentiated from true sediment because they have a curved rather than a flat interface with the urine, they are only seen at the periphery of the lumen perpendicular to the direction of the ultrasound

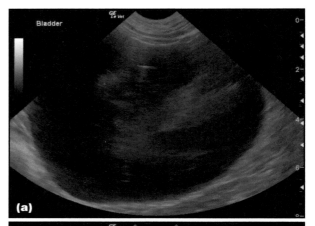

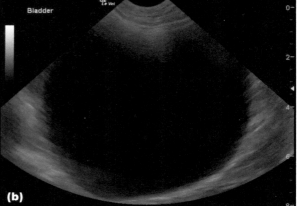

14.5 **(a)** Multiple echoes are seen within the bladder lumen of a Golden Retriever due to secondary lobe artefacts. Note the multiple focal zones depicted by the yellow arrowheads to the right of the image. **(b)** The bladder imaged with a single focal zone (yellow arrowhead) aligned with the middle of the lumen. The secondary echoes are no longer present. (Sagittal plane; cranial is to the left of the image.)

beam, and they do not alter position with gravity (Figure 14.6). Imaging within the focal zone and using a higher frequency transducer results in a thinner beam and therefore fewer slice thickness artefacts.

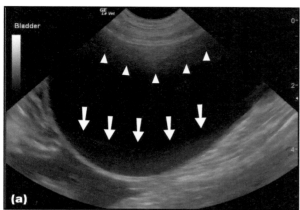

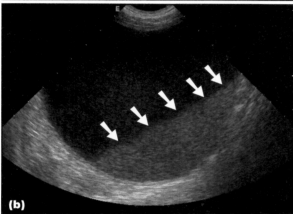

14.6 **(a)** 'Pseudosludge' due to slice thickness artefacts. This can be differentiated from genuine sediment by the curved interface with the urine (arrowed) and the fact that this 'pseudosludge' does not move with gravity. A similar band of echoes due to slice thickness artefacts is seen within the superficial part of the bladder lumen (arrowheads). **(b)** Genuine sediment settled dependently within the bladder of a crossbred dog. Note the straight interface (arrowed) between the urine and sediment. (Sagittal plane; cranial is to the left of the image.) (Courtesy of the University of Bristol)

Intraluminal material

Possible sources of intraluminal material include:

- Bladder sediment
- Calculi
- Air bubbles
- Haemorrhage/blood clots
- Foreign material.

Bladder sediment

Bladder sediment is usually recognized as multiple small echogenic foci within the bladder lumen. The distribution depends mainly on the effects of gravity. Typically, the sediment consists of small quantities of red blood cells, white blood cells, organisms, epithelial cells, crystals and casts which settle dependently against the bladder wall until disturbed into a swirling cloud by ballotting the bladder or reposition-

ing the patient. Fat droplets are a common component of feline urine, and will remain floating within the urine. Whilst a small amount of sediment can be an incidental finding, urinalysis is indicated for further investigation.

Calculi

Although acoustic shadowing deep to the sediment is consistent with mineralized calculi, the lack of shadowing does not rule out calculi. The likelihood of shadowing increases with the size of the calculus and the frequency of the transducer, but does not depend on the type of calculus (Weichselbaum *et al.*, 2000). When examining the patient in dorsal recumbency, it is important to distinguish dependent mineralized material from mineralized faecal material within the colon, which lies immediately adjacent to the bladder wall and casts a similar acoustic shadow (Figure 14.7). Following the extent of the shadowing structure in transverse and longitudinal planes, imaging the bladder from a different angle and repositioning the patient are useful techniques in differentiating intra-luminal material from colonic contents (Berry, 1992). Calculi tend to collect against the dependent bladder wall; small calculi may be resuspended on ballotting the bladder (see **Cystic calculi** clip on DVD), whilst larger calculi are usually dislodged by repositioning the patient.

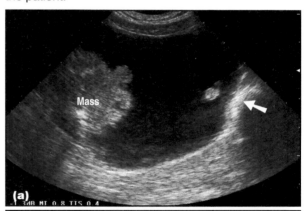

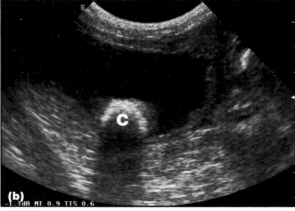

14.7 **(a)** The colon (arrowed) lies immediately adjacent to the bladder and can mimic the appearance of a large calculus. This dog also had a large bladder mass. **(b)** A genuine calculus (C) lying against the bladder wall, casting a strong acoustic shadow. The calculus moves position with gravity. (Transverse plane; right is to the left of the image.) (Courtesy of the University of Bristol)

Air bubbles

Air bubbles may be seen within the bladder lumen secondary to cystocentesis, catheterization or occasionally with emphysematous cystitis. Air bubbles should be recognizable as brightly echogenic foci, usually associated with a localized reverberation artefact and located in the highest (non-dependent) part of the bladder (Figure 14.8).

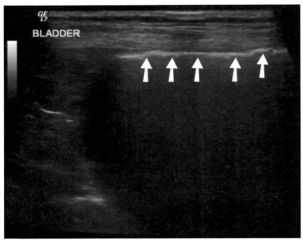

14.8 Emphysematous cystitis. The air is seen as a brightly echogenic line (arrowed) with distal reverberation artefacts located within the highest (non-dependent) part of the bladder. (Sagittal plane; cranial is to the left of the image.) (Courtesy of the University of Liverpool)

Haemorrhage and blood clots

Intraluminal haemorrhage often arises from the bladder itself, but may also originate from the kidneys or ureters. It may occur secondary to trauma, coagulopathy, neoplasia, severe cystitis and occasionally as an idiopathic finding. Recent haemorrhage may be seen as multiple small echoes either swirling within the lumen or settled dependently against the wall (Figure 14.9), and can be difficult to distinguish from bladder sediment.

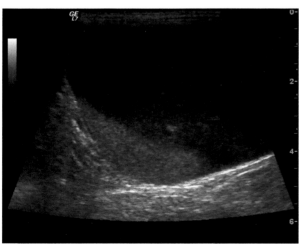

14.9 Haemorrhage settled dependently in the bladder of an adult dog due to a coagulopathy caused by warfarin toxicity. (Sagittal plane; cranial is to the left of the image.) (Courtesy of the University of Liverpool)

Blood clots are usually recognized as variably sized and often irregularly shaped non-shadowing echogenic masses, which may be floating free in the lumen or may be adherent to the bladder wall. The lack of blood flow on Doppler ultrasonography may be useful in distinguishing clots from neoplastic lesions. By repositioning the patient and/or gently ballotting the bladder, it may be possible to dislodge adherent clots into the lumen; however, care should be taken not to cause additional trauma, and, depending on the history, it may be more prudent to re-evaluate the bladder after 24–48 hours.

Foreign bodies

Foreign bodies are occasionally recognized within the bladder lumen. Urinary catheters are readily visible as parallel echogenic lines (Figure 14.10) and suture material may be seen as echogenic foci within or immediately adjacent to the bladder wall.

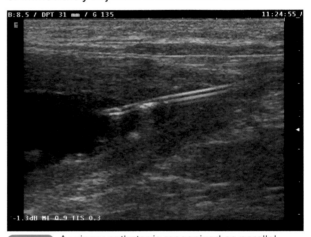

14.10 A urinary catheter is recognized as parallel echogenic lines passing through the urethra into the bladder lumen. (Sagittal plane; cranial is to the left of the image.) (Courtesy of the University of Bristol)

Mural masses

The majority of mural mass lesions identified within the urinary bladder are malignant tumours; however, benign masses, polyps and adherent blood clots mimicking a mass are occasionally seen. If a mass is identified, the kidneys, ureters, local lymph nodes and urethra should be evaluated for the presence of obstructive disease and local metastases.

Transitional cell carcinoma is the most commonly diagnosed bladder tumour. It is typically identified at the trigone or bladder neck as a single, irregular, broad-based mass of complex echogenicity, often hypoechoic to the wall and highly vascular on colour Doppler evaluation (Figure 14.11). Less frequently, it is seen as multiple masses, pedunculated masses or an area of irregularly thickened wall (Leveille *et al.*, 1992).

Smooth muscle tumours arising from the bladder wall are rare in the dog and cat, but may be seen as single, round, well defined, broad-based hypoechoic or mixed echogenic masses, often with little detectable blood flow on colour Doppler examination (Heng *et al.*, 2006). Bladder polyps are usually seen

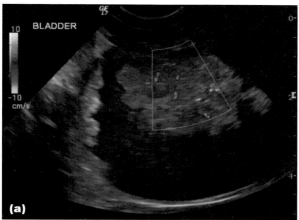

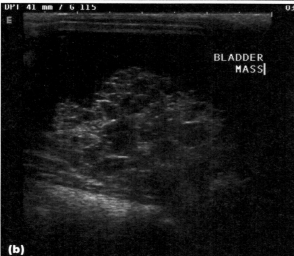

14.11 **(a)** Irregular broad-based mass, confirmed as a transitional cell carcinoma, located at the bladder trigone in a 7-year-old bitch. Colour Doppler ultrasonography demonstrated the mass to be well vascularized. (Transverse plane; right is to the left of the image.) (Courtesy of the University of Liverpool) **(b)** Cystic appearing mass identified arising from the bladder wall in a female neutered Domestic Shorthaired cat. (Sagittal plane; cranial is to the left of the image.) (Courtesy of the University of Bristol)

with polypoid cystitis, a relatively rare condition in dogs, characterized by inflammation of the bladder wall and the development of benign polypoid masses (Martinez *et al.*, 2003). Ultrasonographically, these polyps appear as irregular, pedunculated soft tissue masses (Figure 14.12), typically multiple in number and arising from the cranioventral or craniodorsal bladder wall (Takiguchi and Inaba, 2005). It is not possible to differentiate accurately between neoplastic and non-neoplastic lesions, or between different tumour types without a biopsy.

Although urethral neoplasia most often occurs due to local spread from the bladder (Figure 14.13) or prostate gland, primary tumours are occasionally id-entified. Primary urethral transitional cell carcinoma has been described as a well defined, smooth or irregular non-shadowing hyperechoic line seen at the epithelial margin of the proximal urethra, together with hypoechoic thickening of the urethral

wall (Hanson and Tidwell, 1996). In the male dog, ultrasonography may be useful in the identification or further characterization of distal urethral masses (Figure 14.14).

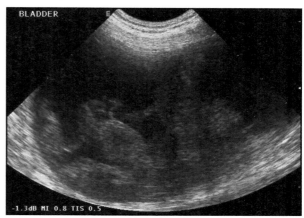

14.12 Multiple polypoid masses seen in a male neutered Cocker Spaniel with polypoid cystitis. Note the adjacent thickened bladder wall. (Sagittal plane; cranial is to the left of the image.) (Courtesy of the University of Bristol)

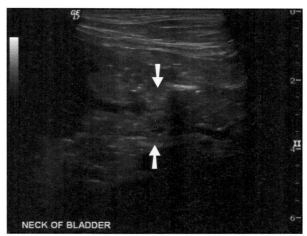

14.13 An irregular broad-based mass in an entire male dog extending beyond the bladder neck (arrowed) to involve the proximal urethra. (Sagittal plane; cranial is to the left of the image.) (Courtesy of the University of Liverpool)

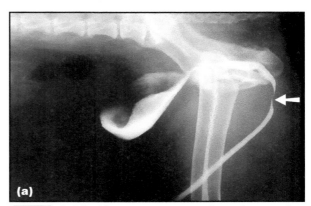

14.14 **(a)** Positive contrast retrograde urethrogram in a male neutered dog demonstrating the presence of a filling defect (arrowed) within the urethra consistent with a urethral mass. (continues) ▶

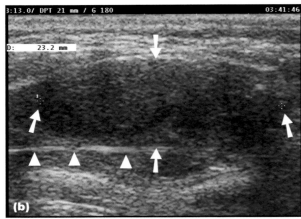

14.14 (continued) **(b)** Ultrasonogram using a high frequency linear transducer confirming the presence of the mass (arrowed). The parallel echogenic lines (arrowheads) seen deep to the mass lesion are echoes from the urethral catheter. A diagnosis of undifferentiated carcinoma was made from an ultrasound-guided fine needle aspirate. (Courtesy of the University of Bristol)

Ureteroceles are uncommon congenital cystic dilatations of the terminal ureter as it passes through the bladder wall. They appear ultrasonographically as anechoic structures within the dorsolateral bladder wall (Figure 14.15), described as a 'cyst within a cyst' (Takiguchi *et al.*, 1997).

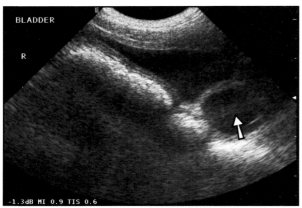

14.15 Ureterocele (arrowed) seen as a 'cyst within a cyst'. (Transverse plane; right is to the left of the image.) (Courtesy of the University of Bristol)

Diffuse lesions
Diffuse mural lesions are recognized as changes to the thickness, shape and echogenicity of the bladder wall. These changes may be generalized or localized to one area of the bladder. A subjective assessment of bladder distension is required to evaluate relative wall thickness; it is difficult to evaluate accurately the wall when the bladder is empty. Bladder wall thickening is most frequently seen due to cystitis or neoplastic infiltration, but may also be caused by intramural haemorrhage.

Cystitis results in wall thickening with irregularity of the mucosal surface, which may be localized (typically cranioventrally) or generalized (Figure 14.16). Emphysematous cystitis, reported most frequently in

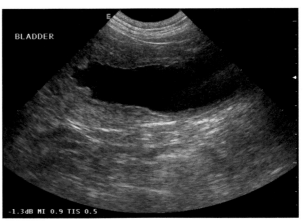

14.16 Irregular cranioventral and craniodorsal wall thickening in a neutered bitch with cystitis. (Sagittal plane; cranial is to the left of the image.) (Courtesy of the University of Bristol)

diabetic animals, results in the collection of small gas bubbles initially within the bladder wall and ultimately within the bladder lumen. Ultrasonography is very sensitive in the detection of mural gas, seen as irregular hyperechoic foci which remain trapped in the same location within the bladder wall, irrespective of patient position (Petite *et al.*, 2006). The presence of reverberation artefacts beyond the gas is useful in distinguishing gas bubbles from mineralization.

Although a sessile mural mass is the most common presentation of transitional cell carcinoma, irregular thickening of the bladder wall in the trigone region without a discrete mass lesion may also be seen. Diffuse infiltrative neoplasia, recognized as local or generalized wall thickening is uncommon but has been seen with diffuse carcinomatous infiltrations (Sutherland-Smith, 2008).

Mural haemorrhage has been reported in three dogs with coagulopathy (O'Brien and Wood 1998), seen as fairly marked diffuse wall thickening that resolved within several days following treatment of the underlying problem.

Ischaemia and partial sloughing of the bladder mucosa is an occasional complication of over-distension of the bladder due to obstruction. Fluid may be seen under-running the bladder mucosa, whilst sloughed portions may be seen within the bladder lumen as linear or irregularly shaped hypoechoic material.

Bladder rupture

Positive contrast retrograde urethrocystography remains the technique of choice for the identification of bladder and urethral rupture in dogs and cats. Although the ultrasonographic identification of bladder rupture has been described (Dubinsky *et al.*, 1999), it is not a very sensitive technique. The most reliable feature is the presence of free abdominal fluid, a sample of which should be obtained by ultrasound-guided aspiration. A concentration of creatinine within this fluid >1.5–2 times the serum concentration confirms urinary leakage. The actual defect within the bladder wall is rarely recognized, and there is often residual urine present within the bladder lumen. The infusion of agitated saline into the bladder via a urinary catheter has been described as a way of increasing the sensitivity of ultrasonography in the identification of bladder rupture (Cote *et al.*, 2002). The microbubbles within the agitated saline are recognized as multiple brightly echogenic foci within the bladder lumen; in cases of rupture, these should subsequently appear in the peritoneal fluid. Although theoretically it should be possible to identify the defect as the bubbles leave the bladder, this has not been demonstrated.

Ectopic ureters

Although intravenous urography and cystoscopy remain the most commonly used techniques, ultrasonography has the potential to allow the reasonably quick and non-invasive diagnosis of ectopic ureters. However, in some cases ultrasonographic identification of the abnormal ureter can be technically challenging, and thus the accuracy of the technique is operator-dependent. The main ultrasonographic features to be recognized are the absence of normal ureteric termination(s) and the presence of abnormal ureteric termination(s). The normal ureteric terminations are identified as small echogenic bumps, symmetrically located in the dorsolateral wall of the bladder trigone. A high frequency probe, time and patience should allow identification of the intermittent jets of urine entering the bladder from the ureteral papillae. If available, power Doppler can be used to enhance the signal from these moving jets of urine, which are displayed as small bursts of colour. Ectopic ureters, which are often abnormally dilated, most frequently terminate on the urethra just distal to the bladder neck. They may be recognized as anechoic tubular structures running within the retroperitoneal space to converge with the urethra just beyond the bladder neck (Figure 14.17; see also **Ectopic ureter** clip on DVD). Occasionally an ectopic ureter may be seen to run within the bladder wall, before terminating in the urethra. Colour Doppler is useful in distinguishing between blood vessels, which show pulsatile or continuous flow, and dilated ureters, which may show intermittent waves of peristalsis. If an ectopic ureter is suspected, it is important to evaluate the kidneys (see Chapter 10) for evidence of pelvic dilatation, which may suggest the presence of ascending infection.

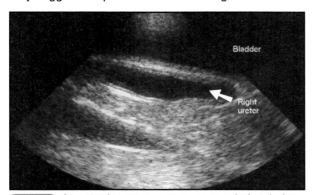

14.17 An ectopic ureter seen as an anechoic tubular structure (arrowed) running dorsal to the bladder before it converges with the urethra just beyond the bladder neck. (Sagittal plane; cranial is to the left of the image.) (Courtesy of the University of Liverpool)

Particular considerations for sampling

Ultrasound-guided cystocentesis is a very useful technique for obtaining non-contaminated urine samples, especially in cats and dogs where the bladder is difficult to palpate. However, ultrasound-guided fine-needle aspiration of bladder masses is not recommended, due to the risk of seeding tumour cells along the needle tract (Nyland *et al.*, 2002). Ultrasound-guided catheter biopsy of the bladder and urethra provides a safe, non-invasive alternative to needle aspiration (Lamb *et al.*, 1996). A urinary catheter is passed and identified on the ultrasonogram within the urethra or bladder lumen. The catheter can then be manipulated to line the side holes up with the lesion and suction applied to draw tissue fragments into the catheter. Limitations of this technique include the potential difficulty of aligning the catheter and the lesion, small sample sizes and the inability to sample deeper lesions.

References and further reading

Barthez PY, Leveille R and Scrivani P (1997) Side lobes and grating lobes artifacts in ultrasound imaging. *Veterinary Radiology and Ultrasound* **38**, 387–393

Berry CR (1992) Differentiating cystic calculi from the colon. *Veterinary Radiology and Ultrasound* **33**, 283–285

Biller DS, Kantrowitz B, Partington BP and Miyabayashi T (1990) Diagnostic ultrasound of the urinary bladder. *Journal of the American Animal Hospital Association* **26**, 397–402

Cote E, Carroll MC, Beck KA, Good L and Gannon K (2002) Diagnosis of bladder rupture using ultrasound contrast cystography: in vitro model and two case-history reports. *Veterinary Radiology and Ultrasound* **43**, 281–286

Dubinsky TJ, Deck A and Mann FA (1999) Sonographic diagnosis of a traumatic intraperitoneal bladder rupture. *American Journal of Roentgenology* **172**, 770

Finn-Bodner ST (1995) The urinary bladder. In: *Practical Veterinary Ultrasound*, ed. RE Cartee *et al.*, pp. 210–235. Lea and Febiger, Philadelphia

Geisse AL, Lowry JE, Schaeffer DJ and Smith CW (1997) Sonographic evaluation of urinary bladder wall thickness in normal dogs. *Veterinary Radiology and Ultrasound* **38**, 132–137

Hanson JA and Tidwell AS (1996) Ultrasonographic appearance of urethral transitional cell carcinoma in ten dogs. *Veterinary Radiology and Ultrasound* **37**, 293–299

Heng HG, Lowry JE, Boston S, Gabel C, Ehrhart N and Stocker Gulden SM (2006) Smooth muscle neoplasia of the urinary bladder wall in three dogs. *Veterinary Radiology and Ultrasound* **47**, 83–86

Lamb CR, Trower ND and Gregory SP (1996) Ultrasound-guided catheter biopsy of the lower urinary tract: technique and results in 12 dogs. *Journal of Small Animal Practice* **37**, 413–416

Leveille R, Biller DS, Partington BP and Miyabayashi T (1992) Sonographic investigation of transitional cell carcinoma of the urinary bladder in small animals. *Veterinary Radiology and Ultrasound* **33**, 103–107

Martinez I, Mattoon JS, Eatone KA, Chew DJ and DiBartola SP (2003) Polypoid cystitis in 17 dogs (1978–2001) *Journal of Veterinary Internal Medicine* **17**, 399–509

Nyland TG, Wallack ST and Wisner ER (2002) Needle-tract implantation following us-guided fine-needle aspiration biopsy of transitional cell carcinoma from the bladder, urethra and prostate. *Veterinary Radiology and Ultrasound* **43**, 50–53

O'Brien RT and Wood EF (1998) Urinary bladder mural haemorrhage associated with systemic bleeding disorders in three dogs. *Veterinary Radiology and Ultrasound* **39**, 354–356

Petite A, Busoni V, Heinen M-P, Billen F and Snaps F (2006) Radiographic and ultrasonographic findings of emphysematous cystitis in four non-diabetic female dogs. *Veterinary Radiology and Ultrasound* **47**, 90–93

Sutherland-Smith J (2008) Bladder and urethra. In: *Atlas of Small Animal Ultrasonography*, ed. D. Penninck and MA d'Anjou, pp. 365–384. Blackwell Publishing, Iowa

Takiguchi M and Inaba M (2005) Diagnostic ultrasound of polypoid cystitis in dogs. *Journal of Veterinary Medical Science* **67**, 57–61

Takiguchi M, Yasude J, Ochiai K, Morita Y and Hashimoto A (1997) Ultrasonographic appearance of orthoptic ureterocele in a dog. *Veterinary Radiology and Ultrasound* **38**, 398–399

Weichselbaum RC, Fenney DA, Jessen CF, Osborne CA, Dreyster V and Holte J (2000) Relevance of sonographic artifacts observed during in vitro characterization of urocystolith mineral composition. *Veterinary Radiology and Ultrasound* **41**, 438–446

Video extras

- Cystic calculi
- Ectopic ureter
- Ureteric jet

Access via QR code or bsavalibrary.com/ultrasound_14

15

Prostate gland

Kate Bradley

Indications

Indications for ultrasonographic examination of the prostate gland in the dog include:

- Recurrent or chronic urinary tract infections
- Haematuria
- Dysuria
- Dyschezia
- Prostatomegaly (palpable or radiographic)
- Pyrexia of unknown origin
- Caudal abdominal pain
- Orchitis
- Haemospermia.

Prostatic disease is rare in cats, but there are similar indications for ultrasonographic examination of the feline prostate gland.

Value of ultrasonography compared with radiography and computed tomography

Ultrasonography

Ultrasonography is a quick, non-invasive and inexpensive way of evaluating the size and parenchyma of the prostate gland; the prostatic urethra may also be assessed. Fine-needle aspirates and core tissue biopsy (CTB) samples may be obtained under ultrasound guidance, and urethral catheters can be guided for prostatic washes.

Radiography

Compared with ultrasonography, plain radiographs provide little extra information; radiography may give a better overview of prostatic position, but is often less helpful for assessment of size due to the superimposition of other structures, especially on the ventrodorsal view. Little information about the parenchyma of the gland is obtained on radiographs, other than identification of any gas accumulations or areas of mineralization. Radiographs are even more limiting if free abdominal fluid is present, or if an animal has little intra-abdominal fat. Contrast studies still have a place in evaluating the prostate gland; retrograde urethrography allows better assessment of the urethral path, diameter and epithelial surface than ultrasonography, and is also valuable for further assessment of cavitating lesions within the prostate gland, particularly with respect to any urethral communication. Radiographs are useful for identifying any reactive bony changes on the lumbar vertebrae and/or pelvis, which may occur secondary to prostatic neoplasia.

Advanced modalities

Cross-sectional imaging techniques (i.e. computed tomography and magnetic resonance imaging) provide more information on the prostatic parenchyma than radiography, and are potentially more valuable than ultrasonography for assessing the local extent and spread of neoplastic lesions. However, cost and limited availability still preclude their use for investigating most cases of suspected prostatic disease.

Scintigraphy is widely used in humans for the detection of osseous metastases from prostatic neoplasms, but these are reported to occur less frequently in dogs and early detection is currently unlikely to alter subsequent treatment or prognosis.

Imaging technique

Patient preparation

Hair is often sparse in this area, so clipping may not be necessary to obtain adequate skin contact for imaging, but should be done to facilitate asepsis if aspirates or biopsy samples are to be taken.

Positioning

For examination of the prostate gland, the dog can be placed in dorsal or lateral recumbency. The transducer should be positioned on the caudal abdominal wall, to one side of the prepuce and just cranial to the pubic bone.

By scanning the area just caudal to the bladder neck, there is usually no difficulty in locating an enlarged prostate gland. Smaller, intrapelvic glands may be harder to find. The easiest way to locate the prostate gland is to identify the bladder neck on a long-axis view and angle the probe caudally following the orientation of the bladder neck. Imaging a dog with a full bladder makes locating the prostate gland easier, as the weight of the urine tends to displace the prostate gland cranially. Imaging a dog in a standing position may have a similar effect, as gravity helps displace the bladder and prostate gland cranially. In placid or sedated animals, an assistant can help locate the prostate gland by digital manipulation *per rectum*, and push it cranially. In this situation, it may be advisable to withdraw the finger before attempting a biopsy procedure. If the prostate gland still proves difficult to locate, a perineal approach may be helpful for identifying and assessing the gland, particularly the more caudal aspects of the parenchyma. A perineal approach is also the method of choice in cases of perineal hernia, to enable identification and evaluation of the hernia contents.

Having identified the prostate gland, it should be systematically examined in both sagittal and transverse planes. For caudally positioned prostate glands, the short-axis plane is more dorsally oriented due to the angulation of the transducer. For a complete examination, the rest of the urinary tract (kidneys, bladder, region of the ureters), the sublumbar area and, in entire males, the testicles should also be examined. The presence or absence of sublumbar lymphadenopathy may be relevant in many clinical scenarios, and aspiration of enlarged nodes may help with diagnosis and staging of disease.

Equipment

As the prostate gland is a relatively superficial structure, it is best examined with a higher frequency transducer. A 7.5–10 MHz probe gives good detail of the prostatic parenchyma. A linear transducer may be used to image a prostate gland lying within the abdomen; however, in many cases a smaller footprint transducer (microconvex or phased array) is better as it allows the beam to be angled caudally into the pelvic canal. Transrectal ultrasonography with a specialized endorectal probe is a standard means of imaging the prostate gland in humans, but is little used in dogs due to the need for specialized equipment and the discomfort of the procedure, which is likely to necessitate sedation or general anaesthesia in most animals.

Doppler ultrasonography

Prostatic perfusion can be assessed using contrast-enhanced Doppler ultrasonography, and has been described in the normal canine prostate gland (Russo *et al.*, 2009). The prostatic artery enters the prostate gland on the dorsolateral surface and branches into parenchymal arteries directed towards the urethra. A normal prostate gland shows homogeneous enhancement with contrast medium. Altered patterns of contrast medium 'wash-in' and 'wash-out' may be useful in the future to differentiate different disease entities.

Normal ultrasonographic appearance

Dogs

The normal canine prostate gland surrounds the proximal urethra; it may encircle the area immediately caudal to the bladder neck or there may be a short portion of urethra between the bladder neck and prostate gland. In a mid-sagittal section, the prostate gland appears ovoid with the urethra running through it as a hypoechoic linear structure (Figure 15.1; see also **Normal prostate gland (1)** clip on DVD). In transverse section, the prostate gland appears bilobed, each lobe being semi-ovoid, with a rounded

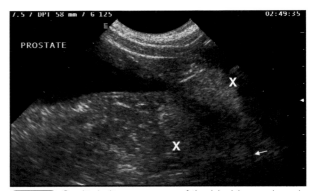

15.1 Sagittal ultrasonogram of the bladder neck and prostate gland (x–x). The urethra is visible as a hypoechoic linear structure running through the prostatic parenchyma. Edge shadowing is seen to the right of the image (arrowed).

ventral margin and more flattened dorsal margin. The bilobed appearance can be subtle in a normal prostate gland, but becomes much more evident when the prostate gland is enlarged (see Figure 15.5). The urethra may be seen as a hypoechoic structure between the lobes, and is centrally to slightly dorsally located.

The size of the prostate gland is variable, increasing with age and decreasing in neutered males. The normal prostatic parenchyma has a homogeneous, finely stippled echotexture. In older, intact males, the prostate gland is typically hyperechoic to the surrounding tissues (Figure 15.2a; see also **Normal prostate gland (2)** clip on DVD), whereas in young and neutered males it appears smaller and hypoechoic (Figure 15.2b). However, the echogenicity in different animals can be variable and depends on the age and hormonal status of the dog, as well as the ultrasound machine settings. Small anechoic cystic lesions (<1 cm), which are thought to represent an accumulation of prostatic secretions, are frequently seen in asymptomatic dogs, and in the absence of other changes are considered normal findings. The capsule may be evident in places, where the ultrasound beam is perpendicular to it, and is seen as a thin echogenic line. Edge shadowing is frequently seen on transverse images of the prostate gland. Acoustic shadowing is commonly

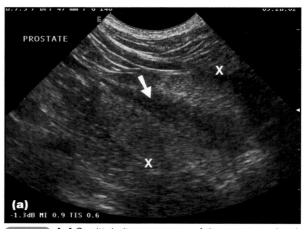

15.2 **(a)** Sagittal ultrasonogram of the prostate gland (x–x) in an entire male dog, showing a homogeneous, relatively echogenic parenchyma. The urethra (arrowed) is visible as a hypoechoic linear structure. (continues) ▶

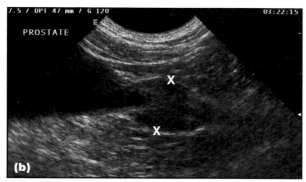

15.2 (continued) **(b)** Sagittal ultrasonogram of a normal prostate gland (x–x) in a young male dog, which is positioned close to the bladder neck. The prostate gland appears relatively small and hypoechoic. The capsule is seen as a thin echogenic line surrounding the prostate gland, and is more obvious than in (a) due to the contrast with the parenchyma.

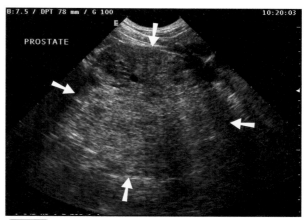

15.3 BPH: the prostatic parenchyma (arrowed) is heterogeneous and contains numerous small cystic areas.

seen deep to the descending colon/rectum and pubic bone, which lie dorsally and ventrally, re-spectively, to the prostate gland.

Cats
In the cat the prostate gland is also bilobed, but only covers the urethra dorsally and laterally. It tends to be more caudally positioned than in the dog, with some prostatic tissue disseminated within the urethral wall caudal to the prostate gland itself.

Diffuse disease

Benign hyperplasia and metaplasia
Benign prostatic hyperplasia (BPH) is so common that it is considered a normal finding in middle-aged to old entire male dogs. Histologically, it can start from around 2 years of age and is present in 100% of male dogs >7 years of age, many of whom will remain completely asymptomatic. It results from diffuse epithelial or glandular proliferation throughout the prostate gland. Variable distension of prostatic acini can occur to form cystic areas.

Squamous metaplasia occurs when the glandular epithelium of the prostate gland becomes stratified squamous in type instead of the columnar epithelium normally present. The main cause of this change in cell type is an increase in circulating oestrogen levels (such as with Sertoli cell tumours), but it can also occur secondary to chronic inflammation. Secretory stasis as a result of squamous metaplasia can lead to cyst or abscess formation.

Ultrasonographically, the prostate gland is usually mildly to moderately enlarged and appears smoothly marginated and symmetrical. The echotexture of the gland is variable; it most commonly appears diffusely hyperechoic but may appear heterogeneous (Figure 15.3; see also **Benign prostatic hyperplasia (1)**, **(2)** and **(3)** clips on DVD). Mineralization is uncommon unless there is concurrent disease. Cystic areas are common and appear as variably sized and shaped anechoic regions, demonstrating distal acoustic enhancement. The capsule remains intact and local lymph nodes are unaffected. It is not possible ultrasonographically to distinguish hyperplasia from metaplasia; however, a complete ultrasound examination may detect an underlying cause of metaplasia, such as a Sertoli cell tumour in a testicle.

As the majority of entire male dogs presenting with suspected prostatic disease have existing BPH, this complicates interpretation of the ultrasonographic findings, as changes due to other disease entities add to those already present due to BPH. Hyperplasia, prostatitis and neoplasia may all be present in the same gland, increasing the importance of biopsy samples for a diagnosis, although it should be remembered that biopsy samples only reflect changes in the small proportion of the gland sampled. Biopsy is necessary to definitively diagnose BPH, but a presumptive diagnosis and monitoring response to treatment is often more practical. Following castration, the prostate gland starts to shrink after 7–14 days and will substantially reduce in size (by ≥50%) within 3–4 months.

Inflammation
There is considerable overlap in the ultrasonographic appearance of BPH and prostatitis. Typically, acute, diffuse prostatitis presents as a symmetrically enlarged gland with an overall hypoechoic parenchyma. However, the ultrasonographic appearance is variable and the parenchyma can also appear coarsely hyperechoic or mottled, presumably reflecting the varying degrees of oedema, haemorrhage and necrosis that may be present within the gland. Small hypoechoic to anechoic cavitary lesions may be seen, representing areas of abscessation. Abscesses may coalesce to give a larger cavitary lesion (Figure 15.4), which may exhibit distal acoustic enhancement.

With chronic disease, the prostate gland is usually smaller and the overall appearance is typically more hyperechoic, which is likely to relate to fibrosis within the gland. Mineralization may be present, but is less common than with neoplasia. Granulomatous prostatitis, resulting from blastomycosis and cryptococcosis, is unlikely to be seen in the UK, but has rarely been reported in endemic areas such as parts of the United States. The prostate gland may appear enlarged and heterogeneous with overall increase in echogenicity.

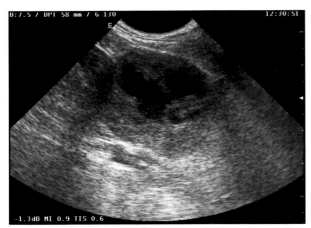

15.4 Irregularly marginated, anechoic cavitary lesion within the prostate gland. The cavity was aspirated and *Escherichia coli* cultured.

Neoplasia

The most common tumours to occur in the canine prostate gland are carcinomas, mainly adenocarcinomas, but also transitional cell carcinomas, squamous cell carcinomas and mixed morphology carcinomas. Other tumour types such as leiomyosarcoma, haemangiosarcoma, osteosarcoma and lymphoma have been reported but are very rare. Prostatic neoplasia is seen in both entire and neutered dogs, usually middle-aged to old, medium to large breeds. Prostatic neoplasia is very rare in the cat, although there are sporadic reports of adenocarcinoma.

On ultrasound examination, the prostate gland is usually asymmetrically enlarged. Asymmetry can be appreciated ultrasonographically, either by identifying the two lobes in the transverse plane (Figure 15.5) or by identifying the urethra (if possible), as this should run centrally to slightly dorsally within the prostate gland. The capsule is frequently disrupted with neoplasia, so particular attention should be paid to assessing the margins of the gland. Many tumours also spread locally to involve the bladder neck, so this should be examined in detail for any thickening

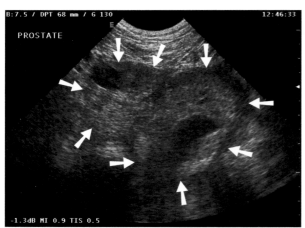

15.5 Transverse image showing asymmetry of the prostate gland. Both lobes (arrowed) contain anechoic cystic areas. A mixed growth was cultured following aspiration of the cavities and the lesions resolved following appropriate antibiotic therapy.

or irregularity. A perineal approach may be helpful to assess whether there is any evidence of caudal extension of the tumour to involve the pelvic canal and rectal area.

The prostatic parenchyma is usually very heterogeneous with neoplasia, and cavitary lesions may be present. Mineralization is another common feature, and this is seen ultrasonographically as hyperechoic foci with distal acoustic shadowing (Figure 15.6; see also **Prostatic carcinoma (1)** clip on DVD). Chances of seeing shadowing are maximized by using a high frequency transducer with the area of interest within the focal zone.

Although there are no ultrasonographic features specific to neoplastic prostatic disease, enlargement of the prostate gland in a neutered male dog, especially if mineralized foci are present, warrants further investigation as neoplasia is the most likely reason.

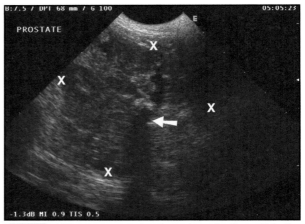

15.6 Ultrasonogram showing mineralization within the prostate gland (x–x), characterized by echogenic foci with distal acoustic shadowing (arrowed). The prostate gland is generally heterogeneous. Histological diagnosis was squamous cell carcinoma.

Metastasis

Metastases to the sublumbar lymph nodes (see **Prostatic carcinoma (2)** clip on DVD) are common and therefore the medial iliac, hypogastric and lumbar aortic nodes should be examined, looking for any increase in size or alteration in echogenicity. The normal medial iliac nodes are relatively easy to locate, as they lie lateral to the caudal aorta and external iliac arteries. The hypogastric nodes lie caudal to this area, between the internal iliac vessels and the median sacral artery. Aortic nodes lie along the length of the aorta. Both the hypogastric and aortic lymph nodes are difficult to identify unless enlarged. For an optimum examination of this area, it is best to scan the dog in both right and left lateral recumbency, with the probe positioned on the uppermost flank, just ventral to the lumbar muscles.

Osteoblastic bone metastases to the pelvis and lumbosacral spine can occur, and it is possible to detect irregularity of the bone surfaces on an ultrasound examination. However, radiography gives a better overview of this area and provides more information on the nature of any new bone production.

Focal disease

Intraprostatic cysts

Focal cysts are frequently seen in the prostate gland and can either be incidental findings or occur in association with other disease entities, such as prostatitis or neoplasia. Most are retention cysts, where cavitary lesions within the prostatic parenchyma fill with prostatic secretions and/or urine. Congenital cysts can result from anatomical abnormalities, for example, persistence of Müllerian duct remnants. Cysts appear ultrasonographically as anechoic structures with thin walls and distal acoustic enhancement (Figure 15.7; see also **Prostatic cysts (1)** and **(2)** clips on DVD). The internal margin of the cavity is typically smooth and regular. Multiple tiny cysts may appear hyperechoic due to the distal enhancement being the predominant feature seen. Cysts may be infected and still appear anechoic on ultrasonography.

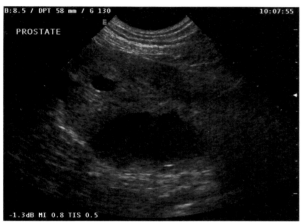

15.7 Sagittal ultrasonogram of a prostate gland showing two anechoic lesions: one small and well defined, and the other larger with slightly irregular margins. The prostate gland otherwise appears homogeneous. Differential diagnoses for these lesions includes cysts and abscesses. Diagnosis in this case was confirmed as cysts associated with BPH.

Paraprostatic cysts

Paraprostatic cysts arise outside the prostatic parenchyma. They are often connected to the prostate gland by a stalk, but otherwise have no contact with the prostatic parenchyma. The origin of these cysts is hard to ascertain; theories include development from remnants of the uterus masculinus or arising subsequent to either haematoma formation or squamous metaplasia and ductal occlusion.

Ultrasonographically, cysts may be located either within the abdomen or in the pelvic/perineal area. Most cysts appear as large anechoic structures with a thin echogenic wall. Their size can be considerable, with cysts reaching diameters of ≥30 cm. Many cysts have internal septations (Figure 15.8), which helps in distinguishing them from the urinary bladder. In some cases echogenic material may be present within a cyst, and it is possible for cysts to contain a proportion of solid-looking material. Mineralization of the wall is a common feature, but this may not always be confirmed ultrasonographically, probably due to a very

thin calcified wall not casting an acoustic shadow when the ultrasound beam crosses it perpendicularly. Radiography may be more sensitive than ultrasonography for detecting cyst wall mineralization, and is also useful for providing an overview of the relative position of the cyst(s), prostate gland and bladder within the caudal abdomen. Concurrent prostatic disease is common, so the prostatic parenchyma should also be fully assessed.

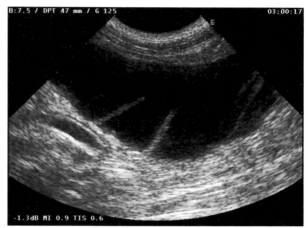

15.8 Ultrasonogram showing a paraprostatic cyst. The contents of the cyst are predominantly anechoic, and echogenic internal septations are present. The prostate gland (not pictured) appeared large, echogenic and contained a small intraprostatic cyst.

Abscesses

Prostatic abscesses may occur due to infection of cysts or as a sequel to acute or chronic prostatitis. Prostatic abscesses are often lobulated, the walls are usually thicker and more irregular than those of cysts, and there may be septated internal margins. Size is variable and it is possible for abscesses to involve the entire prostatic parenchyma (Figure 15.9). Peripherally located lesions may distort the overall shape of the prostate gland. The contents of abscesses are variable in appearance: they may be anechoic or hypoechoic and distal acoustic enhancement may be present. If echoes are present within

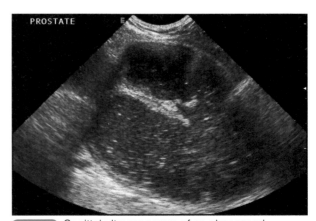

15.9 Sagittal ultrasonogram of an abscessed prostate gland. The abscess appears septated and contains echoes, which were swirling on real-time imaging (see also **Prostatic abscess** clip on DVD). Other than a peripheral rim, little normal prostatic tissue remains.

the cavity it may be possible to see 'swirling' in real-time imaging (see **Prostatic abscess** clip on DVD). Identification of reverberation artefacts within a cavitary lesion indicates the presence of gas; as gas is more likely to be present within an abscess than within other cavitary lesions, this can be a useful diagnostic feature. Radiographs are also useful for detecting any foci of gas within the prostate gland. Differential diagnoses include haematomas, cysts, haematocysts and cystic neoplasia. The necrotic centre of a large neoplasm may also resemble an abscess ultrasonographically.

Calculi
Examination of the prostate gland may aid in the detection and localization of calculi lodged within the prostatic urethra. Calculi may also form directly in the prostatic urethra or in cystic periurethral areas secondary to chronic inflammation. Ultrasonographically, calculi are seen as hyperechoic linear interfaces with distal acoustic shadowing. If there is any obstruction to urine outflow, the prostatic urethra may appear wider and more dilated than normal. As calculi can move between the bladder and prostatic urethra, their position should be confirmed by ultrasonography or radiography prior to any surgical procedure.

Particular considerations for sampling

As there is considerable overlap in the ultrasonographic appearance of different prostatic disease processes, prostatic washes, fine-needle aspiration (FNA) and core tissue biopsy (CTB) are essential in most cases for achieving a diagnosis through cytology and/or histology.

Prostatic wash
When performing a prostatic wash, ultrasound guidance can be useful for positioning the tip of the urinary catheter prior to introducing the sterile saline (Figure 15.10). Having the tip of the catheter in the

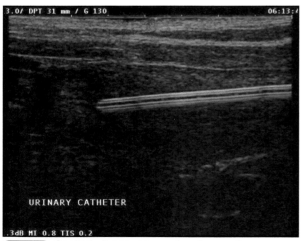

15.10 Sagittal ultrasonogram showing a urinary catheter within the prostatic parenchyma. The catheter was withdrawn slightly prior to a wash sample being taken.

urethra, just distal to the prostate gland, makes the wash more selective. For an optimum sample, the prostate gland should be massaged *per rectum* for about 1 minute prior to the wash being taken. If a transitional cell carcinoma involving the prostate gland is suspected, a traumatic catheterization technique may be used, where a catheter is advanced to the level of the prostatic urethra and several aspirates are taken whilst concurrently massaging the prostate gland *per rectum*. This technique is an alternative to percutaneous FNA and avoids any risk of tumour cells implanting along the needle tract.

Aspiration and biopsy
Fine-needle aspirates and biopsy samples are usually taken from a transabdominal approach with the dog lying in dorsal or lateral recumbency. A transperineal approach is also feasible if the prostate gland is very caudally positioned. Cytological samples may be preferable to larger biopsy samples in some cases, as they are less invasive, usually do not require general anaesthesia, multiple areas of the gland can be easily sampled, and results can be obtained quickly. Individual cell morphology can often be better assessed in a monolayer, and cytology is more sensitive than histology for the detection of sepsis (bacteria are not generally seen in histological sections). Up to 80% agreement between histological and cytological diagnoses has been reported (Powe *et al.*, 2004). Histopathological examination allows a more detailed assessment of tissue architecture; therefore, collection of biopsy samples is indicated following FNA results that are inconclusive, or that are clinically suspected to be unrepresentative.

Both FNA and CTB are relatively easy to perform using ultrasound guidance when the prostate gland is enlarged and lying within the abdomen. Obtaining samples from a smaller, intrapelvic prostate gland can be more challenging in terms of aligning the needle with the plane of the ultrasound beam, and care needs to be taken to ensure the path of the needle is visible at all times.

There are no specific contraindications to taking fine-needle aspirates from the prostate gland. Sedation for the procedure should be considered, both for analgesia and to minimize the likelihood of movement during needle placement, as the aorta and caudal vena cava lie in relatively close proximity to the dorsal border of the prostate gland, and could be inadvertently damaged if the dog moves. Core tissue biopsy samples should only be taken if the prostate gland appears to have a 'solid' parenchyma. Biopsy of a cyst or an abscess is unlikely to yield a useful sample for histology and may lead to peritonitis. Prior to biopsy, it is advisable to check clotting parameters and to have the animal under deep sedation or general anaesthesia. The biopsy needle path should be directed so as to avoid the urethra, but if it inadvertently includes the urethra, haematuria (which may last for a few days) is likely to be the only complication. Other potential complications of FNA and CTB include local haemorrhage and seeding of neoplastic cells and/or bacteria.

Drainage

Ultrasound guidance may also be used therapeutically to drain cavitating prostatic lesions (i.e. cysts and abscesses). More than one drainage procedure is usually necessary and there is no guarantee of permanent resolution, although ultrasound-guided percutaneous drainage has been reported to have a good success rate when used as the primary treatment for prostatic abscessation. Animals should be monitored for 24–48 hours following each drainage procedure, and ultrasound-guided drainage should not be used as the primary treatment if there is any evidence of peritonitis or other severe systemic signs.

References and further reading

Bradbury CA, Westropp JL and Pollard RE (2009) Relationship between prostatomegaly, prostatic mineralization and cytological diagnosis. *Veterinary Radiology and Ultrasound* **50**(2), 167–171

Nyland TG, Wallack ST and Wisner ER (2002) Needle-tract implantation following US-guided fine-needle aspiration biopsy of transitional cell carcinoma of the bladder, urethra and prostate. *Veterinary Radiology and Ultrasound* **43**(1), 50–53

Powe JR, Canfield PJ and Martin PA (2004) Evaluation of the cytological diagnosis of canine prostatic disorders. *Veterinary Clinical Pathology* **33**(3), 150–154

Root Kustritz MV (2006) Collection of tissue and culture samples from the canine reproductive tract. *Theriogenology* **66**, 567–574

Russo M, Vignoli M, Catone G *et al.* (2009) Prostatic perfusion in the dog using contrast-enhanced Doppler ultrasound. *Reproduction in Domestic Animals* **44**(Suppl. 2), 334–335

Smith J (2008) Canine prostatic disease: a review of anatomy, pathology, diagnosis and treatment. *Theriogenology* **70**, 375–383

Video extras

- Benign prostatic hyperplasia (1)
- Benign prostatic hyperplasia (2)
- Benign prostatic hyperplasia (3)
- Normal prostate gland (1)
- Normal prostate gland (2)
- Prostatic abscess
- Prostatic carcinoma (1)
- Prostatic carcinoma (2)
- Prostatic cysts (1)
- Prostatic cysts (2)

Access via QR code or bsavalibrary.com/ultrasound_15

16

Uterus

Frances Barr

Indications

A complete ultrasonographic examination of the abdomen should always include the uterus in the entire bitch or queen. In the neutered animal, the vaginal or uterine stump should be examined where possible. However, specific indications for ultrasonographic examination of the uterus include:

- Pregnancy diagnosis
- Assessment of fetal viability
- Monitoring uterine involution post-partum
- Investigation of infertility
- Vaginal discharge
- Perivulval irritation
- Haematuria
- Evaluation of palpable masses in the caudal abdomen/pelvis
- Evaluation of caudal abdominal or pelvic pain
- Evaluation of abdominal distension
- Systemic signs suggestive of pyometritis.

Value of ultrasonography compared with radiography and computed tomography

Diagnostic ultrasonography has many advantages over alternative imaging techniques for examination of the uterus. It is an imaging modality which is now widely available in small animal practice, and the level of operator expertise is rising all the time. The examination can be performed with the patient conscious, and the owner can safely be present if that is considered to be helpful. The procedure is non-invasive, painless, and, in the light of current knowledge, safe to the patient, to the developing fetus and to the operator. This is in contrast to imaging modalities which make use of ionizing radiation (i.e. computed tomography (CT) and conventional radiography).

Conventional radiography allows evaluation of the uterine silhouette. Thus, the enlarged uterus is visible radiographically, but soft tissues and fluid are of the same radiographic opacity; not until fetal skeletal mineralization occurs during the third trimester of pregnancy can fetal structures be confirmed radiographically. During the last trimester of pregnancy it is often easier to count the number of fetuses on a radiograph, if this information is required, than on ultrasonographic examination.

Radiography can be a useful means of detecting fetal death during late pregnancy; as fluid is resorbed from the dead fetus, the skull bones begin to overlap and the body becomes more tightly curled. Eventually, fetal structures start to disintegrate, and gas may be seen within the fetus, within the uterine lumen or uterine wall. In some instances the dead fetus may become mummified, with the compacted skeletal structures producing a small mineralized ball.

Ultrasonography allows fetal structures to be identified much earlier in pregnancy, and the real-time images allow evaluation of fetal viability. Doppler techniques allow blood flow within the uterus, placenta and fetus to be assessed. In cases of uterine disease, ultrasonography allows differentiation between fluid and soft tissues, thus refining the differential diagnosis list.

CT allows more detailed evaluation of abdominal structures than does conventional radiography, and as technology advances to allow reduced scan times and higher resolution, it is likely that CT will be used more for the diagnosis of uterine disease. In particular, CT may be useful in the staging of uterine malignancies. However, the hazards of ionizing radiation mean that ultrasonography remains the diagnostic procedure of choice for patients who are, or may be, pregnant.

Imaging technique

Ultrasonographic examination of the uterus may be performed with the patient in either dorsal or lateral recumbency. If the patient is reluctant to lie, then the examination may be carried out with the animal standing. Hair is clipped from the ventral abdomen, extending from the umbilicus back to the pubic brim, and extending several centimetres each side of the midline. Clipping is not usually necessary in animals with pronounced mammary gland development, but if clipping is required in such patients, then care should be taken not to damage this sensitive region.

After cleaning the skin and applying a water-soluble acoustic gel, a high frequency (usually 7.5–10 MHz) microconvex or linear array transducer should be placed on the skin in the midline, just cranial to the pubic brim. The ultrasound beam should be oriented in a sagittal plane. A useful initial landmark is the fluid-filled bladder. The colon, which often contains gas and/or faecal material, lies dorsal and often to the left of the bladder. The proximal vagina, cervix and uterine body should be looked for first dorsal to the bladder and ventral to the colon. If not apparent, then look to the right and to the left of the bladder. Once the uterus is identified, it can then be examined in both sagittal and transverse planes. It is not usually possible to follow normal, non-gravid uterine horns cranial to the bladder, but if the uterus is enlarged or there is free abdominal fluid, then this may become possible.

Normal ultrasonographic appearance

The normal, non-gravid uterus may be difficult to identify in dogs, and is often not seen in cats. When imaged during late dioestrus or anoestrus, the uterus is a narrow, uniformly hypoechoic tube. The uterine wall does not usually show any layering, in contrast to the distinct layering of the wall of the normal small intestine. However, during pro-oestrus, oestrus and early dioestrus there may be a hyperechoic streak in the centre of the uterus (Figure 16.1; see also **Normal uterus in a dog** clip on DVD), and the wall may variably show a hypoechoic inner layer. The cervix is usually only obvious during this time, and has multiple layers which are best appreciated on transverse section. Absolute diameter of the uterus will vary according to species/breed, parity and the stage of the oestrous cycle. The diameter of the uterine body is said to range from 3 mm in small breeds of dog to 8 mm in larger breeds, with an increase in diameter of 1–3 mm during oestrus. The uterine stump is not usually recognized in neutered animals, although a narrow, blind-ending tubular structure may be identified lying between the bladder and the colon.

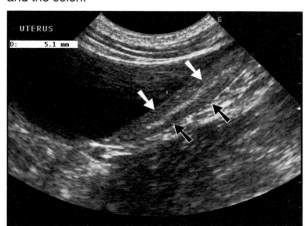

16.1 Sagittal image of the caudal abdomen of an entire Springer Spaniel bitch. The uterus (arrowed) lies dorsal to the bladder. A central hyperechoic line is visible.

Pregnancy

Normal ultrasonographic appearance
Ultrasonography is a well established technique for the diagnosis of pregnancy in the bitch and queen. There have been numerous ultrasonographic studies following normal gestation in the bitch, and most of these determine the length of gestation according to

the preovulatory surge in luteinizing hormone (LH). This should be borne in mind when using the published data, as most owners will only be aware of the dates of mating. When gestation is timed from the LH surge, the fluid-filled gestational sac is usually first identified at around day 20, with the embryo and its heartbeat evident at day 23–25. Since confirmation of a viable pregnancy relies on positive identification of the embryo, it is common to perform ultrasonographic examinations for this purpose around 4 weeks after the last known mating (Figure 16.2; see also **4-week pregnancy in a Jack Russell Terrier** clip on DVD). Although it is often possible to diagnose pregnancy earlier than this, a confident negative diagnosis is difficult. If no embryonic structures are seen at 4 weeks, a repeat examination a week later can be performed to conclusively rule out pregnancy. The canine fetus develops rapidly after day 30, with individual fetal organs differentiating and becoming visible (Figure 16.3). Fetal movements are usually visible from day 34–36 onwards.

In the queen, gestational age is defined as the number of days after mating, which makes interpretation of the published data more straightforward. Positive identification of gestational sacs may be possible as early as 10 days after mating, with the

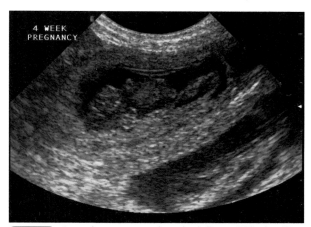

16.2 4-week pregnancy in a Jack Russell Terrier. The fetus is clearly visible, surrounded by fetal fluids and fetal membranes, within the uterus.

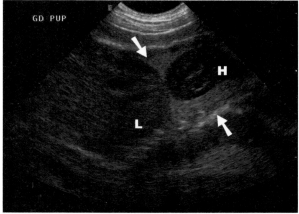

16.3 A Great Dane pup *in utero* near term. The heart (H) is visible to the right of the image, surrounded by the lungs (arrowed). The hypoechoic liver (L) is visible to the left of the image.

embryo visible from day 16–18 (Figure 16.4; see also **4-week pregnancy in a cat** clip on DVD). Pregnancy diagnosis is thus usually possible at an earlier stage in the queen than in the bitch.

Doppler techniques have been used to monitor uterine and fetal blood flow as gestation progresses in dogs and cats. Theoretically, such baseline information could be used to monitor high risk pregnancies, but the technique is not yet widely applied.

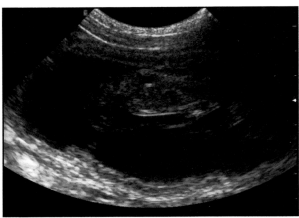

16.4 4-week pregnancy in a Domestic Shorthaired cat.

Prediction of parturition date

During early and mid pregnancy in the bitch and queen, the internal diameter of the gestational sac may be measured and used to predict the number of days to parturition. In late pregnancy the gestational sac loses its spherical shape and is less easy to measure. A number of fetal dimensions may then be recorded as gestation progresses; biparietal head diameter has been found to be the most accurate parameter for estimation of gestational age in the bitch, and thus for prediction of parturition date, but body diameter or crown–rump length may also be used. Measurement of head diameter or body diameter may used to predict the parturition date in the queen.

Prediction of fetal numbers

Ultrasonography is not an accurate means of assessing fetal numbers in either the dog or cat, and accuracy diminishes as litter size increases. If an approximate estimate of litter size is required, then this is most readily achieved between 25 and 35 days' gestation, when the gestational sacs are large enough to be clearly seen but remain separate from each other. However, embryonic resorption or fetal loss may subsequently occur, so estimation of final litter size can only be approximate.

Abnormalities

Embryonic or fetal loss

Death of the embryo before day 25 of gestation leads to a collapse of the normally spherical gestational sac. The contents may become echoic and the wall may thicken. The embryo itself becomes indistinct and no heartbeat is visible. In the bitch, dead embryos usually resorb, although a focal thickening of the uterus may persist at the site of resorption until the end of gestation. In the queen, although the dead embryo progressively decreases in size, the surrounding membranes and fluid may persist and even increase in volume until the end of gestation.

Late fetal death is recognized by the absence of a fetal heartbeat and of any fetal movements. The fetal structures become less distinct as disintegration occurs, and the surrounding fetal fluids become echogenic and reduced in volume. If gas forms within or around the fetus, then echogenic foci with streams of reverberations may be seen. However, gas as a result of fetal death may be easier to recognize radiographically.

Fetal distress

The normal fetal heart rate is around twice the maternal heart rate. Slowing of the fetal heart rate is an indicator of fetal hypoxia and thus fetal distress. This can be a useful parameter in trying to determine whether intervention is appropriate in an overdue pregnancy or a prolonged parturition, although other factors including the wellbeing of the bitch or queen are also relevant.

Fetal development

Whilst a wide range of developmental abnormalities may occur in the dog or cat, these are rarely diagnosed *in utero*. A case report (Allen *et al.*, 1989) described the ultrasonographic diagnosis of hydrops fetalis in a Bichon Frise bitch.

Uterine torsion

Uterine torsion is a rare but serious condition, which may occur in cats and dogs. Although torsion of the non-gravid uterus may occur, most reported cases in cats occur in mid to late pregnancy. Ultrasonographic examination is likely to reveal fetal death (see above), whilst the uterine wall may appear thickened and of increased echogenicity. Vascular perfusion of the affected segment of the uterus would be expected to be reduced or absent. In the bitch, most published reports of uterine torsion do not involve pregnant animals.

Post-partum uterus

In the immediate post-partum period, the uterus remains enlarged, due to both residual fluid contents and thickening of the uterine wall. However, the uterus should then progressively reduce in size as involution takes place. A study of 6 normal queens post-partum (Ferretti *et al.*, 2000) showed a mean total uterine thickness of 16.5 mm on day 1, whilst on day 14 the mean total uterine thickness was 6.2 mm, with individual wall thickness of 2.1 mm. Involution was considered ultrasonographically complete by 24 days post-partum. In the bitch, normal uterine involution (Figure 16.5) is reported to take a little longer. Involution is usually largely complete within 3–4 weeks, although focal enlargements may persist at placental sites for up to 15 weeks (Yeager and Concannon, 1990; Pharr and Post, 1992).

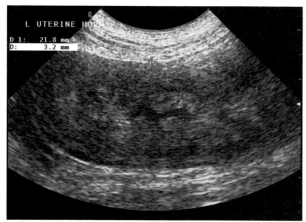

16.5 One uterine horn of a Great Dane bitch, which had undergone a Caesarean operation 5 days previously. The uterus is involuting well, with residual luminal fluid at a minimum, but remains enlarged with an overall diameter of approximately 2 cm.

Uterine diseases

Pyometra

Pyometra results in the accumulation of fluid within the uterine lumen. This fluid may be anechoic (Figure 16.6) or variably echoic (Figure 16.7), and

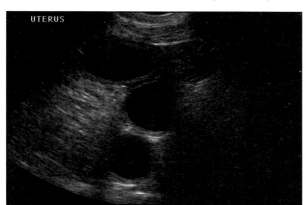

16.6 Transverse section through the distended uterus of a 9-year-old German Shepherd Dog presented for persistent vaginal bleeding since oestrus. The uterus contains fluid with few echoes. The final diagnosis was pyometra.

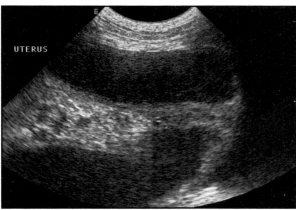

16.7 Rough Collie bitch with pyometra. The uterine horns are distended with fluid, which contains echoes that could be seen to swirl in real-time images.

may contain amorphous accumulations of debris. The uterine wall may appear thickened or be thin and barely visible; however, when the wall is visible, it may be distinguished from intestinal wall by the lack of visible layering and the absence of peristaltic activity. Mucometra, hydrometra and haematometra are also characterized by intraluminal uterine fluid, but cannot be distinguished from pyometra based on ultrasonographic criteria alone.

Cystic endometrial hyperplasia

Cystic endometrial hyperplasia (CEH) most commonly develops as a result of prolonged exposure of the endometrium to progesterone. Although cats are not generally spontaneous ovulators, and thus might be expected to have a lower incidence of CEH than the bitch, in fact there is a significant incidence of CEH in the older queen. In both dogs and cats with CEH, the uterine wall becomes thickened and irregular (Figure 16.8), and proliferation of the endometrial glands may result in multiple tiny cystic lesions within the uterine wall (Figure 16.9). There is sometimes a small volume of fluid within the uterine lumen. CEH may progress to pyometra or mucometra.

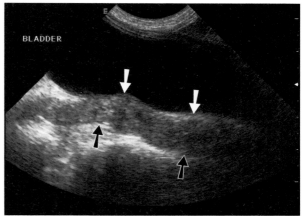

16.8 Sagittal image of the caudal abdomen of a 13-year-old entire Cocker Spaniel bitch, presented with a persistent vaginal discharge since oestrus 2 months previously. There is irregular thickening of the uterus (arrowed), which lies dorsal to the bladder. The uterus is also mildly heterogeneous in echogenicity.

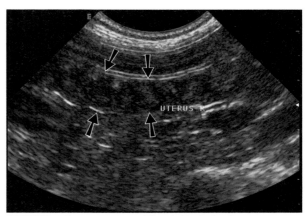

16.9 Ultrasonogram of the right uterine horn (arrowed) of a 10-year-old Cocker Spaniel bitch with CEH. Note the multiple small hypoechoic foci within the thickened horn.

175

Uterine stump lesions

The uterine stump normally lies between the bladder and descending colon, and is usually a slender, inconspicuous structure. Images of the uterine stump in the days immediately following ovariohysterectomy may show an irregular mass-like lesion of mixed echogenicity around the stump (Figure 16.10). Such a mass is likely to represent a blood clot and/or sterile surgical reaction at the site, and should progressively decrease in size.

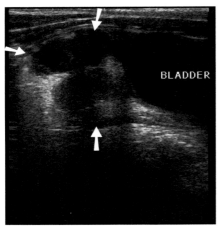

16.10 A 3-year-old Springer Spaniel crossbred dog presented with pyrexia of unknown origin. The bitch had undergone ovariohysterectomy 5 days previously. A mass of mixed echogenicity (arrowed) is visible cranial to the bladder. The mass was considered most likely to be a result of the recent surgery, and thus an incidental finding.

When a mass is detected in the region of the uterine stump without a history of surgery in the preceding few days, then a stump abscess or granuloma (Figure 16.11), or less commonly a neoplasm, should be considered. The presence of localized fluid and hyperechoic fat around the lesion is suggestive of an inflammatory process, but differentiation of inflammatory and neoplastic lesions is not usually possible using ultrasonographic findings alone. Enlargement of the medial iliac lymph nodes may be seen whether the disease process is inflammatory or neoplastic.

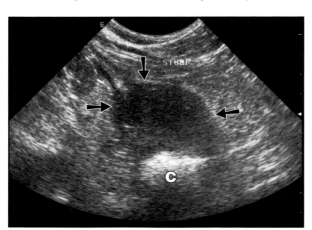

16.11 A 10-month-old neutered Border Collie bitch presented with pyrexia and lethargy. A rounded hypoechoic mass (arrowed) in the caudal abdomen, ventral to the colon (C), was identified. The mass was confirmed as a uterine stump granuloma.

Neoplasia

Uterine neoplasms are not common in dogs and cats. When they occur, they may be benign or malignant, of variable size, and of uniform or complex echogenicity. The histological type cannot be determined from the ultrasonographic appearance, although a lack of distinct margins may indicate local infiltration, and enlarged, rounded medial iliac lymph nodes may signal metastatic spread. Benign uterine polyps can occur, and may be small structures outlined by fluid within the lumen or large masses. Vaginal masses may be imaged ultrasonographically if they extend cranial to the pubic brim (Figure 16.12).

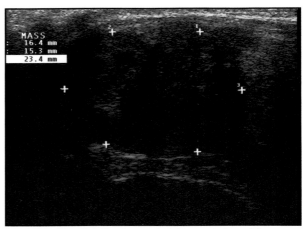

16.12 This ill defined, rounded, hypoechoic, mildly heterogeneous mass in the caudal abdomen of an 11-year-old entire Cocker Spaniel bitch was confirmed as a vaginal mass, which extended just cranial to the pubic brim.

References and further reading

Allen WE, England GCW and White KB (1989) Hydrops foetalis diagnosed by real time ultrasonography in a Bichon Frise bitch. *Journal of Small Animal Practice* **30**, 465–467

Ferretti LM, Newell SM, Graham JP *et al*. (2000) Radiographic and ultrasonographic evaluation of the normal feline postpartum uterus. *Veterinary Radiology and Ultrasound* **41**, 287–291

Luvoni GC and Grioni A (2000) Determination of gestational age in medium and small size bitches using ultrasonographic fetal measurements. *Journal of Small Animal Practice* **41**, 292–294

Pharr JW and Post K (1992) Ultrasonography and radiology of the canine postpartum uterus. *Veterinary Radiology and Ultrasound* **33**, 35–50

Thilagar S, Yew YC, Dhaliwal GK *et al*. (2005) Uterine horn torsion in a pregnant cat. *The Veterinary Record* **157**, 558–560

Voges AK and Neuwirth L (1996) Ultrasound diagnosis – cystic uterine hyperplasia. Veterinary Radiology and Ultrasound 37, 131–132

Yeager AE and Concannon PW (1990) Serial ultrasonographic appearance of post partum uterine involution in Beagle dogs. *Theriogenology* **34**, 523–533

Yeager AE, Mohammed HO, Meyers-Wallen V *et al*. (1992) Ultrasonographic appearance of the uterus, placenta, fetus and fetal membranes throughout accurately timed pregnancy in Beagles. *American Journal of Veterinary Research* **53**, 342–351

Zambelli D and Prati F (2006) Ultrasonography for pregnancy diagnosis and evaluation in queens. *Theriogenology* **66**, 135–144

Video extras

- **Normal uterus in a dog**
- **4-week pregnancy in a cat**
- **4-week pregnancy in a Jack Russell Terrier**

Access via QR code or bsavalibrary.com/ultrasound_16

17

Ovaries and testes

Gawain Hammond

Ovaries

Indications

Indications for ultrasonography of the ovaries include:

- Derangement of the normal oestrous cycle (e.g. prolonged oestrus or anoestrus)
- Investigation of hormonal disorders such as diabetes mellitus and acromegaly, which may be linked to progesterone secretion during the luteal phase
- Investigation of an abdominal mass that may have an ovarian origin.

In addition, the use of ultrasonography may be considered if the neutering history of the patient is unknown; however, it may be easier to identify the uterus than the ovaries.

Value of ultrasonography compared with radiography and advanced imaging techniques

Ultrasonography is the most convenient imaging modality for the investigation of ovarian disease in small animals. Unless there is severe enlargement and/or mineralization of the ovarian tissue, the ovaries are extremely unlikely to be visualized on abdominal radiography. Whilst the ovaries may be seen on computed tomography (CT) or magnetic resonance imaging (MRI), the cost, limited availability and requirement for deep sedation or anaesthesia for these modalities limits their use in practice.

Imaging technique

The patient may be positioned in either dorsal or lateral recumbency, and the hair coat should be clipped (ideally) or soaked down over the area of the kidneys on both sides. The ovaries are peritoneal organs located caudally to the kidneys and close to the abdominal wall. The blood supply to the ovaries arises directly from the aorta caudal to the renal arteries, whilst the ovarian veins drain into the left renal vein (left ovary) or directly into the caudal vena cava (right ovary). The left and right ovaries are found by identifying the ipsilateral kidney and then interrogating the area caudal and ventral to the caudal pole of the kidney (Figure 17.1). This should be performed in both transverse and sagittal planes.

Ultrasonographic investigation of the ovaries is best performed with a high frequency transducer. Due to the superficial position of the ovaries, optimal

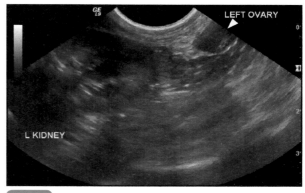

17.1 Normal left ovary located caudal to left kidney.

images are likely to be obtained with a linear transducer due to the excellent near-field resolution. However, in some patients use of a linear transducer may be limited by the conformation or the presence of gas in the adjacent gastrointestinal tract; in these cases a microconvex or curvilinear array transducer may be required. Not infrequently, the ovaries cannot be visualized due to interference by the gastrointestinal tract contents or due to the large amount of fat in the surrounding ovarian pedicle.

Normal ultrasonographic appearance

The ovaries are ovoid structures of about 1.5 x 0.7 x 0.5 cm in the dog, and slightly smaller in the cat. Although the ovary has a medulla and a cortex, it is difficult to clearly distinguish these on an ultrasonogram (Figure 17.2). However, the ultrasonographic appearance of the ovary does vary during the

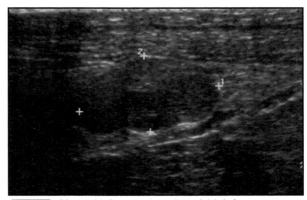

17.2 Normal left ovary in a dog. A high frequency linear array transducer was used to examine the superficially located ovary.

oestrous cycle, and the stages of the cycle and appearance of the ovary are summarized in Figure 17.3. It should be noted that the detection of ovulation in the dog using ultrasonography is of debatable accuracy, and requires serial scanning during oestrus. Even then the ultrasonographic appearance of the early corpus luteum is very similar to that of the ripe follicle.

Oestrous cycle stage	Ovarian changes	Ultrasonographic appearance
Anoestrus		Small, ovoid. Echogenicity similar to renal cortex
Early pro-oestrus	Developing follicular cysts (small)	Similar to anoestrus
Pro-oestrus (days 2–7)	Enlarging follicular cysts. May approach approximately 1 cm in diameter as ovulation nears	Increasing size, irregular shape as cysts enlarge. Identification of cysts. Many small cysts may give hyperechoic appearance
Ovulation		Decrease in number of visible cysts
Dioestrus	Development of corpus luteum	Hypoechoic 6 days following ovulation, returning to more rounded shape. Anechoic to hypoechoic corpus luteum may also be identified

17.3 Correlation of the changes in the ovary during the oestrous cycle with ultrasonographic appearance.

Ovarian cystic disease

Ovarian cysts typically have a rounded, well defined appearance with anechoic content, and may show distal acoustic enhancement (Figure 17.4). Cysts may be solitary or multiple, and be variable in size, although the ovary often shows generalized enlargement. Cysts may be follicular or luteal, but ultrasonography cannot distinguish between the forms. Follicular cysts may be associated with prolonged oestrus, and luteal cysts may be implicated in extended anoestrus. Cysts are often seen in conjunction with uterine diseases such as cystic endometrial hyperplasia and pyometra.

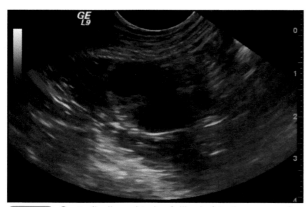

17.4 Cysts (believed to be follicular) in the ovary of a dog.

Ovarian neoplasia

Ovarian tumours fall into four broad categories:

- Epithelial cell neoplasia (carcinomas, cystadenomas, adenocarcinomas and papillary carcinomas)
- Germ cell neoplasia (dysgerminoma, teratoma and teratocarcinoma)
- Sex-cord stromal neoplasia (granulosa cell tumours)
- Metastatic neoplasia.

Ultrasonographically, the tumour appears as a mass in the area of the ovary, and the architecture may be largely solid, largely cystic, or heterogeneous and complex (Figure 17.5). In addition, in some ovarian tumours (especially teratomas) areas of mineralization with distal acoustic shadowing may be identified within the mass (Figure 17.6).

Other ovarian diseases

Ovarian haematomas and hydrovarium are rarely reported conditions of the ovary, which may be identified on ultrasonographic examination. In addition, ovarian stump granulomas have been reported following ovariohysterectomy, producing complex mass lesions seen in the area of the ovary on ultrasonographic examination.

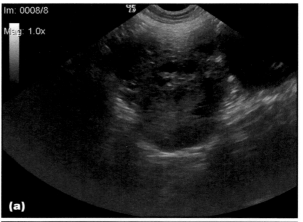

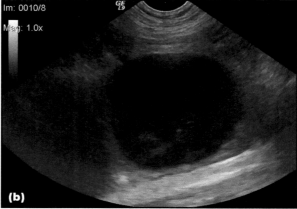

17.5 Granulosa cell tumour in the ovary of a dog showing **(a)** solid and **(b)** cystic components.

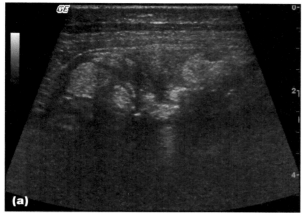

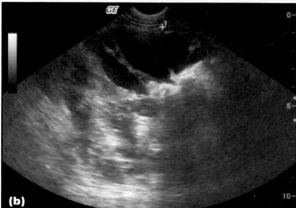

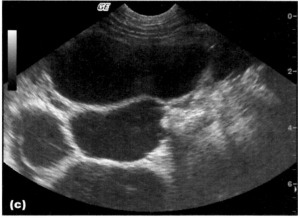

17.6 Teratoma with a highly complex nature in the ovary of a dog. **(a)** Solid components.
(b) Mineralized tissue with distal acoustic shadowing.
(c) Cystic components.

Testes

Indications

Indications for ultrasonography of the testes include:

- When there is evidence of prostatic or urinary tract disease or reproductive dysfunction
- Endocrine dysfunction
- Testicular enlargement
- Testicular mass
- Testicular or scrotal pain
- Investigation of cryptorchidism
- As part of the diagnostic work-up in cases of infertility.

Value of ultrasonography compared with radiography and advanced imaging techniques

Ultrasonography provides a quick and convenient method for examining the scrotal testes, and is generally possible without patient sedation. Radiography, CT and MRI are unlikely to offer any significant benefits in the examination of the descended testis; however, CT could be considered in cases of cryptorchidism where the undescended testis cannot be located by conventional imaging or palpation. CT may also be useful in the investigation of more disseminated systemic disease associated with testicular abnormalities. Thoracic radiography should be performed in cases with suspected testicular neoplasia (although distant metastasis from testicular neoplasia is uncommon), but radiography is unlikely to offer much information on the testes themselves that cannot be obtained by ultrasonography.

Imaging technique

For the descended testes, the ultrasound transducer is simply applied to the scrotal skin, with the testis immobilized manually. A high frequency linear probe is optimal, as this allows greater coverage of the testicular parenchyma than a microconvex or phased array probe. In addition, due to the thin layer of scrotal skin interposed between the testis and the transducer, a stand-off pad may improve visualization of the testicular parenchyma. Colour Doppler ultrasonography is useful for assessing blood flow through the testicular parenchyma.

Normal ultrasonographic appearance

The normal testis has a central hyperechoic mediastinum (Figure 17.7a), which has a linear appearance in sagittal plane images, with the surrounding parenchyma having a medium echogenicity. The tunics give a thin hyperechoic outer margin. The epididymis lies mainly around the dorsal aspect of the testis, with the tail caudally and the head craniodorsally (Figure 17.7b). The tail of the epididymis is hypoechoic compared with the normal testis, and the body and head are isoechoic compared with the testicular parenchyma. The epididymis can be visualized in both sagittal and transverse planes.

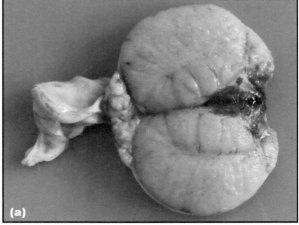

17.7 **(a)** Section through the testis of a dog showing the central mediastinum. (continues) ▶

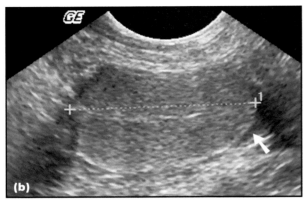

17.7 (continued) **(b)** Ultrasonogram of a normal testis in a dog showing the faintly hyperechoic central mediastinum and hypoechoic epididymis (arrowed) wrapping around the far side of the testis.

Testicular abnormalities

Testicular descent

During development of the reproductive tract, the testes are drawn through the inguinal canal into the scrotal sac from their original intra-abdominal location by contraction of the gubernaculums. When testicular descent fails, the cryptorchid testis may be found within the abdominal cavity (Figure 17.8) or, more commonly, in the area of the inguinal canal (often between the superficial inguinal ring and the scrotum). Therefore, in cases of cryptorchidism, these areas should be interrogated during the ultrasonographic examination. However, the retained testis is often small and flaccid, and may be easily missed or mistaken for other structures such as inguinal lymph nodes.

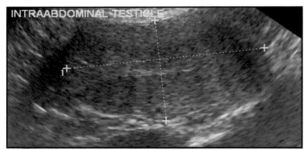

17.8 Intra-abdominal cryptorchid testicle. This mass can be recognized as a testicle due to the central hyperechoic mediastinum.

Testicular neoplasia

Testicular neoplasia is rare in the cat. In the dog most tumours fall into one of three categories:

- Sertoli cell tumour (most common)
- Seminoma
- Interstitial or Leydig cell tumour.

They are most common in older dogs and the majority do not metastasize (<10% of seminomas and Sertoli cell tumours, and almost no interstitial cell tumours show metastatic spread). The ultrasonographic appearance of testicular neoplasia is not indicative of the tumour type. A mass of mixed echogenicity may be seen within the testicular parenchyma, possibly distorting or obliterating the mediastinum (Figure 17.9). Alternatively, with very large tumours, the entire testicle may be occupied by neoplastic tissue (Figure 17.10). Multiple nodules are common and the testis is frequently enlarged. The contralateral testicle may atrophy (particularly with Sertoli cell tumours). Cryptorchid testes are predisposed to development of neoplasia, and in these cases a rounded heterogeneous mass may be found in the area of the inguinal canal or within the abdominal cavity (Figure 17.11).

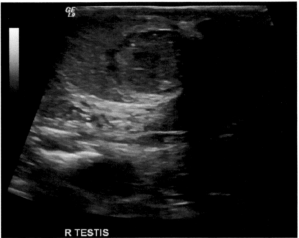

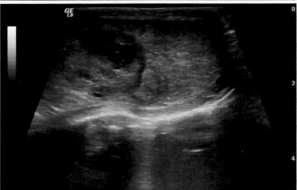

17.9 Sertoli cell tumour of the testis showing heterogeneous echogenicity. Note that the tumour has caused distortion of the normal testicular architecture.

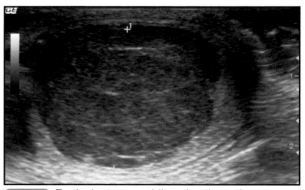

17.10 Testicular tumour obliterating the entire parenchyma.

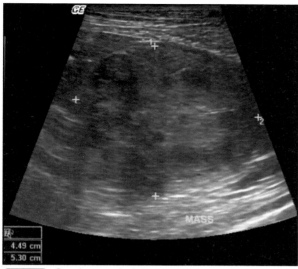

17.11 Caudoventral abdominal mass identified as a Sertoli cell tumour in a retained testicle.

Orchitis

Orchitis (inflammation of the testis) may arise from infectious agents ascending the vas deferens, and may be associated with prostatic or lower urinary tract infections. Orchitis generally results in a hypoechoic patchy appearance to the testicular parenchyma (Figure 17.12). The testicle may appear swollen, with a cross-section that is more rounded than usual. Abscessation can also occur, with an irregular cavitated area within the testicular parenchyma. Orchitis is frequently seen in conjunction with epididymitis (see below). Chronic orchitis may lead to testicular atrophy, with the parenchyma having a heterogeneous echotexture. Inflammation of the testicle and/or epididymis is frequently associated with peritesticular fluid or oedema of the scrotal wall.

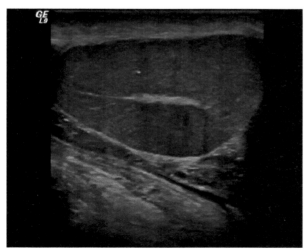

17.12 Orchitis in the testicle of a dog. Note the diffusely hypoechoic testis, resulting in increased prominence of the mediastinum. Culture following castration confirmed infection with *Escherichia coli*. Note the hyperechoic and thickened scrotal skin in the near-field due to the associated scrotal oedema.

Testicular torsion

Torsion of the testis typically results in an enlarged testicle with diffuse hypoechogenicity of the parenchyma and swelling of the epididymis and spermatic cord. On colour Doppler ultrasonography no blood flow is identified in the abnormal testis. A small volume of peritesticular fluid may be noted.

Other testicular abnormalities

Testicular cysts and haematomas have been reported. Cysts typically appear as rounded thin-walled structures with anechoic content and possible distal acoustic enhancement. A haematoma may have the appearance of a heterogeneous nodule, and could appear similar to a testicular neoplasm.

Localized testicular infarcts may occur as a result of injury or disease. In common with infarcts in other parenchymal organs, recent infarcts may appear hypoechoic or isoechoic to the normal testicular parenchyma, whilst older, organized infarcts are typically hyperechoic and wedge-shaped.

Epididymitis

Epididymitis arises from the same routes as orchitis (from an infection of the vas deferens, lower urinary tract or prostate gland), and can occur in the absence of orchitis. Typical ultrasonographic findings are dilatation of the epididymis, which has a more hypoechoic appearance than normal, and possible dilatation of the ductus deferens (Figure 17.13). In addition, peritesticular fluid is also commonly identified.

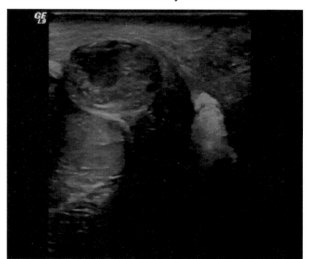

17.13 Ultrasonogram of the same dog as in Figure 17.12 showing epididymitis. Note the marked enlargement of the head of the epididymis and dilatation of the epididymal duct.

Scrotal disease

Disease affecting the scrotal wall generally presents ultrasonographically as thickening and hyperechogenicity (especially with oedema) (see Figure 17.12). In cases of inflammatory disease, peritesticular fluid may also be seen.

Hydrocele, or accumulation of fluid within the scrotal sac, is uncommon in the dog. However, it may occur secondary to conditions resulting in fluid accumulation within the peritoneal cavity (i.e. a dog with ascites may also have hydrocele), or be localized to the scrotal sac (e.g. due to venous obstruction). Haematocele refers to blood within the scrotal sac; trauma is the most common cause, but any condition leading to haemorrhage should be considered.

Herniation of abdominal organs (especially small intestinal loops) into the scrotal sac via the inguinal canal can easily be detected using ultrasonography, particularly if intestinal wall layering or peristalsis can be identified. Rarely, scrotal haematomas may be identified following castration; these typically have an irregular shape and a heterogeneous echotexture, and no blood flow is evident on colour Doppler ultrasonography.

References and further reading

Cooley DM and Waters DJ (2001) Tumours of the male reproductive system. In: *Small Animal Clinical Oncology, 3rd edn*, ed. SJ Withrow and EG MacEwen, pp. 478–489. WB Saunders, Philadelphia

Costello M (2009) The male reproductive system. In: *BSAVA Manual of Canine and Feline Abdominal Imaging*, ed. R O'Brien and F Barr, pp 237–245. BSAVA Publications, Gloucester

Davidson AP, Nyland TG and Tsutsui T (1986) Pregnancy diagnosis with ultrasound in the domestic cat. *Veterinary Radiology and Ultrasound* **27**, 109–114

Dennis R, Kirberger RM, Wrigley RH and Barr FJ (2001) *Handbook of Small Animal Radiological Differential Diagnosis*. WB Saunders, Philadelphia

Diez-Bru N, Garcia-Real I, Martinez EM *et al.* (1998) Ultrasonographic appearance of ovarian tumours in 10 dogs. *Veterinary Radiology and Ultrasound* **39**, 226–233

Durant BS, Ravida N, Spady T and Cheng A (2006) New technologies for the study of carnivore reproduction. *Theriogenology* **66**, 1729–1736

Dyce KM, Sack WO and Wensing CJG (2010) The pelvis and reproductive organs of the carnivores. In: *Textbook of Veterinary Anatomy, 4th edn*, ed. KM Dyce *et al.*, pp. 429–441. WB Saunders, Philadelphia

England GCW (1999) Diseases of the reproductive system. In: *Textbook of Small Animal Medicine*, ed. JW Dunn, pp. 574–611. WB Saunders, Philadelphia

Feeney DA and Johnston GR (2007) The uterus, ovaries and testes. In: *Textbook of Veterinary Diagnostic Imaging, 5th edn*, ed. DE Thrall, pp. 738–749, WB Saunders, Philadelphia

Gunzel-Apel AR, Mohrke C and Poulsen Nautrup C (2001) Colour-coded and pulsed Doppler sonography of the canine testis, epididymis and prostate gland: physiological and pathological findings. *Reproduction in Domestic Animals* **36**, 236–240

Hammond G (2009) The female reproductive system. In: *BSAVA Manual of Canine and Feline Abdominal Imaging*, ed. R O'Brien and F Barr, pp. 222–236. BSAVA Publications, Gloucester.

Hecht S, King R, Tidwell AS and Gorman SC (2004) Ultrasound diagnosis: intra-abdominal torsion of a non-neoplastic testicle in a cryptorchid dog. *Veterinary Radiology and Ultrasound* **45**, 58–61

Johnston GR, Feeney DA, Johnston SD and O'Brien TD (1991) Ultrasonographic features of testicular neoplasia in dogs: 16 cases (1980–1988). *Journal of the American Veterinary Medical Association* **198**, 1779–1784

Johnston GR, Feeney DA, Rivers B and Walter PA (1991) Diagnostic imaging of the male canine reproductive organs: methods and limitations. *Veterinary Clinics of North America: Small Animal Practice* **21**, 553–589

Klein MK (2001) Tumours of the female reproductive system. In: *Small Animal Clinical Oncology, 3rd edn*, ed. SJ Withrow and EG MacEwen, pp. 445–454. WB Saunders, Philadelphia

Mattoon JS and Nyland TG (2001) *Small Animal Diagnostic Ultrasound, 2nd edn*. WB Saunders, Philadelphia

Nagashima Y, Hoshi K, Tanaka R *et al.* (2000) Ovarian and retroperitoneal teratomas in a dog. *Journal of Veterinary Medical Science* **62**, 793–795

Rivers W and Johnston GR (1991) Diagnostic imaging of the reproductive organs of the bitch: methods and limitations. *Veterinary Clinics of North America: Small Animal Practice* **21**, 437–466

Sforna M, Brachalente C, Lepri E and Mechelli L (2003) Canine ovarian tumours: a retrospective study of 49 cases. *Veterinary Research Communications* **27(Suppl 1)** 359–361

18

Eyes

Susanne A.E.B. Boroffka

Indications

Ultrasonography has become a standard imaging modality in ophthalmology and is routinely used as the first imaging technique for evaluation of ocular and orbital structures. Ultrasonography allows:

- Detection and evaluation of intraocular or orbital neoplastic and non-neoplastic lesions
- Detection of intraocular changes such as lens luxation and/or retinal detachment in opaque eyes
- Measurement of the dimensions of the lens, anterior chamber and globe
- Evaluation of traumatic injuries to the eye and orbit.

A-mode ultrasonography, Doppler techniques and ultrasound biomicroscopy are also used to examine ocular and orbital structures for clinical and research purposes.

Value of ultrasonography compared with radiography and advanced imaging techniques

Conventional radiography provides limited diagnostic information about the eye and orbit. Disruption of the bony structures of the orbit may be appreciated to some extent on good quality radiographs. Radiopaque foreign material may be visible radiographically, and multiple radiographic views allow an approximate three-dimensional (3D) localization.

Ultrasonography, computed tomography (CT) and magnetic resonance imaging (MRI) are excellent and complementary cross-sectional diagnostic modalities for imaging the ocular and orbital structures. The choice of the imaging modality depends on availability, experience of the operator and cost. Ultrasonography is a non-ionizing and cost-effective imaging technique, which can be performed without general anaesthesia. B-mode ultrasonography provides biometric and detailed morphological and vascular information about the ocular structures, but information on the orbital structures is limited. Fine-needle aspiration may be performed under ultrasound guidance.

CT and MRI require general anaesthesia, are more expensive and their availability is limited. However, both techniques provide outstanding morphological detail of the orbital structures. MRI provides excellent contrast resolution of the soft tissues (with no radiation exposure) and has multiplanar imaging capability; whereas CT is superior for imaging the bony structures and mineralization in the soft tissues.

Imaging technique

Ocular structures

The patient is positioned in either sternal or lateral recumbency with the diseased eye uppermost. It is preferable to avoid sedation of the patient, so that rotation and retraction of the eye is minimized. After topical corneal anaesthesia, the eyelids are retracted manually and the transducer is placed gently on to the corneal surface in conjunction with water-soluble lubricating acoustic gel. After the examination the gel should be flushed from the eye.

B-mode ocular ultrasonography is performed using a high resolution 10–20 MHz sector or linear transducer. Both eyes are imaged in horizontal, vertical and transverse planes. The entire globe is evaluated, beginning from the central axis (an imaginary line from the centre of the cornea to the centre of the scleroretinal rim) and then angling the transducer gently from one side to the other in each scan plan. The following biometric measurements are routinely obtained:

- Anteroposterior depth of the eye, including the scleroretinal rim
- Anteroposterior depth of the anterior chamber
- Anteroposterior depth and mediolateral/dorsoventral diameter of the lens.

Orbital structures

An orbital ultrasonographic examination can be performed using either the corneal contact method (described above) or the temporal approach. With the temporal approach the patient is positioned in lateral recumbency with the diseased orbit uppermost. The procedure can be performed with or without sedation. The temporal fossa is shaved caudal to the orbital ligament and a high frequency (7.5–8.5 MHz) phased or curved array transducer is used.

Both eyes are imaged in longitudinal and transverse planes. For longitudinal images, the transducer is aligned rostrocaudally, with a slight rotation of the caudal sector medially to adjust to the normal course of the periorbita, including the optic nerve. The transducer is then angled gently medially and laterally for evaluation of the entire orbit. For transverse images, the transducer is rotated 90 degrees placed caudal to the orbital ligament, and then moved gently caudally. Longitudinal images provide most information on the orbital soft tissues, whereas the bony orbit can be evaluated more clearly on transverse images. The zygomatic salivary gland may be imaged from the area ventral to the zygomatic arch and caudoventral to the globe.

Normal ultrasonographic appearance

Ocular structures
The normal canine and feline eye is a nearly spherical, well delineated structure with anechoic contents and echogenic interfaces with the cornea, iris, lenticular capsules and scleroretinal rim (Figure 18.1). Depending on the breed, the eye is between 18 and 23 mm in diameter. The cornea appears as two discrete parallel hyperechoic curvilinear lines, representing ultrasound beam reflection from the anterior epithelial and posterior endothelial corneal layers, with the anechoic stroma inbetween. The anterior part of the sclera is visible as a continuation of the cornea without the anechoic stroma, resulting in a homogeneous echogenic appearance.

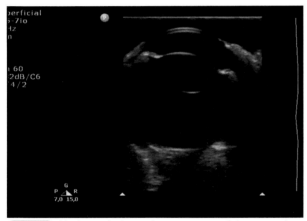

18.1 Horizontal plane ultrasonogram of the normal eye of a 5-year-old Standard Poodle.

The iridocorneal angle is formed by the corneoscleral junction and the iris, and represents the most important site for aqueous humour outflow (Figure 18.2). The anterior and posterior areas of the lenticular capsule are visible as discrete hyperechoic convex/concave curvilinear interfaces, lying symmetrically between the ciliary body. The lens is supported by zonular fibres, which appear as striations that attach to the lens contour. The normal lens nucleus is anechoic. The highly vascular ciliary body appears as a circumferential echogenic structure at the periphery of the lens and forms the ora serrata at the junction with the choroid. The iris is

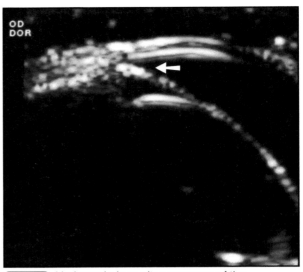

18.2 Horizontal plane ultrasonogram of the iridocorneal angle (arrowed) of the normal eye of a 5-year-old Standard Poodle.

an elongated echogenic contractile structure, continuous with the ciliary body and located anterior to the lens. The central opening in the iris, the pupil, is circular in dogs and elliptical in cats. It has a variable size depending on the amount of light shining on the eye. It is best imaged using a dorsal or lateral approach to the conjunctiva.

The anterior chamber is delineated by the posterior aspect of the cornea, the iris and the anterior lens capsule, and is distended by anechoic aqueous humour. The posterior chamber is a triangular, anechoic space bound by the anterior lenticular surface, iris and ciliary body. The anechoic vitreal body fills the vitreous cavity and attaches primarily at the region of the optic disc and at the ora serrata. The echogenic choroid, retina and sclera cannot be identified separately and are referred to as the scleroretinal rim. The optic disc may be visible in the ventrolateral aspect of the posterior wall of the globe, as an indistinct focal, slightly recessed and hyperechoic area.

Orbital structures
The optic nerve appears as an undulating, hypoechoic linear structure bound by hyperechoic lines extending caudoventrally from the optic disc towards the optic foramen. The extraocular rectus muscles and retractor bulbi are very thin hypoechoic bands and are visible dorsal, ventral, lateral and medial to the optic nerve. The oblique muscles have not been identified with ultrasonography. The shape of the muscles may change with eye movement due to contraction or lengthening. The orbital fat is hyperechoic and visible between the extraocular muscles and optic nerve and surrounding the cone-shaped periorbita. The zygomatic salivary gland is located in the ventrolateral aspect of the orbit and appears as a slightly more hypoechoic structure than the ventromedially located medial pterygoid. The bony orbit is represented on ultrasonograms as a hyperechoic line with distal acoustic shadowing and interruptions for the optic canal and orbital fissure.

Intraocular abnormalities

Cornea

Corneal disease may be caused by inflammation, trauma, degeneration, oedema or neoplasia. Irrespective of the precise aetiology, there is a change in depth and/or echogenicity of the cornea. The cornea becomes thicker and the normally anechoic stroma becomes echogenic (Figure 18.3).

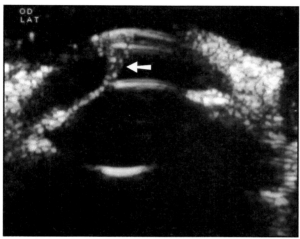

18.3 Horizontal plane ultrasonogram of the eye of a 3-year-old mixed-breed dog with corneal oedema following injury to the eye. There is thickening of the mid-region of the cornea with increased echogenicity of the corneal stroma. Note also the echogenic strand (arrowed) connecting the posterior aspect of the cornea with the anterior lens capsule.

Anterior chamber

An increased depth of the anterior chamber may be caused by glaucoma, posterior lens luxation or aphakia (absence of the lens). A shallower anterior chamber may be created artificially due to compression by the transducer, or may be due to anterior lens luxation caused by trauma, glaucoma or neoplasia. Cells and fibrin debris may be seen as echogenic foci moving within the aqueous of the anterior chamber. Free-moving masses may represent blood clots, perforated lens material or neoplasia arising from the iris, ciliary body or cornea. Doppler examination may be helpful for differentiation between vascularized and non-vascularized tissue.

Uveal tract
Cysts

Iridociliary cysts (Figure 18.4a) are usually congenital and may occur in both dogs and cats. Golden Retrievers, Great Danes, Rottweilers and Labrador Retrievers are predisposed. Depending on the location, these cysts may cause uveitis or glaucoma, but are usually incidental. Arising from the iris and/or ciliary body, the cysts may extend into the anterior and/or posterior chamber or the vitreous body, and may be attached to the cornea or free-floating. They appear as single or multiple, thin-walled, anechoic, round structures. Only the wall of the cyst is vascularized, which can be seen on Doppler examination (Figure 18.4b).

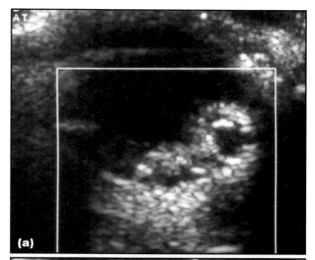
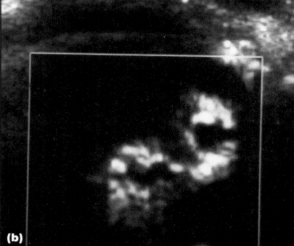

18.4 **(a)** Transverse image obtained from the dorsal aspect of the anterior section of the eye of a 10-year-old Domestic Shorthaired cat. Two cysts are visible at the anterior aspect of the iris, appearing as anechoic, round structures with an echogenic wall. **(b)** Power Doppler ultrasonogram showing only vascularization of the walls of the cysts and not of the centre.

Uveitis

Uveitis refers to inflammation of the uveal tract; in small animals most commonly the entire uveal tract (panuveitis) is involved. In some patients only the anterior (iriditis/iridocyclitis) or posterior (choroiditis/chorioretinitis) uvea are diseased. Ultrasonographically, the diseased structures appear thickened and more hypoechoic than normal. The aetiology may be either ocular or systemic. Ocular causes include corneal ulceration, lens-induced (immune-mediated or metabolic), ocular trauma or a primary ocular tumour. Systemic causes include bacteraemia (leptospirosis, brucellosis, *Borelia*), fungal (blastomycosis, cryptococcosis, coccidiomycosis, histoplasmosis), viraemia (distemper, infectious canine hepatitis) and septicaemia.

Neoplasia

Occasionally neoplasms may be identified which involve the uveal tract (see below).

Lens
Congenital
Many congenital abnormalities of the lens have been reported in a wide range of dog breeds, including:

- Aphakia (absence of the lens)
- Microphakia (abnormally small lens)
- Lenticonus (abnormally shaped lens)
- Lentiglobus (abnormally shaped lens)
- Coloboma (abnormally shaped lens)
- Vascular.

These changes seldom occur, but when they do they may be associated with other ocular changes, including retinal detachment or dysplasia, microphthalmia and microcornea. In cats sporadic cases have been reported in Siamese kittens. Ultrasonographically, aphakia, microphakia, lenticonus, lentiglobus and coloboma may be seen, possibly in combination with a small eye and/or retinal detachment. With posterior lenticonus the lens has a localized cone-shaped protrusion of the mid-region of the thin posterior capsule, which may appear irregular and thickened on an ultrasonogram. These changes may be associated with a retrolenticular membrane and a persistent hyperplastic primary vitreous, with or without a persistent hyaloid artery. In patients with vascular abnormalities, blood flow may be seen within the normally avascular lens with colour flow or power Doppler imaging.

Nuclear sclerosis
Nuclear sclerosis is often found in dogs >7 years old. This condition may be confused with cataracts, since the lens is no longer anechoic. However, on ultrasonography only a thin hyperechoic curvilinear line is seen running parallel with the lens capsule and the nucleus remains anechoic (Figure 18.5).

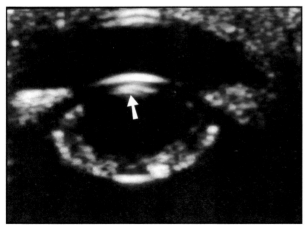

18.5 Horizontal plane ultrasonogram showing nuclear sclerosis in a 9-year-old mixed-breed dog. The nuclear sclerosis is visible as a curvilinear hyperechoic line running parallel with the anterior (arrowed) and posterior lens capsule.

Cataracts
A cataract is defined as any opacification of the lens and/or its capsule regardless of cause, location or size. In dogs, inherited congenital defects are the most common cause of cataracts, but nutritional deficiencies, toxic substances, uveal adhesions and diabetes mellitus may also cause cataracts. In cats, cataracts occur more often secondary to chronic inflammation and rarely because of an inherited abnormality. However, congenital cataracts have been described in Persian, British Shorthair, Himalayan and Birman cats, suggesting an autosomal recessive trait. Ultrasonographically, the echogenicity, shape and size of the lens may vary with the type and duration of the cataract. With cortical cataracts (anterior and posterior or equatorial) the anterior and posterior cortices of the lens become echogenic, and the entire capsule may be apparent (Figure 18.6ab). With nuclear cataracts, the central nucleus becomes echogenic and the entire lens may be involved. Diabetic or immature cataracts usually show an increased axial thickness of the lens, whereas hypermature cataracts may show a decreased axial depth. Prognosis in patients with posterior cataracts and irregularity is guarded because more complications during surgery may occur.

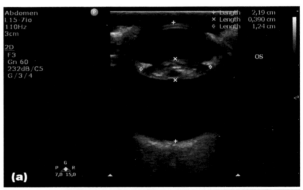

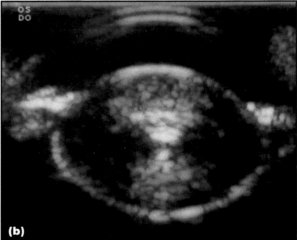

18.6 **(a)** Vertical plane ultrasonogram of the eye of a 1-year-old Golden Retriever with a juvenile cataract. Note the decreased anterior–posterior diameter (between the callipers) and the increased echogenicity of the lens nucleus. The other intraocular structures are within normal limits. Biometric measurements have been performed. **(b)** Horizontal plane ultrasonogram of the eye of a 5-year-old Cavalier King Charles Spaniel with diabetes mellitus and secondary cataract formation. Note the increased anterior–posterior diameter and the increased echogenicity of the lens nucleus.

Rupture

Lens rupture may occur anteriorly, posteriorly or peripherally, and may be associated with anterior uveitis, proliferation of granulation or fibrous tissue, and adherence to the pupil. Ultrasonographically, the lens capsule appears irregular and lenticular tissue is visible adjacent to the capsule (Figure 18.7).

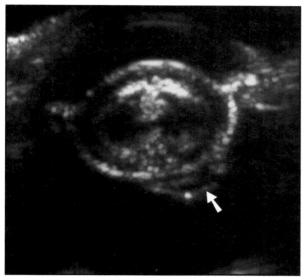

18.7 Vertical plane ultrasonogram of the eye of a 7-year-old Golden Retriever presented with a cataract. Note the increased echogenicity of the nucleus of the lens. There is a rupture of the posterior lens capsule indicated by the presence of lenticular tissue (arrowed) adjacent to the posterior lens capsule with interruption of the posterior lens capsule.

Luxation

In patients with subluxation of the lens, there is partial rupture of the lens zonule. The position of the lens may be asymmetrical, but is still posterior to the iris and anterior to the vitreous (Figure 18.8a). With complete lens luxation there is total rupture of the zonule, and the lens luxates anteriorly into the anterior chamber or posteriorly into the vitreal cavity (Figure 18.8b). The luxated lens receives no nutrition and is therefore often cataractous. Lens luxation may occur due to trauma, glaucoma, secondary to chronic uveitis (especially in cats), neoplasia, secondary to a hypermature cataract, senile zonular degeneration or hereditary predisposition. Potential complications of lens (sub-) luxation are corneal damage, corneal oedema, secondary glaucoma, anterior uveitis and retinal detachment.

Vitreous and scleroretinal rim

Ultrasonographic changes of the vitreous include changes in the shape of the eyeball, vitreous opacities (degeneration, asteroid hyalosis, synchysis scintillans, haemorrhage, inflammation), posterior vitreous detachment, persistent and hyperplastic primary vitreous and/or remnant of the hyaloid artery, retinal detachment, and presence of neoplasia or a foreign body. Alteration of the shape and size of the globe may be caused by developmental anomalies, trauma, endophthalmitis, intraocular mass lesions, glaucoma or pressure from orbital mass lesions.

Vitreal degeneration

Degenerative changes often occur in the vitreous of older patients and include:

- Asteroid hyalosis caused by calcium-containing lipids (pinpoint reflectors with faint small comet tails, which are dispersed throughout the vitreous)
- Synchysis scintillans caused by cholesterol crystals, which sink to the bottom of the liquefied vitreous body
- Vitreal degeneration (increase in echogenicity of the normal anechoic vitreous).

Vitreal degeneration is often seen during the presurgical cataract ultrasound examination, with the frequency depending on the cataract stage (in 100% of patients with hypermature cataracts). Fibrin tags, vitreal membranes and a detached vitreous may appear as faint or clear hyperechoic lines or curvilinear convex structures in the vitreal body. Vitreal membranes usually appear less echogenic than retinal detachments, but may be difficult to differentiate.

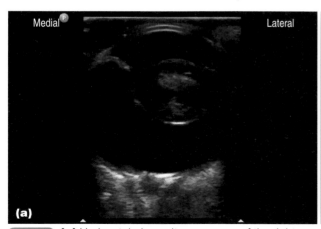
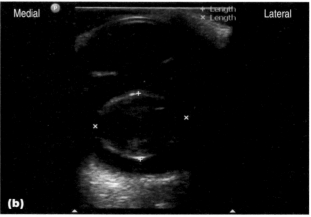

18.8 **(a)** Horizontal plane ultrasonogram of the right eye of an 8-year-old mixed-breed dog presented with cataracts and suspected lens luxation. Subluxation of the lens is indicated by its asymmetrical position within the anterior segment. The distance between the cornea and anterior lens capsule is wider at the medial aspect compared with the lateral aspect. **(b)** Horizontal plane ultrasonogram of the left eye. There is complete posterior luxation of the lens, which is located in the posterior chamber.

Haemorrhage

Haemorrhage may appear as multiple point-like echoes in a liquefied vitreous (Figure 18.9), but the appearance depends on the duration, severity and location of the bleeding. Acute haemorrhage may not be visible with ultrasonography for several days or until clots form. Vitreal haemorrhage is resolved slowly and a blood clot may present as a mass, mimicking a tumour. Fibrous strands may develop after resorption of the blood and can cause tractional retinal detachment. Haemorrhage is often traumatic in origin, although coagulopathies should be considered. A persistent hyaloid artery may bleed into the vitreous in young animals.

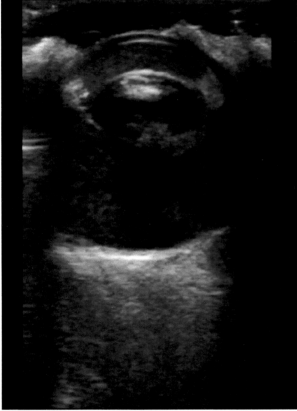

18.9 Ultrasonogram of the eye of a 9-year-old Golden Retriever presented with hyphaema. The anterior chamber and the vitreous body are echogenic due to the presence of blood cells. The echogenic structures visible within the anterior and posterior aspect of the lens are compatible with a cataract.

Retina

Many retinal diseases show no ultrasonographic changes. However, retinal detachment has a characteristic appearance. The retina is normally firmly attached to the optic nerve and the ora serrata, so in patients with retinal detachment, the retinal layers will always stay attached to these two points. Ultrasonographically, focal or entire retinal detachment is visible as a curvilinear hyperechoic line(s) separated from the choroid by anechoic or echogenic fluid. Focal retinal detachment can occur in various locations and may be only a few millimetres long. A total retinal detachment is V-shaped, and is often descriptively

referred to as 'seagull wings' or 'morning glory' (Figure 18.10). Over time the detached retinal membrane becomes thickened, rigid and more echogenic, and moves towards the centre of the vitreous (funnel retinal detachment). Echogenic subretinal fluid (Figure 18.11) may be caused by haemorrhage or exudate due to chorioretinitis. Causes for retinal detachment include trauma, inflammation, tumours or systemic hypertension. Patients with hypermature cataracts may develop retinal detachment due to traction and tearing caused by the shrinking lens.

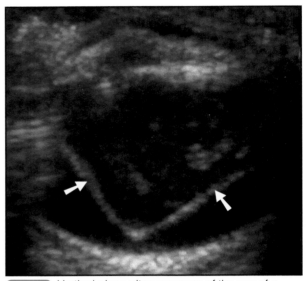

18.10 Vertical plane ultrasonogram of the eye of a 5-year-old Labrador Retriever with a cataract presented for preoperative evaluation. There is a total V-shaped retinal detachment (arrowed). Within the anterior segment of the eye, an oblique section of the complete opacified lens is visible.

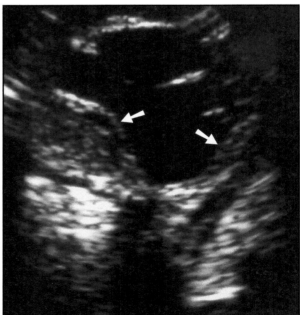

18.11 Horizontal plane ultrasonogram of the eye of a 6-year-old Boxer presented with glaucoma. There is an elevation of the retina visible on the medial and lateral aspects of the globe (arrowed). The subretinal material appears echogenic, compatible with subretinal bleeding.

Endophthalmitis and scleritis

Endophthalmitis is inflammation of all intraocular structures. The ultrasonographic appearance may be similar to haemorrhage, with echoes within either the vitreous or the echogenic subretinal fluid. In follow-up examinations the inflammatory echoes appear to become organized faster then those associated with haemorrhage and produce vitreous membranes more often.

Persistent hyperplastic tunica vasculosa lentis/hyperplastic primary vitreous

In this congenital disease, the primary vitreous (hyaloid artery and posterior tunica vasculosa lentis) fails to regress completely after birth. It has been reported to be an inherited disease in the Dobermann and Miniature Schnauzer, but has also been described in other breeds and in cats. The lens shows a hyperechoic nucleus with a triangular-shaped, echodense, retrolenticular structure (Figure 18.12a). A persistent hyaloid artery appears as a very thin or funnel-shaped retrolenticular hyperechoic strand, which is visible penetrating the anechoic vitreous from the retrolenticular tissue to the area of the optic nerve. Using colour or power Doppler imaging, blood flow may be evident in parts of the retina and the hyperechoic strand (Figure 18.12b). Concurrent microphthalmia, cataract formation and retrolenticular connective tissue have been reported in these patients.

Foreign bodies

The ultrasonographic appearance of an intraocular foreign body depends on the type and shape of the foreign material and its location. Most foreign bodies found in animals are plant materials (grass awns, wooden pieces), recognizable as hyperechoic structures with acoustic shadowing. However, not all foreign bodies show acoustic shadowing and normal intraocular structures may mimic foreign bodies. Metal, such as bullets, show the typical comet-ring artefact.

Neoplasia

Intraocular neoplasia occurs regularly in dogs and cats and may mimic or induce ocular inflammatory disease, and can cause hyphaema and/or secondary glaucoma. Early diagnosis is important for successful management and choice of therapy. Intraocular tumours may present as focal echogenic mass lesions or as diffuse infiltrative disease. They may arise from the conjunctiva, including the nictitating membrane, from the cornea, iris and ciliary body, or from the scleroretinal rim; the iris and ciliary body are the most common sites of origin. The iris is most often affected by limbal or uveal tract melanoma, whereas ciliary body neoplasia is more often caused by lymphoma, adenocarcinoma, adenoma, medulloepithelioma or metastatic disease. Limbal mass lesions (Figure 18.13a) may be evaluated ultrasonographically for depth and extension to the ciliary body or iris. Differentiation of neoplasms from blood clots and granulomas may be made by colour Doppler examination, since neoplasms are vascularized (Figure 18.13b).

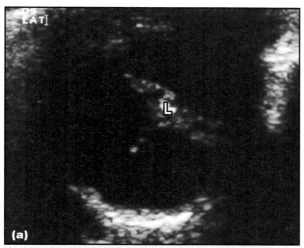

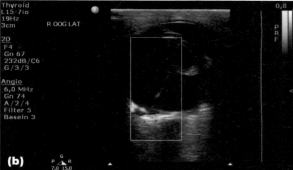

18.12 **(a)** Horizontal plane ultrasonogram of the eye of a 1-year-old Dobermann presented with a left-sided cataract and suspected microphthalmia. A small hyperechoic lens (L) is visible with a linear hyperechoic strand running from the posterior aspect of the lens to the optic nerve head. Note the triangular-shaped posterior lens capsule showing mild lenticonus. **(b)** Horizontal plane ultrasonogram of the eye of a 9-month-old mixed-breed dog with a cataract and suspected microphthalmia. There is a hyperechoic linear strand running from the posterior aspect of the lens to the optic nerve head. Note the increased echogenicity at the medial aspect of the posterior lens nucleus and the power Doppler signal within the hyperechoic strand. These findings are compatible with a cataract and patent hyaloid artery.

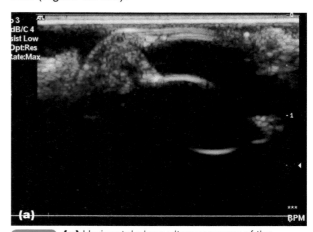

18.13 **(a)** Horizontal plane ultrasonogram of the anterior aspect of the eye of a 7-year-old Flat-coated Retriever. Note the echogenic thickening of the medial aspect of the iris, extending to the ciliary body. The echogenic and enlarged iris/ciliary body are compatible with neoplasia, such as melanoma or adenocarcinoma. (continues) ▶

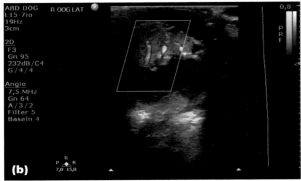

18.13 (continued) **(b)** Horizontal plane ultrasonogram of the eye of a 4-year-old Shih Tzu suspected of having a ciliary tumour. Colour flow Doppler demonstrates vascularization within a limbal mass at the lateral aspect of the ciliary body. Pathology confirmed a limbal melanoma.

Orbital abnormalities

The location and extent of a soft tissue or cystic lesion, deviation and/or changes in the shape of the globe and orbital structures, appearance of the normal orbital structures, and in some cases bone destruction may be evaluated ultrasonographically. Identification of an enlarged optic nerve sheath complex on ultrasonography may be used to diagnose increased intracranial pressure. Ultrasonography can also be used to guide real-time fine-needle aspiration or core tissue biopsy of orbital lesions, as well as to aid removal of orbital foreign bodies.

Cellulitis, abscess formation and foreign bodies

Tooth root abscesses, trauma, foreign bodies and extension of sinusitis may result in orbital inflammation, with or without abscess formation. Inflammation may also occur from haematogenous, trans-scleral, or transmucosal disease or laceration. Diffuse orbital cellulitis results in a generalized loss of definition of the hypoechoic optic nerve, extraocular muscles and other orbital tissues (Figure 18.14). Cellulitis can also

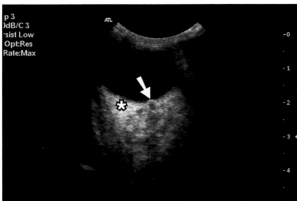

18.14 Horizontal plane ultrasonogram of the orbit of a 7-year-old mixed-breed dog presented with painful unilateral exophthalmos. The orbital fat (*) is more hyperattenuating and the optic nerve and extraocular muscles are less well defined than usual. The optic head is mildly elevated (arrowed). These changes are suggestive of orbital inflammation.

produce focal mass lesions which may be mistaken for neoplasms. Hypoechoic and homogeneous mass lesions with well delineated margins, proven on histological examination to be granulomatous inflammation, have been described as orbital pseudotumours. Abscesses are variable in appearance and may be seen as mass lesions with well defined or ill defined echogenic walls, smooth or ragged internal margins, and echogenic to hypoechoic fluctuant content (Figure 18.15). Fungal cellulitis, such as that due to aspergillosis, has been associated with bone lysis.

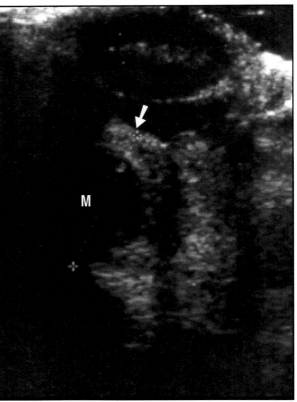

18.15 Transverse image of the orbit of a 3-year-old Domestic Shorthaired cat from a dorsal approach. The near-field shows an indention (arrowed) of the posterior aspect of the scleroretinal rim. Note the mass lesion (M), which has a thick and irregular echogenic wall surrounding a more hypoechoic centre. These changes are compatible with an abscess.

Myositis

Masticatory muscle myositis produces similar ultrasonographic changes to those described for orbital cellulitis, but is more often bilateral. The history and clinical examination may help to differentiate these diseases. In extraocular polymyositis, one or more extraocular muscles may be severely thickened and hypoechoic (Figure 18.16). Unilateral or bilateral thickening of the extraocular muscles usually only occurs with immune-mediated myopathy, but a case of infiltrative lymphoma has been reported. Optic neuritis is the inflammation of one or both optic nerves, and may be a primary disease or secondary to systemic central nervous system disease. The optic nerve often has a normal appearance on ultrasonography, but may also appear thickened and hypoechoic.

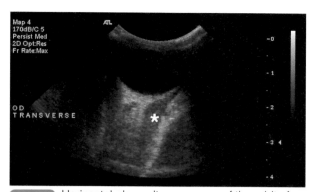

only alter the echogenicity of the orbital structures and may be difficult to recognize. Bone lysis is diagnosed when the hyperechoic delineation of the orbital wall shows interruptions (Figure 18.18) and new bone formation is recognized when the bone margins are irregular. Optic nerve or optic nerve sheath tumours (meningioma, glioma) have been described as round, well defined echogenic to hypoechoic mass lesions caudal to the posterior aspect of the globe, sometimes also causing enlargement of the optic disc (Figure 18.19).

18.16 Horizontal plane ultrasonogram of the orbit of a 3-year-old mixed-breed dog presented with painful bilateral exophthalmos. Note the severe thickening and hypoechoic appearance of the extraocular muscles (*), together with the ill defined margins. In addition, the orbital fat appears more hyperattenuating than usual. These changes are compatible with extraocular polymyositis. Differential diagnosis includes lymphoma of the extraocular muscles. (Courtesy of the Department of Surgical and Radiological Sciences, University of California-Davis)

Cystic disease and haematomas

Orbital cysts, arising from epithelial or glandular tissue (lacrimal gland, gland of the nictitating membrane, zygomatic gland or mucosa of the paranasal sinus, conjunctiva or nasolacrimal apparatus), may be caused by trauma, blocked salivary ducts or infection. On ultrasonography, the orbital cyst or haematoma shows an echogenic thin wall with echogenic to anechoic fluctuant contents. The surrounding structures may show loss of definition.

Zygomatic sialocele and sialoadenitis

Ultrasonograms of zygomatic sialoadenitis and sialocele show the enlarged gland with a mixed echogenic or mainly hypoechoic pattern. Depending on the severity of the disease there may be ocular involvement with signs of endophthalmitis. In severe cases abscess and/or mucocele formation may be appreciated as fluctuant contents within the gland. Possible causes are immune-mediated disease, trauma, systemic or localized infection.

Neoplasia

Orbital tumours may be primary, arising from the soft tissues within the orbital space or from the adjacent skull, or secondary to local extension into the orbit from the nasal cavity, paranasal sinuses, or oral cavity. These tumours are mostly unilateral, whereas metastatic orbital neoplasia from distant sites may be unilateral or bilateral. Differentiation between neoplastic and non-neoplastic disease may be difficult. However, typically, neoplastic disease appears as a well defined hypoechoic to echogenic, non-fluctuant mass lesion. Depending on the extension and location of the orbital tumour, indentation of the globe may also be appreciated (Figure 18.17). Osteogenic tumours or chondrosarcoma of the skull appear as very echogenic mass lesions with distal acoustic shadowing. Diffusely growing neoplasms

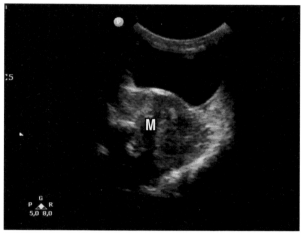

18.17 Longitudinal plane ultrasonogram, from a dorsal approach, of the orbital space of a 9-year-old Irish Terrier presented with non-painful unilateral left-sided exophthalmos. There is a well defined hypoechoic mass (M) visible at the caudal aspect of the eye with indention of the posterior aspect of the globe. The well defined margins and hypoechoic aspect should raise suspicion for neoplasia.

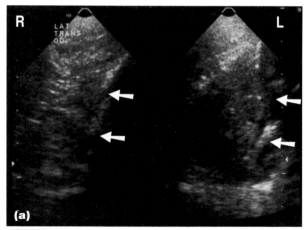

18.18 (a) Transverse image, from a dorsal approach caudal to the eye, of a 10-year-old Siberian Husky presented for mild unilateral left-sided nasal discharge and exophthalmos. **Left:** the normal right orbital space is shown using the temporal muscles as an acoustic window. Note the hyperechoic line (arrowed) representing the medial orbital wall. **Right:** the abnormal left orbital space. Note the irregular hypoechoic mass extending medially beyond the margins of the medial orbital wall. There are interruptions within the hyperechoic margin of the medial orbital wall (arrowed), representing severe osteolysis. (continues) ▶

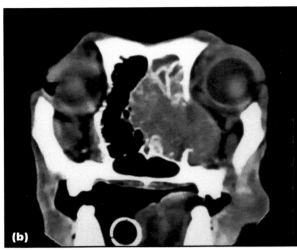

18.18 (continued) **(b)** Transverse CT image illustrating the extension of the bony lysis and mass lesion. Pathology confirmed an adenocarcinoma.

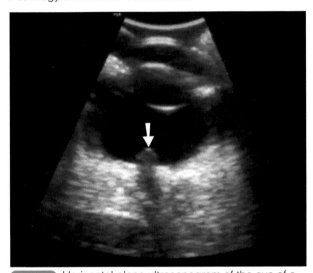

18.19 Horizontal plane ultrasonogram of the eye of a 4-year-old Welsh Springer Spaniel showing a severe hypoechoic thickening of the optic nerve head (arrowed) and proximal optic nerve. Differential diagnoses include granulomatous optic nerve neuritis and neoplasia. Pathology confirmed the diagnosis of a meningioma.

References and further reading

Anderson J and Harvey CE (1993) Masticatory muscle myositis. *Journal of Veterinary Dentistry* **10(1)**, 6–8

Attali-Soussay K, Jegou JP and Clerc B (2001) Retrobulbar tumors in dogs and cats: 25 cases. *Veterinary Ophthalmology* **4**, 19–27

Boroffka SA, Verbruggen AM, Boeve MH *et al.* (1998) Ultrasonographic diagnosis of persistent hyperplastic tunica vasculosa lentis/persistent hyperplastic primary vitreous in two dogs. *Veterinary Radiology and Ultrasound* **39(5)**, 440–444

Boroffka SA, Verbruggen AM, Grinwis GC *et al.* (2007) Assessment of ultrasonography and computed tomography for the evaluation of unilateral orbital disease. *Journal of the American Veterinary Medical Association* **230(5)**, 671–680

Boroffka SA and Voorhout G (1995) In search of the optic nerve. *Veterinary Radiology and Ultrasound* **36**, 436

Boroffka SA, Voorhout G, Verbruggen AM *et al.* (2006) Intraobserver and interobserver repeatability of ocular measurements obtained by means of B-mode ultrasonography in dogs. *American Journal of Veterinary Research* **67**, 1743–1749

Cottrill NB, Banks WJ and Pechman RD (1989) Ultrasonographic and biometric evaluation of the eye and orbits of dogs. *American Journal of Veterinary Research* **50**, 898–903

Deehr AJ and Dulbielzig RR (1998) A histopathological study of iridociliary cysts and glaucoma in Golden Retrievers. *Veterinary Comparative Ophthalmology* **1**, 153–156

Hager DA, Dziezyc J and Millichamp NJ (1987) Two-dimensional real-time ocular ultrasonography in the dog. *Veterinary Radiology* **27**, 24–29

Kern TJ (1985) Orbital neoplasia in 23 dogs. *Journal of the American Veterinary Medical Association* **186**, 489–491

Labruyere JJ, Hartley C, Rogers K *et al.* (2008) Ultrasonographic evaluation of vitreous degeneration in normal dogs. *Veterinary Radiology and Ultrasound* **49**, 165–171

Lee H-C, Choi H-J, Choi M-C *et al.* (2003) Ultrasonographic measurement of the optic nerve sheath diameter in normal dogs. *Journal of Veterinary Science* **4(3)**, 265–268

Mason DR, Lamb CR and McLellan GJ (2001) Ultrasonographic findings in 50 dogs with retrobulbar disease. *Journal of the American Animal Hospital Association* **37**, 557–562

Mattoon JS and Nyland TG (2002) Eye. In: *Small Animal Diagnostic Ultrasound, 2nd edn*, ed. TG Nyland and JS Mattoon, pp. 305–323. WB Saunders, Philadelphia

Mendenhall WM and Lessner AM (2010) Orbital pseudotumor. *American Journal of Clinical Oncology* **33(3)**, 304–306

Miller PE and Dubielzig RR (2001) Ocular tumors. In: *Small Animal Clinical Oncology, 3rd edn*, ed. SJ Withrow and EG MacEwan, pp. 532–545. WB Saunders, Philadelphia

Morgan RV (1989) Ultrasonography of retrobulbar diseases in dogs and cats. *Journal of the American Animal Hospital Association* **25**, 393–399

Morris J and Dobson JM (2000) The eye and orbit. In: *Small Animal Oncology*, ed. J Morris and JM Dobson, pp. 252–261. Blackwell Science, Massachusetts

Penninck D, Daniel GB, Brawer R *et al.* (2001) Cross-sectional imaging techniques in veterinary ophthalmology. *Clinical Techniques in Small Animal Practice* **16**, 22–39

Spaulding K (2008) Eye and orbit. In: *Atlas of Small Animal Ultrasonography*, ed. D Penninck and M-A d-Anjou, pp. 49–90. Blackwell Publishing, Iowa

Spiess BM, Bolliger JO, Guscetti F *et al.* (1998) Multiple ciliary body cysts and secondary glaucoma in the Great Dane: a report of 9 cases. *Veterinary Comparative Ophthalmology* **1**, 41–45

Spiess BM and Wallin-Hakanson N (1999) Diseases of the canine orbit. In: *Veterinary Ophthalmology, 3rd edn*, ed. KN Gelatt, pp. 511–533. Lippincott, Williams & Wilkins, Philadelphia

Stades FC, Djajadiningrat-Laanen SC, Boroffka SA *et al.* (2003). Suprascleral removal of a foreign body from the retrobulbar muscle cone in two dogs. *Journal of Small Animal Practice* **44(1)**, 17–20

Stuhr C and Scagliotti RH (1996) Retrobulbar ultrasound in the mesaticephalic and doliocephalic dog using a temporal approach. *Veterinary Comparative Ophthalmology* **6**, 91–99

Tobias G, Tobias TA and Abood SK (2000) Estimating age in dogs and cats using ocular lens examination. *Compendium on Continuing Education for the Practicing Veterinarian* **22**, 1085–1091

Williams DL (2004) Lens morphometry determined by B-mode ultrasonography of the normal and cataractous canine lens. *Veterinary Comparative Ophthalmology* **7**, 91–95

Woerdt A, Wilkie DA and Myer CW (1993) Ultrasonographic abnormalities in the eyes of dogs with cataracts: 147 cases. *Journal of the American Veterinary Medical Association* **203(6)**, 838–841

Zeiss CJ and Dubielzig RR (2004) A morphologic study of intravitreal membranes associated with intraocular hemorrhage in the dog. *Veterinary Comparative Ophthalmology* **7**, 239–243

19

Thyroid and parathyroid glands

Olivier Taeymans

Indications

The indications for ultrasonography of the thyroid and parathyroid glands include:

- The presence of a space-occupying lesion of unknown origin
- To differentiate solid from cystic thyroid masses
- To stage a thyroid mass
- To search for ectopic thyroid tissue
- To document primary hypothyroidism in dogs
- To differentiate canine primary hypothyroidism from euthyroid sick syndrome
- To document a goitre
- To assess thyroid size before radioiodine treatment of thyroid tumours
- Treatment planning and monitoring of thyroid tumours
- Hypercalcaemia (and hypocalcaemia).

Value of ultrasonography compared with radiography and advanced imaging techniques

Ultrasonography has numerous advantages compared with other imaging techniques. It is readily available, relatively inexpensive, usually does not require any sedation or general anaesthesia, is safe, and has a high inherent spatial and contrast resolution. It is possible to identify the thyroid and parathyroid glands ultrasonographically in normal dogs and cats, given careful technique and the availability of high resolution technology. In cases of disease, the size and structure of the thyroid and parathyroid glands can be evaluated and the relationship with adjacent anatomical structures (including major blood vessels) determined.

However, image quality and interpretation is operator-dependant. Ultrasonography provides a limited field of view, resulting in difficulties determining the origin of large space-occupying lesions, and as the ultrasound beam does not penetrate gas-containing structures, the evaluation of the soft tissues dorsal to the trachea is limited. Similarly, ultrasonography has limited value in searching for intrathoracic ectopic thyroid tissue and pulmonary thyroid carcinoma metastases. Although ultrasonography has its limitations, it is routinely used as a first line imaging modality and often provides a diagnosis, especially when combined with ultrasound-guided aspiration.

Radiography has limited scope in the investigation of thyroid and parathyroid disease, but allows the detection of pulmonary metastases, as well as the skeletal changes which may occur with primary hyperparathyroidism. Computed tomography (CT) and magnetic resonance imaging (MRI) are less widely available, but offer advantages in the detailed evaluation of the margins of a thyroid neoplasm, particularly when there is extension into the thoracic cavity and/or invasion of the surrounding tissues (trachea, oesophagus, major blood vessels). CT is also more sensitive than conventional radiography in the detection of pulmonary metastases. Scintigraphy is an imaging modality that allows detection of functional thyroid tissue, and so offers advantages when searching for ectopic thyroid tissue or evaluating hyperthyroidism when there is no palpable goitre.

Imaging technique

Positioning
The patient should be positioned in dorsal recumbency with the neck in maximal extension. Maximal extension of the neck is obtained by having the dorsal aspect of the skull resting on the table. The patient's front legs need to be pulled backwards to obtain good access to the more caudal aspect of the neck. Care should be taken to align the neck with the rest of the body, and to straighten the neck and head. This considerably helps in recognizing the normal symmetrical anatomy of the neck. A high frequency (>10 MHz) linear transducer is recommended for ultrasonography of the neck.

Protocol
Both thyroid lobes are located along the dorsolateral aspect of the trachea, just caudal to the larynx and medial to the common carotid arteries. The sternothyroid, sternocephalic and sternohyoid muscles delineate the thyroid lobes ventrally. The oesophagus can often be found just dorsal to the left thyroid lobe, although its location may be variable in the cranial neck. An isthmus, connecting the caudal aspect of both lobes and spanning the trachea ventrally, is almost never seen ultrasonographically but has been described on CT and MRI in dogs.

Location of the thyroid lobes is best achieved in the transverse plane. Once found, the thyroid lobe can be scanned along its long axis by rotating the transducer through 90 degrees. This requires dexterity, as the relatively small thyroid lobe is easily lost from the image during rotation of the probe. Alternatively, once the craniocaudal location of the thyroid lobe is identified on transverse images, the transducer can be placed in a longitudinal plane at this level within the jugular groove. Once the common carotid artery is identified and displayed in its entire length, the probe is slowly fanned medially. The thyroid lobe subsequently appears in a long-axis view. If the probe is fanned too far medially, a longitudinal image of the trachea is obtained. Minimal transducer pressure should be applied to avoid distortion of the anatomy. Care should be taken to scan the entire neck, including both the tongue base and thoracic inlet, for possible ectopic thyroid tissue.

Normal ultrasonographic appearance

In long-axis views, both thyroid lobes are fusiform in shape with a rounded cranial pole and a pointed caudal end (Figure 19.1; see also **Normal thyroid gland (1)** clip on DVD). In transverse images, the lobes appear triangular to polygonal in shape (Figure 19.2; see also **Normal thyroid gland (2)** clip on DVD).

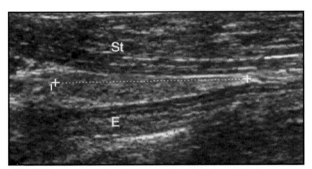

19.1 Longitudinal image of the left thyroid lobe (between the callipers) in a healthy Beagle. The thyroid lobe has a rounded cranial pole and a pointed caudal pole. Note the homogeneous, hyperechoic gland parenchyma compared with the surrounding musculature, and the hyperechoic smooth capsule. E = oesophagus; St = sternothyroid muscle.

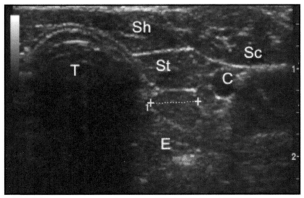

19.2 Transverse image of the left thyroid lobe (between the callipers) in a healthy Beagle. The thyroid lobe has a polygonal to almost triangular shape. C = common carotid artery; E = oesophagus; Sc = sternocephalic muscle; Sh = sternohyoid muscle; St = sternothyroid muscle; T = trachea.

Normal thyroid lobes have a homogeneous parenchyma, being slightly to moderately hyperechoic compared with the surrounding musculature. A well defined and smooth hyperechoic capsule outlines each lobe. The size of the lobe is directly correlated to the size of the patient. In Beagles the average size is 2.5 cm (L) x 0.5 cm (W) x 0.6 cm (H). On MRI, the thyroid lobe diameter corresponds to twice the diameter of the common carotid artery in healthy dogs. Thyroid lobes in cats measure approximately 2.0 cm (L) x 0.2 cm (W) x 0.3 cm (H).

There are usually four parathyroid glands in dogs and cats, two on each side. The two most cranial glands are often seen in the extrathyroidal fascia of the thyroid gland (external parathyroid), and colour Doppler should be used to differentiate them from the cranial thyroid vein and artery. The two most caudal glands are commonly embedded within the thyroid parenchyma (internal parathyroid), and should not be confused with small thyroid cysts. Their location and number may vary significantly. The parathyroid glands appear as discrete, well defined, small (2–3 mm), oval to round, hypoechoic to almost anechoic structures (Figure 19.3).

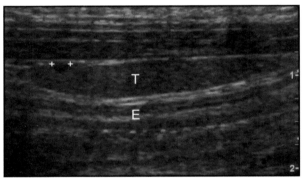

19.3 Longitudinal image of an external parathyroid gland (between the callipers) in a healthy dog. The gland measures 2 mm. E = oesophagus; T = thyroid lobe.

Thyroid gland abnormalities

Euthyroid sick syndrome
Ultrasonography is an extremely helpful tool in differentiating euthyroid sick syndrome from true hypothyroidism. Dogs with euthyroid sick syndrome have abnormal thyroid hormone levels as a result of a variety of diseases other than primary hypothyroidism. It may be very difficult to differentiate euthyroid from hypothyroid patients, based on clinical findings and serum thyroid levels alone. In comparison with dogs with hypothyroidism, the thyroid gland in dogs with euthyroid sick syndrome has a normal appearance on ultrasonography.

Hypothyroidism
A variable combination of diffusely small, irregular, hypoechoic and/or heterogeneous thyroid lobes characterize primary canine hypothyroidism (Figure 19.4). Using a combination of these parameters, ultrasonography has a sensitivity of 94% in detecting

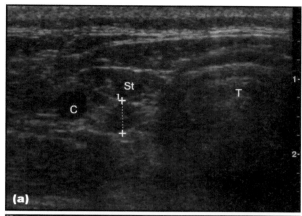

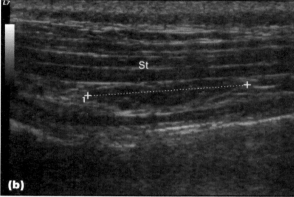

19.4 **(a)** Transverse and **(b)** longitudinal images of a thyroid lobe (between the callipers) of a dog with primary hypothyroidism. The lobe is mildly decreased in size, is isoechoic to almost hypoechoic compared with the surrounding muscles, has a heterogeneous parenchyma, an undulating and ill defined capsule, and has a rounded shape on transverse section. C = common carotid artery; St = sternothyroid muscle; T = trachea.

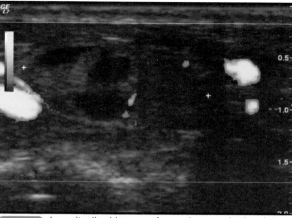

19.5 Longitudinal image of an adenoma in the right thyroid lobe (between the callipers) in a cat. Note the multiple anechoic areas in the cranial aspect of the diffusely enlarged lobe. The remainder of the lobe is normal in echotexture and echogenicity. Power Doppler indicates mildly increased vasularization within the gland. The larger blood vessels at the cranial and caudal poles of the thyroid lobe represent the normal cranial and caudal thyroid arteries and veins.

hypothyroidism. Thus, it is recommended that ultrasonography be utilized as an additional diagnostic tool in the often challenging diagnosis of hypothyroidism. After initiating treatment with thyroid hormone supplementation, the thyroid lobes decrease in size over time and the ultrasonographic abnormalities remain unchanged.

Neoplasia

Thyroid tumours (adenoma or carcinoma) in both dogs and cats are vascularized, hypoechoic and heterogeneous masses deforming the contour of the affected lobes. Almost all thyroid tumours in cats are adenomas (Figure 19.5), and anechoic necrotic centres are frequently seen in these often bilaterally occurring hypersecreting tumours.

In dogs, adenomas and carcinomas are equally distributed and can have the same ultrasonographic appearance. However, adenomas tend to remain undetected during life because they do not result in serum thyroid hormone abnormalities and are often small in size. Consequently, adenomas are often not palpated by the dog's owner, do not tend to compress adjacent organs, resulting in the absence of respiratory or swallowing abnormalities, and do not

result in hyperthyroidism or hypothyroidism. On the other hand, rapid growth, large size, local tissue invasion, capsule disruption and foci of dystrophic mineralization are characteristic of malignancy (Figure 19.6). Unilateral carcinomas are found twice as often as bilateral carcinomas. When bilateral carcinomas are present, clinical signs of hypothyroidism may occur as a result of destruction of the majority of the gland.

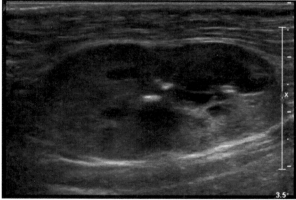

19.6 Longitudinal image of a compact cellular thyroid carcinoma of the right thyroid lobe in a 10-year-old Golden Retriever. The lobe contains multiple areas of dystrophic mineralization, suggesting the malignant nature of this neoplasm. Note the multiple anechoic areas of necrosis throughout the gland parenchyma. No capsule disruption or local tissue invasion were detected. The lobe measured 24 mm x 11 mm.

Cysts

Thyroid cysts appear as anechoic cavities of variable size, with or without septations. If small, the cysts can be confused with parathyroid glands. Thyroid cysts are rare and often considered incidental, but have been observed in dogs being treated for hypothyroidism (Figure 19.7).

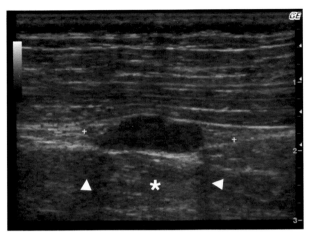

19.7 Longitudinal image of a thyroid lobe (between the callipers) containing a cyst. The cyst was noted in a dog being treated for primary hypothyroidism. Note the faint distal enhancement dorsal to the cyst (*), together with side lobe artefacts (arrowheads).

Parathyroid gland abnormalities

Diseases affecting the parathyroid glands include:

- Diffuse hyperplasia
- Adenoma
- Adenomatous hyperplasia
- Adenocarcinoma (less common).

All these conditions are characterized by one or more enlarged parathyroid glands. Parathyroid tumours are usually solitary and >4 mm in diameter (average is 7 mm), whilst diffuse hyperplasia (seen in secondary hyperparathyroidism; Figure 19.8) involves

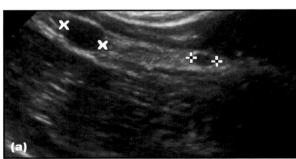

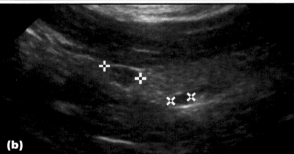

19.8 Longitudinal images of the **(a)** left and **(b)** right thyroid lobes with the corresponding external and internal parathyroid glands (between the callipers) in a 9-year-old Weimaraner with renal secondary hyperparathyroidism. The largest parathyroid gland measures 7.0 mm, the smallest measures 3.5 mm.

all parathyroid glands and results in a less pronounced enlargement (range of 3–6 mm). Both adenomas and adenocarcinomas usually have a slightly increased echogenicity compared with the normal parathyroid tissue, but remain hypoechoic to the surrounding thyroid tissue (Figure 19.9). Accuracy of ultrasonography for detecting a single adenoma in cases of primary hyperparathyroidism has been reported to be >90%. Due to overlap in size and appearance between secondary hyperplasia and primary adenomas, histopathology is necessary to make a definitive diagnosis.

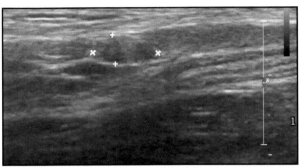

19.9 Longitudinal image of the left external parathyroid gland (between the callipers) in an 11-year-old Samoyed with primary hyperparathyroidism. The parathyroid gland measures 8 mm. Note the mildly increased echogenicity of the lesion compared with the normal parathyroid tissue. Histopathology confirmed the lesion was an adenoma.

References and further reading

Brömel C, Pollard RE, Kass PH *et al.* (2005) Ultrasonographic evaluation of the thyroid gland in healthy, hypothyroid and euthyroid Golden Retrievers with non-thyroidal illness. *Journal of Veterinary Internal Medicine* **19**, 499–506

Brömel C, Pollard RE, Kass PH *et al.* (2006) Comparison of ultrasonographic characteristics of the thyroid gland in healthy small-, medium- and large-breed dogs. *American Journal of Veterinary Research* **67**, 70–77

Reese S, Breyer U, Deeg C *et al.* (2005) Thyroid sonography as an effective tool to discriminate between euthyroid sick and hypothyroid dogs. *Journal of Veterinary Internal Medicine* **19**, 491–498

Reusch CE, Tomsa K, Zimmer C *et al.* (2000) Ultrasonography of the parathyroid glands as an aid in differentiation of acute and chronic renal failure in dogs. *Journal of the American Veterinary Medical Association* **217**, 1849–1852

Taeymans O (2009) Thyroid ultrasound in dogs: a review. *Ultrasound* **17(3)**, 137–143

Taeymans O, Daminet S, Duchateau L and Saunders JH (2007) Pre- and post-treatment ultrasonography in hypothyroid dogs. *Veterinary Radiology and Ultrasound* **48**, 262–269

Taeymans O, Dennis R and Saunders JH (2008) Magnetic resonance imaging features of the normal canine thyroid gland. *Veterinary Radiology and Ultrasound* **49**, 238–242

Taeymans O, Duchateau L, Schreurs E *et al.* (2005) Intra- and inter-observer variability of ultrasonographic measurements of the thyroid gland in healthy Beagles. *Veterinary Radiology and Ultrasound* **46**, 139–142

Taeymans O and O'Marra SK (2009) Imaging diagnosis – transient goitrous acquired hypothyroidism in a young dog, following treatment with trimethoprim sulfamethoxazole. *Veterinary Radiology and Ultrasound* **50**, 442–444

Taeymans O, Peremans K and Saunders JH (2007) Thyroid imaging in the dog: current status and future directions. *Journal of Veterinary Internal Medicine* **21**, 673–684

Taeymans O, Schwarz T, Duchateau L *et al.* (2008) Computed tomographic features of the normal canine thyroid gland. *Veterinary Radiology and Ultrasound* **49**, 13–19

Wisner ER, Mattoon JS, Nyland TG and Baker TW (1991) Normal ultrasonographic anatomy of the canine neck. *Veterinary Radiology and Ultrasound* **32**, 185–190

Wisner ER and Nyland TG (1998) Ultrasonography of the thyroid and parathyroid glands. *Veterinary Clinics of North America: Small Animal Practice* **28**, 973–991

Wisner ER, Nyland TG and Mattoon JS (1994) Ultrasonographic examination of cervical masses in the dog and cat. *Veterinary Radiology and Ultrasound* **35**, 310–315

Wisner ER, Penninck D, Biller D *et al*. (1997) High-resolution parathyroid sonography. *Veterinary Radiology and Ultrasound* **38**, 462–466

Video extras

- **Normal thyroid gland (1)**
- **Normal thyroid gland (2)**

Access via QR code or bsavalibrary.com/ultrasound_19

20

Musculoskeletal structures

Martin Kramer

Indications

Ultrasonography is an established method for the detection of muscle and tendon pathology. The ultrasonographic evaluation of joints and associated ligaments can also be performed in dogs and cats but is more technically challenging. Indications for ultrasonographic examination of musculoskeletal structures include:

- Diffuse or focal soft tissue swelling around a joint, long bone, tendon or muscle belly
- Atrophy of muscle
- Palpable thickening of a tendon
- Palpable defect in a tendon or muscle belly
- Abnormal range of movement of a joint
- Pain on manipulation of a joint
- Discharging sinus tract.

Value of ultrasonography compared with radiography and advanced imaging techniques

Radiography and ultrasonography are complementary techniques in the examination of the musculoskeletal system. Radiography allows evaluation of the bony structures, whereas ultrasonography can reveal changes in the soft tissues. Radiographic evaluation of joint pathology is limited to the detection of increased soft tissue swelling, bony sclerosis or lucency, and osteophyte or enthesophyte formation. Ultrasonography allows the evaluation of the soft tissue structures, especially the ligamentous and tendinous components of the joints. Differentiating subcutaneous oedema or cellulitis from limb swelling involving the muscles, tendons or joints is a major advantage of ultrasonography. Fracture healing assessment is typically reserved for radiography; however, ultrasonography can be used to assess callus development in certain fractures.

Computed tomography (CT) remains the method of choice for examining skeletal structures. It is also an excellent tool for scanning the musculoskeletal system as part of the pre-surgical planning for mass resection, in order to determine the margination and extent of the soft tissue mass and the possible involvement of the skeleton. For example, large lipomas can be better assessed with CT than with ultrasonography to determine their extent and invasiveness.

Magnetic resonance imaging (MRI) is an excellent diagnostic tool to examine the musculoskeletal system. Usage of different imaging pulse sequences facilitates examination of tissues with variable contrast, tissue signal and slice orientation. It allows evaluation of all components of the joint, including bone and soft tissue structures (e.g. muscles, tendons, ligaments, menisci and joint fluid). Disadvantages of MRI are the high costs, the need for general anaesthesia and the current limited accessibility.

Imaging technique

Individual structures should be scanned in their entirety in both longitudinal and transverse planes. The examination should begin with the evaluation of structures that are easy to identify (so-called orientation points, e.g. muscle belly, tendon body, insertion of a tendon), in order to determine the origin and extent of abnormalities. The unaffected contralateral limb can be of great value for making comparisons when examining an unfamiliar structure, as well as to rule out normal variations. In general, anaesthesia or sedation of the patient is not necessary to perform standardized examinations for most of the larger joints (e.g. shoulder and stifle) unless they are painful to manipulate.

A high frequency (≥7.5 MHz) linear transducer is required to perform examination of tendons, ligaments and joints. The scan format and excellent near-field resolution of the linear probe are ideal for visualization of the fine structure of tendons, small superficial structures and ligaments. Curved array probes are generally reserved for deeper muscular structures.

Muscles

Normal ultrasonographic appearance
In longitudinal images the structure of normal muscle appears hypoechoic with fine, oblique, hyperechoic striations. In cross-section, the appearance is hypoechoic with uniformly distributed hyperechoic foci (Figure 20.1). The overlying muscle fasciae are visible as a thin hyperechoic band.

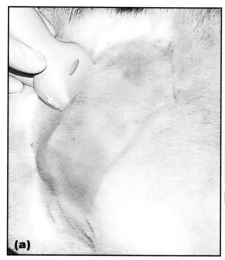

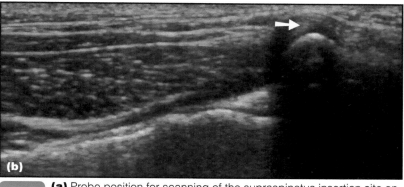

20.1 **(a)** Probe position for scanning of the supraspinatus insertion site on the major tubercle of the humerus in a longitudinal plane. **(b)** Longitudinal image of the normal supraspinatus muscle. Note the normal echotexture of the muscle; hypoechoic with hyperechoic stipples throughout. The short tendon (arrowed) is the hypoechoic structure above the hyperechoic, concave surface of the major tubercle (with acoustic shadowing).

Muscular trauma

The appearance of muscular trauma depends on the age and severity of the injury. With complete muscle rupture, the uniform, striated echotexture of the muscle structure is lost at the site of trauma (Figure 20.2). In an area of acute haemorrhage, the tissue can appear hypoechoic. If the rupture is more chronic, the region appears heterogeneous and has a mixed echotexture, indicating organization of the haematoma. The muscle stumps have been described as cob-like, thickened, heterogeneous structures that are more echogenic than the surrounding tissue. A partial muscle rupture is visible as an incomplete loss of the normal echotexture. The changes are best interpreted in comparison with other unaffected muscle groups.

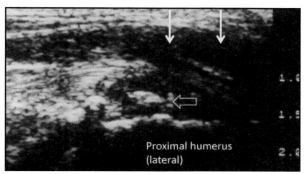

20.2 Infraspinatus muscle rupture. Note the complete rupture of the muscle (thin arrows represent the muscle stump) with small hyperechoic structures representing the avulsed bone at the lateral aspect of the humerus (open arrow). The muscle has a complex, heterogeneous appearance at the rupture site.

Muscle fibrosis and atrophy

In fibrotic myopathies (e.g. gracilis, infraspinatus or quadriceps muscle) the normal echotexture disappears almost completely, depending on the stage of the disease. The muscle becomes hyperechoic and shows a varying degree of heterogeneity. The surrounding fascia is usually difficult to differentiate from the adjacent tissue. Muscle atrophy due to denervation or inactivity, on the other hand, is associated with only minimal changes in the echotexture. The echogenicity of the atrophic muscle is increased, but remains homogeneous.

Cellulitis

Inflammation of the connective tissue can lead to focal or diffuse hypoechoic areas in the subcutaneous tissue, which exhibit a heterogeneous echogenicity with indistinct borders (Figure 20.3).

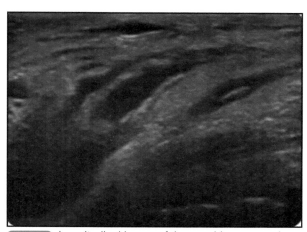

20.3 Longitudinal image of the quadriceps muscle. Cellulitis is present in this dog, seen as a characteristic complex pattern of hypoechoic areas between hyperechoic bands of tissue.

Neoplasia

Soft tissue tumours of the musculoskeletal system can be differentiated into benign (e.g. lipoma) and malignant (e.g. leiomyosarcoma, fibrosarcoma, mast cell tumour). Both benign and malignant tumours can be detected using ultrasonography and are classified as solid, cystic or mixed lesions. Tumours often show mixed echogenicity, but can range from anechoic to hyperechoic with a homogeneous to heterogeneous echotexture. The tumour margins may or may not be clearly visible. When using Duplex or colour Doppler, malignant tumours tend to be hypervascular and the vessels within the tumour have a random distribution (Figure 20.4). Despite these findings, ultrasound-guided fine-needle aspiration or biopsy is strongly recommended for any heterogeneous mass within the musculature to differentiate an organizing haematoma or abscess from neoplasia.

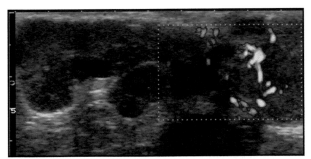

20.4 Longitudinal image in the region of the perineal musculature. An adenocarcinoma (hypoechoic, heterogeneous mass with well defined margins) was diagnosed. Power Doppler ultrasonography shows the irregular tortuous pattern of the vessels, which raises the suspicion of malignancy.

Abscesses

Soft tissue abscesses of the musculoskeletal system appear as focal hypoechoic to anechoic, round to irregularly shaped structures. The content may be anechoic or of mixed echogenicity with hyperechoic foci floating within the fluid. Depending on the age of the abscess, a hyperechoic capsule of variable thickness may be visible. Foreign bodies in the muscular tissue, such as wooden sticks, grass awns (Figure 20.5) or metal objects (e.g. needles) are easily identified as hyperechoic structures if their size exceeds 2–3 mm. In some cases abscesses appear as a hyperechoic double line with a more or less distinct hypoechoic, irregular area surrounding the foreign body (reactive tissue).

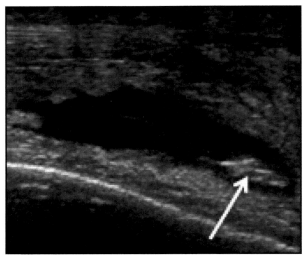

20.5 Longitudinal image of the quadriceps muscle. An abscess (well delineated, hypoechoic fluid pocket) with a hyperechoic foreign body (arrowed) is present. Plant material was diagnosed.

Tendons

Biceps brachii muscle and tendon

Imaging technique

To examine this region, the animal should be placed in lateral recumbency with its legs toward the ultrasonographer, and the affected limb in a non-dependent position. To obtain a perpendicular scan plane of the biceps tendon, the shoulder must be rotated outwards and abducted. This requires the aid of additional personnel to position both the patient and the limb properly.

Normal ultrasonographic appearance

In the longitudinal plane, the muscle (located distal to the shoulder joint) appears hypoechoic with a hyperechoic central line, representing the border between the two fused muscle bellies of the biceps. Hyperechoic lines extend from this central line and run at a slightly oblique angle to the longitudinal axis (fishbone pattern). In cross-section the shape of the muscle resembles a slice of tangerine.

After identification of the biceps muscle, the transducer should be moved proximally to the muscle–tendon interface. This interface appears continuous with the muscle because the typical hypoechoic pattern of the musculature extends a few millimetres beyond the beginning of the tendon structure. The next and most important step in the examination of the biceps tendon is imaging the tendon in the intertubercular groove of the humerus. The intertubercular ligament cannot be distinguished from the surrounding soft tissue. The transverse plane is preferred for assessing changes in the tendinous tissue texture, the tendon sheath and the intertubercular groove.

The transducer should be rotated 90 degrees to the long axis of the limb, so that the lateral structures are displayed on the left side of the image and the medial structures on the right. A thin hypoechoic halo is visible surrounding the oval tendon, defined by the hyperechoic structure of the tendon sheath wall facing the transducer and the hyperechoic surface of the humerus on the side opposite the transducer (Figure 20.6). The greater tubercle appears as a hyperechoic convex, smooth line on the left side of the image. It is more distinct than the lesser tubercle on the right side of the image, which is seen only as a small elevation of the reflective line on the surface of the bone. The intertubercular groove is visible as a mildly concave hyperechoic, smooth line continuous with the border of the tubercles.

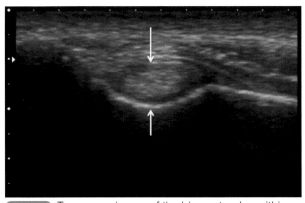

20.6 Transverse image of the biceps tendon within the intertubercular sulcus. The tendon (between the arrows) has a somewhat elliptical shape, is homogeneous and hyperechoic with a thin hypoechoic rim surrounding it.

The final step is the longitudinal examination, performed by following the tendon across the joint to its origin on the supraglenoid tubercle (hyperechoic, convex structure) (Figure 20.7). Distally, the small hypoechoic to anechoic area of the joint space can be distinguished. Due to the tendon curvature, its hyperechoic margins can only be visualized when the transducer is positioned perpendicular to the tendon.

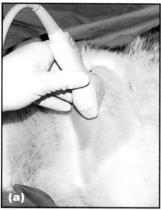

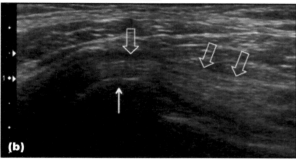

20.7 **(a)** Biceps muscle and tendon. The probe is positioned to scan the origin of the biceps brachii muscle over the supraglenoid tubercle.
(b) Longitudinal scan of the origin of the normal biceps brachii muscle at the supraglenoid tubercle of the shoulder (thin arrow represents proximal humerus). The normal echotexture of the biceps tendon is seen. Note the uniform and parallel tendon fibre alignment and homogeneity of the tendon structure (open arrows).

Tenosynovitis

Tenosynovitis of the biceps brachii tendon can be due to trauma, degeneration or neoplasia of the tendon. It can also occur secondary to osteoarthritis or osteochondrosis of the shoulder joint.

Tendon sheath effusion appears as a hypoechoic to anechoic area surrounding the affected tendon. The effusion can range from mild to severe and is well visualized in cross-sectional scans at the level of the intertubercular groove. The tendon appears mildly to severely thickened. Assessment of tendon size is aided by examination of the unaffected contralateral limb. The wall of the tendon sheath is clearly visible as a hyperechoic line, representing the border between the fluid and the surrounding musculature (Figure 20.8).

The intertubercular groove should be examined for the presence of osteophytes. These lie on the ventral aspect of the tendon and appear as hyperechoic, more or less concave, smooth, curved structures with

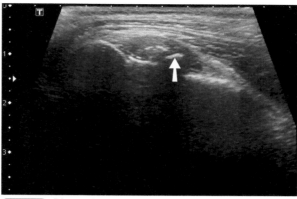

20.8 Biceps brachii tenosynovitis caused by a partial tendon rupture. Transverse scan at the level of the intertubercular groove. The fluid-filled tendon sheath and the heterogeneous tendon are visible. A small piece of bone (arrowed) (from the supraglenoid tubercle) is visible as a hyperechoic structure with acoustic shadowing in the tendon sheath.

acoustic shadowing. These osteoarthritic changes can be found in almost one-third of dogs with tenosynovitis and indicate the chronicity of the disease.

Complete and partial tendon rupture

Most tendon ruptures are secondary to trauma. However, approximately 5–10% of dogs with ultrasonographically diagnosed tenosynovitis have complete rupture of the tendon. With complete rupture, the homogeneous parallel, fibrillar structure of the tendon is lost. An anechoic to hypoechoic region (haematoma) between the tendon stumps is a frequent finding. The distal stump appears oedematous, hypoechoic to hyperechoic (mixed echotexture) and heterogeneous. A moderate to severe tendon sheath effusion may also be observed.

Partial ruptures occur most frequently in the area of the supraglenoid tubercle. Slightly >10% of the cases have underlying tenosynovitis (Figure 20.9). Multiple, small hyperechoic bone fragments with acoustic shadowing are visible within the tendon at the site of avulsion. The tendon tissue appears oedematous, hypoechoic and mildly to moderately heterogeneous. In contrast to a complete rupture, areas of tendon tissue displaying a normal fibrillar

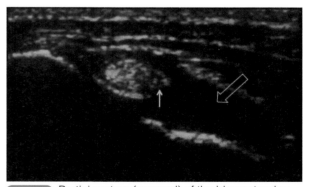

20.9 Partial rupture (arrowed) of the biceps tendon. Transverse scan of the biceps brachii tendon over the intertubercular groove. Accumulation of anechoic fluid in the tendon sheath (open arrow) is consistent with chronic tenosynovitis and synovitis.

echotexture can be found in the transverse image. The partial rupture appears as an anechoic focus in the rounded tendon. Tendon sheath effusion is visible as an anechoic margin surrounding the tendon. The prognosis of a partial or complete rupture of the biceps brachii tendon in medium sized and large dogs is good with surgical repair.

Luxation of the biceps tendon

Rupture of the transverse ligament results in luxation of the tendon over the lesser tubercle. In the transverse plane, the tendon is not located in the intertubercular groove. The round tendon with its typical fibrillar echotexture can be seen medially, in the region of the lesser tubercle. During a dynamic examination (rotating the limb internally and externally) the tendon slides back into the groove. The ruptured ligament itself cannot be visualized ultrasonographically.

Achilles tendon

Imaging technique

Ultrasonographic examination of the Achilles tendon is performed in a standardized fashion with the tarsocrural joint slightly flexed, thus increasing the tension in the tendon.

Normal ultrasonographic appearance

Initially, a longitudinal scan is performed by placing the probe over the calcaneus at the insertion site of the tendon (Figure 20.10a). The transducer is then moved proximally in order to examine the whole structure as well as the musculotendinous junction and the muscles. Cross-sectional plane images are generally obtained at the site where abnormalities are detected. A longitudinal image taken directly over the tuber calcanei shows the surface of the calcaneus as a convex hyperechoic line with distal acoustic shadowing (Figure 20.10b). Immediately proximal to this bony point of orientation, a 5 mm x 5 mm hypoechoic, ill defined area comes into view, which represents the bursa calcanei with its surrounding tissue and the insertion of the tendon. The tendon appears as an echogenic, homogeneous structure with parallel hyperechoic lines (fibrillar texture). The peritendon is visible as a hyperechoic smooth band. Due to the hyperechoic borders, differentiation of the superficial from the deep portions of the tendon is easy. Further proximally, the muscles display the typical echotexture (see above). In transverse images, the Achilles tendon is seen as a moderately echogenic round structure with multiple small hyperechoic dots. The peritendon is visible as a hyperechoic line.

Rupture

Achilles tendon injuries are uncommon in small animals, and are usually the result of direct trauma. A partial or complete rupture of the Achilles tendon looks similar to that of the biceps brachii tendon (Figure 20.11).

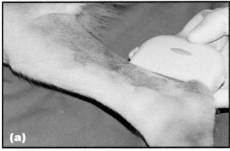
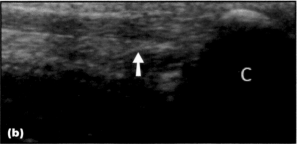

20.10 **(a)** The probe is positioned to scan the insertion region of the Achilles tendon over the calcaneus. **(b)** Longitudinal scan of the normal insertion site of the Achilles tendon. The normal tendon echotexture of the deep and superficial parts of the Achilles tendon is clearly seen proximal to the hyperechoic surface of the calcaneus (C; acoustic shadowing behind the bony surface). The hypoechoic region in the area of the insertion of the deep part of the tendon to the calcaneus represents the bursa (arrowed).

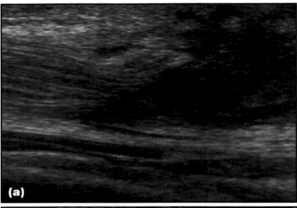
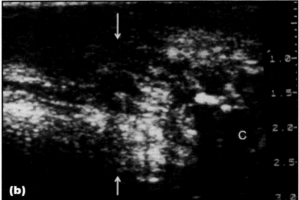

20.11 **(a)** Achilles tendon rupture. There is complete interruption of the tendon echotexture. On the right side of the image a hypoechoic, irregular mass (haematoma) is visible. **(b)** Longitudinal scan over the calcaneus (C) showing a chronic ruptured Achilles tendon (between the arrows). Heterogeneous, hypoechoic zones of tendon healing and small calcifications are visible and are indicative of the chronic nature of the disease.

Monitoring healing: Using ultrasonography, the healing process of the Achilles tendon with or without surgical intervention can be readily observed. In the first 24 hours post-trauma, the haematoma between the ends of the tendon stumps appears hypoechoic to anechoic. Organization of the haematoma during the 1st and 2nd week leads to a more heterogeneous mass with echogenic areas. From the 2nd to 6th week, the diameter and the heterogeneity of the injured area increase. After 8 weeks, replacement tissue begins to grow in a longitudinal direction and there is a decrease in both diameter and heterogeneity. The decrease in diameter is accompanied by the reappearance of the typical tendinous fibrillar echotexture. The healing process is generally completed 10–12 weeks post-trauma. However, the injured Achilles tendon remains much less homogeneous in comparison with the unaffected tendon for a long period of time.

Displacement and luxation

Displacement of the superficial digital flexor tendon (medially or laterally) is mostly caused by trauma. Mild to severe lameness is seen clinically. The displacement can be visualized ultrasonographically by obtaining a transverse image above the hyperechoic convex structure representing the tuber calcanei and locating the malpositioned tendon. Nearly 10% of dogs with an injury of the Achilles tendon also have a luxation. Surgical repair consists of fixing the tendon over the tuber calcanei with sutures.

Calcifying tendinopathies and myopathies

In the condition referred to as calcifying tendinopathy of the abductor pollicis longus or the supraspinatus muscle, the calcium deposits are visible as hyperechoic, irregular dots displaying acoustic shadowing within the tendon tissue.

Bones

Imaging technique

In some instances, ultrasonography can be a helpful tool in gaining additional information on diseased bone. Images obtained with a linear probe are easier to assess than those gained with sector or convex transducers because the field of view is larger. The surface of a long bone is examined by placing the probe along the long axis of the bone. Compared with a transverse image this longitudinal view enables the examiner to assess a larger area of bone.

Normal ultrasonographic appearance

Due to the reflection and absorption of sound waves, bone appears as a very hyperechoic, continuous, smooth line with acoustic shadowing. The bony surface of the sites of origin and insertion of the tendons and ligaments, appears as an irregularly delineated, hyperechoic area with acoustic shadowing. In the near-field the image of the skin–transducer interface can be seen as a hyperechoic zone. Superficial to the bony surface the typical echotexture of the soft tissue structures (muscles and tendons) comes into view.

Inflammation

Inflammatory processes (e.g. periostitis or osteomyelitis) appear as hypoechoic, heterogeneous areas in the surrounding soft tissue, and if the cortex is destroyed, the bony surface (periosteum) appears uneven with multiple indentations, giving it a pallisading appearance. Although the alterations in the periosteum and underlying cortical bone are mainly assessed with ultrasonography, the underlying spongy bone can also be visualized when larger cortical defects are present. Radiography is crucial for assessing the depth of the lytic zone detected at the bony surface on ultrasonograms.

Fractures

Fractures of the long bones and the healing process, as well as the associated soft tissue damage (muscle rupture, haematoma), can be assessed ultrasonographically (Figure 20.12). As there are no points of orientation, the exact relationship between the fractured ends is difficult to determine, and radiography is required for complete assessment. Ultrasonography can be used to evaluate secondary fracture healing in uncomplicated fractures and in instances of non-union and delayed union fractures. Power Doppler can be used to show neovascularization in callus formation.

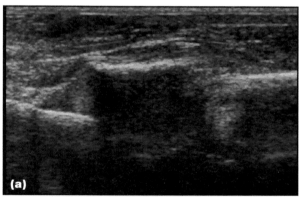

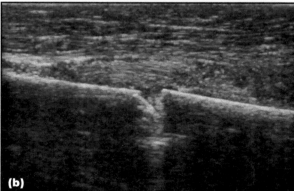

20.12 Longitudinal images showing fracture healing (grades 1–5) in a femur. **(a)** Grade 1. A fracture gap is present with a sharply defined, linear, hyperechoic bone fragment. Note the homogeneous, hypoechoic to anechoic areas of haematoma formation adjacent to the bone fragment and in the fracture gap. **(b)** Grade 2. Haematoma resorption is evident at the fracture site and heterogeneous tissue remains adjacent to the fracture. Note the margins of the fracture remain fairly sharp. ▶

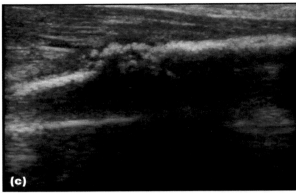

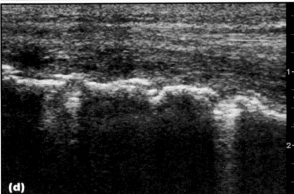

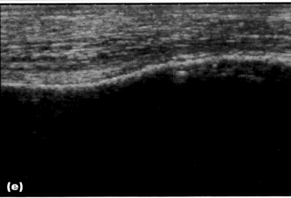

20.12 (continued) **(c)** Grade 3. Fracture margins are irregular and blunted due to resorption. The early, non-ossified callus has a heterogeneous appearance and irregular contours. (continues) Longitudinal images showing fracture healing (grades 1–5) in a femur. **(d)** Grade 4. The callus is increasingly echogenic, continuous and laminar in appearance. The callus is still heterogeneous, which is consistent with immaturity and incomplete ossification. The callus surface is irregular. **(e)** Grade 5. The fracture is completely healed and a continuous hyperechoic contour can be identified bridging the fracture.

Neoplasia
Bone tumours that extend into the surrounding soft tissue can also be assessed ultrasonographically. They have a variable appearance ranging from anechoic to hyperechoic, and homogeneous to heterogeneous. Occasionally, detachment of the periosteum (Codman's triangle) is seen. If the bony surface is destroyed the deeper portions of the bone can be visualized. Whether bone proliferation or bone lysis predominates, the surface of the bone is often markedly irregular (Figure 20.13).

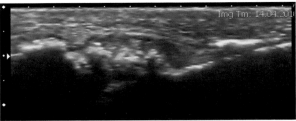

20.13 Longitudinal image of the dorsal bony surface of the distal radial metaphysis. An irregular bony surface with lysis and proliferation is seen. The soft tissue involvement is visible as a hypoechoic, heterogeneous area directly over the bone. The diagnosis was confirmed as osteosarcoma.

Articular ligaments
Imaging technique
The articular ligaments of dogs and cats are usually very small and normally located close to the uneven bony surfaces of the joints, making ultrasonographic assessment difficult. Transducers with a frequency >12 MHz should be used and the examination must be performed directly perpendicular to the ligament.

Normal ultrasonographic appearance
In longitudinal images, ligaments appear as hyperechoic structures with a fibrillar echotexture (with the exception of the cranial cruciate ligament, which appears hypoechoic because of its tortuous structure). The articular surface is visible as an anechoic rim (cartilage and synovial fluid) above the hyperechoic, mostly convex, bony surface.

Ligament disorders
An acute rupture cannot always be seen ultrasonographically, due to the small size of the ligaments in cats and dogs. However, a small anechoic haematoma in the traumatized area may be seen. If the injury is associated with avulsion, a bone fragment may be visible as a hyperechoic structure with acoustic shadowing within the reactive tissue. With chronic injuries, the ruptured end appears as a hyperechoic, irregular structure in the area of the insult (e.g. rupture of the cranial cruciate ligament).

Joints

Joint examination has to be performed with a high frequency (>10 MHz) linear transducer. It is necessary to clip the hair from the whole region of the joint to be examined. For the shoulder, elbow, hip and stifle joints, a standardized examination procedure should be used to visualize the important structures and their diseases.

Shoulder
The standardized examination begins with scanning the supraspinatus and infraspinatus muscles down to their attachment sites at the major tubercle. Then the biceps brachii muscle is examined with maximum outward rotation of the shoulder (see above). In the final step, the intra-articular structures are examined

by positioning the transducer craniocaudally and immediately distal to the acromion. The limited space usually does not allow a second image (perpendicular to the first) to be made. The joint is scanned by slowly adducting and simultaneously rotating the limb, whilst the probe remains in the same position. Subchondral defects caused by osteochondritis on the caudal part of the humeral head can be visualized as concave irregular defects in the hyperechoic convex bone surface. Associated joint effusions appear as distended and hypoechoic areas between the hyperechoic margins of the capsule and the bone surface (Figure 20.14). In chronic osteoarthritis the capsule is seen as a hyperechoic thickened structure, and joint effusion is seen as a hypoechoic to anechoic area between capsule and bone surface.

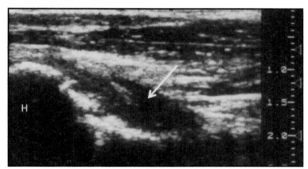

20.14 Longitudinal image of a septic shoulder joint. Osteomyelitis and synovitis are present. The normally hyperechoic convex surface of the humeral head (H) is now irregular and interrupted. It is surrounded by hypoechoic tissue, representing the inflamed synovium (arrowed).

Elbow
The first step of the examination focuses on the lateral and caudal region of the elbow joint. The patient is placed in lateral recumbency with the elbow of interest in a non-dependent position. The patient is then turned over, allowing assessment of the medial and cranial structures. In a normal joint the capsule and the synovial fluid cannot be visualized. In coronoid disease, kissing lesions and osteochondritis defects are seldom visualized with ultrasonography. Secondary osteoarthritic changes such as thickening of the capsule, joint effusion and osteophytes are easier to detect. Ununited anconeal processes, as well as metaplasia of the deep digital flexor muscle, are seen as hyperechoic structures with an acoustic shadow.

Hip
For ultrasonographic imaging of the hip joint, the animal is placed in lateral recumbency. The probe is placed laterally and longitudinally over the joint dorsal to the major trochanter. With a dynamic examination (slight movement in a cranial and caudal direction), the femoral head and adjacent structures can be examined (Figure 20.15a). Signs of osteoarthritis appear as for other joints, and occur most commonly secondary to hip dysplasia in the dog. In an infected, degenerative or traumatized joint, the hyperechoic capsule can be thickened and displaced away from

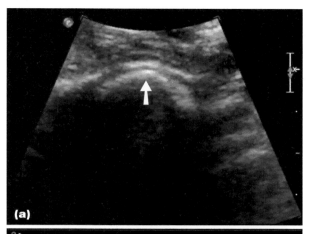

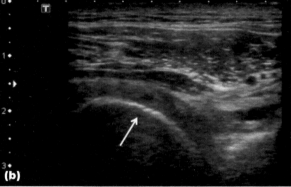

20.15 **(a)** Longitudinal image of the normal hip joint. The smooth rounded hyperechoic surface of the femoral head is shown (arrowed). The joint space appears as a thin hypoechoic rim adjacent to the hyperechoic bony surface of the femoral head. **(b)** Longitudinal image of a hip joint with septic arthritis. Note the presence of heterogeneous, hypoechoic synovitis above the hyperechoic, convex line, which represents the bony surface of the femoral head (arrowed).

the bony margins of the joint due to synovial effusions (Figure 20.15b). In the case of subluxation, the femoral head can be identified as a convex hyperechoic structure located dorsolaterally to the acetabulum. Avascular necrosis of the femoral head results in an irregular, disrupted, convex, hyperechoic structure where the femoral head would generally be located.

Stifle
The patient is initially placed in lateral recumbency with the affected limb in a non-dependent position. The stifle joint is examined from proximal to distal. After scanning the cranial, caudal and lateral aspects of the joint, the patient is turned over to examine the medial aspect of the joint. A dynamic examination follows with flexion and extension, as well as inward and outward rotation, of the knee in the area of the menisci. The stifle examination can be divided into five main regions:

- Suprapatellar (quadriceps tendon, patella, proximal recess)
- Infrapatellar (patella and patellar ligament, medial and lateral femoral condyle, fat pad, cranial and caudal cruciate ligaments, synovium, capsule)

- Lateral (lateral collateral ligament, lateral meniscus, long digital extensor tendon, lateral fabella)
- Caudal (popliteal lymph node and popliteal vessels)
- Medial (medial collateral ligament, medial meniscus, medial fabella).

Osteoarthritis appears as in other joints and is best seen in the suprapatellar and infrapatellar regions. Osteochondrosis of the lateral femoral condyle appears as an irregular concave defect in the convex hyperechoic structure of the condyle. The cruciate ligaments are best seen using a flexed infrapatellar probe position. The normal cranial cruciate ligament is hypoechoic. With chronic cruciate rupture, a hyperechoic area can be seen close to the insertion on the tibia (Figure 20.16). This structure represents part of the ligament and the surrounding hypoechoic haematoma and inflammation.

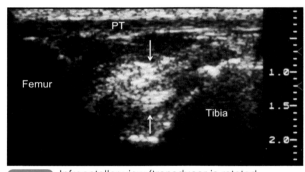

20.16 Infrapatellar view (transducer is rotated approximately 20 degrees laterally) of cruciate rupture. The ligament stump is seen as a small hyperechoic area with irregular margins (bottom arrow). The hypoechoic area around the stump represents the inflamed synovial tissue surrounding the ligament rupture. The top arrow indicates the area of the changed fatty body. PT = patellar ligament.

In the medial and lateral regions, the medial and lateral menisci can be visualized. A normal meniscus appears as a triangular structure of homogeneous, medium echogenicity located between the femoral condyle and the tibial plateau. Degeneration characteristically results in a heterogeneous meniscus with hyperechoic and hypoechoic areas. Due to the difficulty in seeing all parts of the medial and lateral menisci (internal portions), it is difficult to visualize partial or complete tears. The presence of a hyperechoic double line in the parenchyma often correlates with a mensical tear.

References and further reading

Arnault F, Cauvin E, Viguier E *et al.* (2009) Diagnostic value of ultrasonography to assess stifle lesions in dogs after cranial cruciate ligament rupture: 13 cases. *Veterinary Compendium Orthopedic Traumatology* **22**, 479–485

Floeck A, Kramer M, Tellhelm B *et al.* (2003) Die sonographische Untersuchung des Hueftgelenks beim Deutschen-Schaeferhund-Welpen. *Tieraerztliche Praxis* **31**, 82–91

Gnudi G, Volta A, Bonazzi M *et al.* (2005) Ultrasonographic features of grass awn migration in the dog. *Veterinary Radiology and Ultrasound* **46**, 423–426

Greshake RJ and Ackerman N (1992) Ultrasound of the coxofemoral joints of the canine neonate. *Veterinary Radiology and Ultrasound* **33**, 99–104

Kramer M and d´Anjou M-A (2008) Musculoskeletal system. In: *Atlas of Small Animal Ultrasonography*, ed. D Penninck and M-A d´Anjou, pp. 465–510. Wiley-Blackwell, Iowa

Kramer M, Gerwing, M, Hach V *et al.* (1997) Sonography of the musculoskeletal system in dogs and cats. *Veterinary Radiology and Ultrasound* **38**,139–149

Kramer M, Gerwing M, Michele U *et al.* (2001) Ultrasonographic examination of injuries to the Achilles tendon in dogs and cats. *Journal of Small Animal Practice* **42**, 531–535

Kramer M, Gerwing M, Sheppard C *et al.* (2001) Ultrasonography for the diagnosis of diseases of the tendon and tendon sheath of the biceps brachii muscle. *Veterinary Surgery* **30**, 64–71

Kramer M, Schimke E, Schachenmayr W *et al.* (1996) Diagnostic and therapy of special tendon and muscle diseases in the dog. Part I: contracture of the gracilis and infraspinatus muscle. *Kleintierpraxis* **41**, 889–896

Kramer M, Stengel H, Gerwing M *et al.* (1999) Sonography of the canine stifle. *Veterinary Radiology and Ultrasound* **40**, 282–293

Lamb C and Duvernois A (2005) Ultrasonographic anatomy of the normal canine calcaneal tendon. *Veterinary Radiology and Ultrasound* **46**, 326–330

Lamb C and Wong K (2005) Ultrasonographic anatomy of the canine elbow. *Veterinary Radiology and Ultrasound* **46**, 319–325

Long C and Nyland TG (1999) Ultrasonographic evaluation of the canine shoulder. *Veterinary Radiology and Ultrasound* **40**, 372–379

Mueller S and Kramer M (2003) Die Eignung der Sonographie für die Diagnostik von Meniskusläsionen beim Hund. *Tieraerztliche Praxis* **31**, 10–15

Reed AL, Cook CR, Payne JT *et al.* (1997) Ultrasonographic findings in dogs with stifle abnormalities. *Veterinary Radiology and Ultrasound* **38**, 249

Reed AL, Payne JT and Constaninescu GM (1995) Ultrasonographic anatomy of the normal canine stifle. *Veterinary Radiology and Ultrasound* **36**, 315–321

Risselada M, Kramer M, de Rooster H *et al.* (2005) Ultrasonographic and radiographic assessment of uncomplicated secondary fracture healing of long bones in dogs and cats. *Veterinary Surgery* **34**, 99–107

Risselada M, Kramer M, Saunders JH *et al.* (2006) Power Doppler assessment of the neovascularization during uncomplicated fracture healing of long bones in dogs and cats. *Veterinary Radiology and Ultrasound* **47**, 301–306

Risselada M, Kramer M and van Bree H (2003) Approaches for ultrasonographic evaluation of long bones in the dog. *Veterinary Radiology and Ultrasound* **44**, 214–220

Rivers B, Wallace L and Johnston GR (1992) Biceps tenosynovitis in the dog: radiographic and sonographic findings. *Veterinary Compendium Orthopedic Traumatology* **5**, 51–57

Rivers BJ, Walter PA, Kramek B *et al.* (1997) Sonographic findings in canine common calcaneal tendon injury. *Veterinary Compendium Orthopedic Traumatology* **10**, 45–53

Siems JJ, Breur GJ, Blevins WE *et al.* (1998) Use of two-dimensional real-time ultrasonography for diagnosing contracture and strain of the infraspinatus muscle in a dog. *Journal of American Veterinary Medical Association* **212**, 77–80

Swiderski J, Fitch RB, Staatz A *et al.* (2005) Sonographic assisted diagnosis and treatment of bilateral gastrocnemius tendon rupture in a Labrador retriever repaired with fascia lata and polypropylene mesh. *Veterinary Compendium Orthopedic Traumatology* **18**, 258–263

Vandevelde B, Saunders JH, Kramer M *et al.* (2006) Ultrasonographic evaluation of osteochondrosis lesions in the canine shoulder: comparison with radiography, arthrography and arthroscopy. *Veterinary Radiology and Ultrasound* **47**, 174–184

21

Superficial soft tissues

Federica Rossi

Indications

Ultrasonography of the superficial soft tissues is indicated in order to:

- Further examine cutaneous and subcutaneous nodules or masses
- Differentiate nodules and masses from lymph nodes
- Examine the body wall
- Search for foreign bodies
- Examine the mammary glands
- Assess the body wall for defects (congenital or acquired).

Value of ultrasonography compared with radiography

Ultrasonography of the soft tissues is generally indicated when a soft tissue swelling is palpated or recognized radiographically. High frequency ultrasonography is a valuable tool for the evaluation of the skin and other superficial soft tissues affected by focal or diffuse conditions. A high frequency (10–15 MHz) linear transducer is required to obtain detailed images of these very superficial structures.

Imaging technique

Clipping of the hair and the application of an abundant quantity of coupling gel is necessary to obtain high quality images.

Normal ultrasonographic appearance

The normal ultrasonographic appearance of the superficial tissues is variable, depending on the location, body condition and hydration status. Usually, some layering is recognized in the skin, corresponding to the epidermal interface, the sum of the epidermis and dermis, and the subcutaneous tissue. The subcutaneous layer, composed of a mixture of fat and connective tissue, can be identified due to its heterogeneous hypoechoic pattern with linear hyperechoic bands. The fat is normally in contact with the deeper layer of the thoracic/abdominal wall or with the skeletal musculature, which shows variable thickness and a typical longitudinal striated pattern (Figure 21.1). Depending on the area being examined, additional structures such as bones (e.g. ribs), glandular structures (e.g. mammary or salivary glands), lymph nodes, vessels and nerves can be identified.

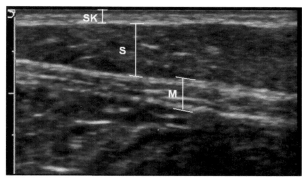

21.1 Ultrasonogram of the normal superficial soft tissues at the level of the caudal abdominal ventral wall. The normal skin (SK), hypoechoic subcutaneous tissue (S) and abdominal wall musculature (M) are visible.

Mammary glands

Normal ultrasonographic anatomy

The non-lactating mammary gland appears as a very thin layer of hypoechoic, homogeneous tissue without evidence of vessels or mammary ducts. During pregnancy, the amount of glandular tissue progressively increases, becoming clearly visible at the beginning of lactation. The margins of the lactating gland are more visible and the parenchyma shows a medium echogenicity with a coarse granular pattern (Figure 21.2; see also **Lactating mammary gland** clip on DVD), due to small hypoechoic areas separated by hyperechoic thin lines corresponding to stroma. In addition, anechoic milk-filled ducts can be observed. Branches of the supplying arteries and veins are easily visualized and can be distinguished from the ducts using colour Doppler ultrasonography.

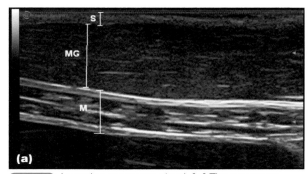

21.2 Lactating mammary gland. **(a)** The mammary gland tissue (MG) extends between the skin (S) and the abdominal wall musculature (M). It has a medium echogenicity with a coarse granular echotexture. (continues) ▶

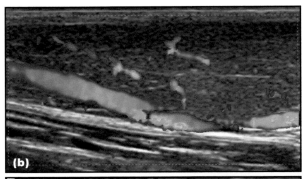

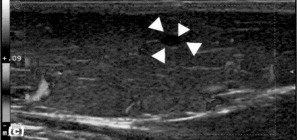

21.2 (continued) Lactating mammary gland.
(b,c) Colour Doppler ultrasonograms showing the abundant vasculature, and one round small structure without flow signal representing a dilated milk duct (arrowheads).

Cysts

Cysts are anechoic, well marginated structures that are sometimes divided by thin septae (Figure 21.3; see also **Mammary cysts** clip on DVD). These lesions are sometimes visualized as incidental findings in the mammary gland; however, they can also be found with tumours. If a cyst is identified, careful examination of the surrounding parenchyma is required to exclude more complex disease. Differentiating cystic tissue from mastitis is typically based on the absence of clinical findings of infection and inflammation.

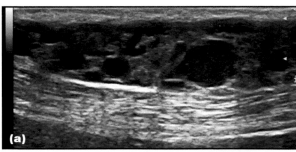

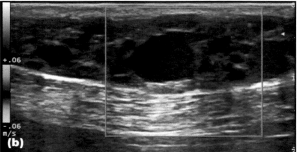

21.3 Mammary gland cysts. **(a)** These cysts appear as round anechoic structures. **(b)** There is no evidence of blood flow on colour Doppler ultrasonography.

Neoplasia

Ultrasonography can be used to evaluate tissue composition and vascularity of mammary gland neoplasia (Figure 21.4). A good correlation between the two-dimensional (2D) greyscale ultrasonogram, colour Doppler appearance, and histopathological changes of benign and malignant lesions has been shown. Size, shape, echogenicity and echotexture, the presence of acoustic enhancement or shadowing, and the density and distribution of supplying vessels can be accurately represented.

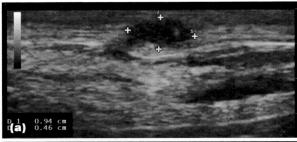

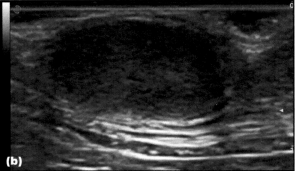

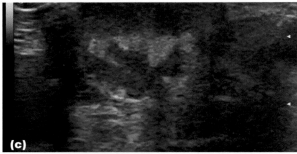

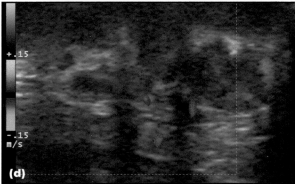

21.4 Ultrasonographic findings of mammary gland neoplasia can be variable. **(a)** Small hypoechoic nodule with irregular margins. Diagnosis was confirmed as a mixed benign tumour. **(b)** Well marginated homogeneous nodule with some edge shadowing. Diagnosis was confirmed as an adenocarcinoma. **(c,d)** Irregular, heterogeneous mass with low vascularization. Diagnosis was confirmed as an inflammatory carcinoma.

Compared with benign lesions, malignant tumours tend to be larger masses of more variable echogenicity and heterogeneous pattern, and show more evident acoustic enhancement due to the frequent presence of necrotic areas. The distribution of vessels is variable with both central and peripheral flow being possible. Malignant tumours tend to have smaller total flow area with evidence of bifurcations and trifurcations of the vessels. However, definitive differentiation between benign and malignant tumours is not possible on the basis of the ultrasonographic appearance alone; tissue sampling for cytology or histopathology is required. Cystic areas and foci of mineralization with shadowing can be observed with both benign and malignant lesions. Evaluation of local invasiveness to the surrounding tissue is another limitation of ultrasonography compared with histopathology.

In young intact queens with single or multiple mammary gland masses, benign fibroepithelial hyperplasia should be considered and differentiated from mastitis and malignant neoplasia. Ultrasonography can be helpful to recognize the benign nature of this condition. Fibroepithelial hyperplasia appears as homogeneous, hypoechoic lesions with regular margins and edge shadowing.

Mastitis

Mastitis is characterized by an increase in size and overall hypoechogenicity of the gland with heterogeneous areas. There is loss of regular architecture and of distinction of the gland from the surrounding subcutaneous tissue and musculature. The presence of anechoic pockets and echogenic content is found in instances of abscess formation.

Superficial swellings and masses

Imaging a superficial swelling or mass is very useful to identify the location and involvement of adjacent tissue layers, and to evaluate its composition. This information is often sufficient to reach a final diagnosis. If not, ultrasound-guided aspiration or biopsy can be easily performed, allowing samples to be obtained from specific areas of the lesion. Ultrasonography is a focused examination technique that does not always allow the extent of a swelling or mass to be determined. In these instances, computed tomography (CT) is often necessary to determine the margination of a mass and its potential invasiveness.

Cavitary lesions

Subcutaneous cysts arising from sebaceous or other superficial glands are a frequent clinical finding; they can be differentiated from solid tumours by ultrasonography. Abscesses can originate from infected cysts or tissues. In dogs and cats, they are often the consequence of a migrating foreign body. The typical appearance of a cavitary lesion is a well marginated structure, delineated by an echogenic peripheral wall of variable thickness. The echogenicity of the content ranges from anechoic to hyperechoic foci or particles depending on the cellular density (Figure 21.5; see also **Abscess** clip on DVD). If an abscess is suspected, careful evaluation of the content is important to identify the foreign body.

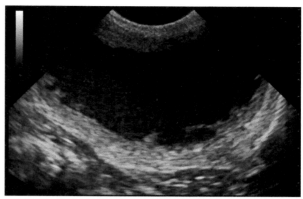

21.5 Typical ultrasonographic appearance of a subcutaneous abscess. The abscess was located in the cervical region. The lesion is well marginated and has a thick, slightly irregular hyperechoic wall and scattered echogenic content.

Foreign bodies

The ultrasonographic appearance of foreign bodies varies depending on size, shape and acoustic properties of the surface. Plant awns are visualized as linear spindle-shaped hyperechoic structures surrounded by a hypoechoic halo, representing oedematous tissue or collection of fluid. Often, two or three parallel reflecting interfaces are seen, corresponding to seeds and seed covers (Figure 21.6; see also **Foreign body (1)** and **(2)** clips on DVD).

The presence of acoustic shadowing is an important feature to distinguish a foreign body from other hyperechoic bands or lines formed by fibrin or connective tissue septae. A very careful examination of the area involved is important in these cases. Frequently, fistulous tracts are visualized as hypoechoic tubular bands, extending out into the surrounding tissue and possibly communicating with the skin surface. They should be followed until the lesion is completely explored. This can be difficult, especially in chronic cases, when the lesion involves a large portion of the thoracic wall or sublumbar region. In these situations, performing a CT scan of the area before or after the ultrasonographic examination is very useful to identify the extent of the condition.

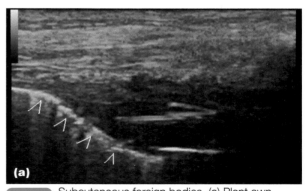

21.6 Subcutaneous foreign bodies. (a) Plant awn located under the 10th rib. The foreign body is visible as a linear spindle-shaped hyperechoic structure with multiple parallel reflecting interfaces, surrounded by a hypoechoic halo representing oedematous tissue. The hyperechoic interface on the left of the image corresponds to the pleural surface of the left caudal lung lobe (arrowheads). (continues) ▶

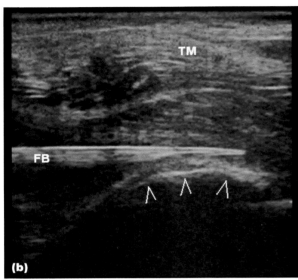

21.6 (continued) Subcutaneous foreign bodies. **(b)** Porcupine spine located in the deep part of the temporal muscle. The dog was presented with a fistula in the skin in the zygomatic region. The foreign body (FB) appears as a hyperechoic pointed structure with sharp margins. The tip of the foreign body (on the right) is in contact with the hyperechoic bone surface of the coronoid process of the mandible (arrowheads). The temporal muscle (TM) is heterogeneous due to the inflammatory process.

Wooden, glass and metallic foreign bodies are less frequently encountered and their appearance ranges from medium echogenicity (wooden) to hyperechoic (glass, metal) with acoustic shadowing. They may also be associated with comet tail artefacts (metal). If a foreign body is identified, its retrieval and drainage of the abscess can sometimes be performed under direct ultrasonographic guidance. In other cases, intraoperative ultrasonography may be necessary to assist the surgeon and visualize the position of the foreign body during dissection of the soft tissues.

Trauma and surgical wounds
Trauma (Figure 21.7; see also **Abdominal wall injury (1)** and **(2)** clips on DVD) and previous surgery are indications to investigate superficial swell-

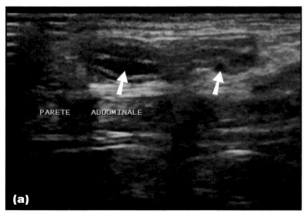

21.7 Lateral abdominal wall of a dog following a bite injury. **(a)** The subcutaneous tissue is thickened and heterogeneous. Note that there are small bowel loops visible just under the skin (arrowed). (continues) ▶

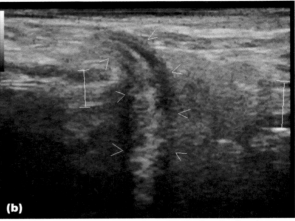

21.7 (continued) Lateral abdominal wall of a dog following a bite injury. **(b)** The muscular wall is interrupted. The two vertical white lines indicate the ends of the ruptured muscular wall. Through the gap, a small bowel loop is visible extending toward the subcutis (arrowheads).

ing of the thoracic or abdominal wall. Ultrasonography is useful to identify complications in wound healing, including infection, suture failure and dehiscence with possible herniation of organs. Recent haemorrhage or subcutaneous haematoma appears as irregular anechoic to hypoechoic areas. The organization of the haematoma produces a heterogeneous appearance with mixed echogenicity. The integrity of the abdominal or thoracic wall musculature can be assessed by ultrasonography. A gap in the continuous longitudinal hyperechoic muscular layer is an indication of an interruption of the musculature due to direct trauma or following dehiscence of a suture. Mesenteric fat or abdominal organs (e.g. intestinal loops) can be observed extending into the subcutaneous tissue if present.

Neoplasia
The role of ultrasonography in the evaluation of soft tissue superficial neoplasia is still under investigation in small animals. It is clear that 2D greyscale and Doppler ultrasonography are able to represent the morphology of the tumour with high accuracy, showing its shape, size, echogenicity, echotexture, margination and the presence and distribution of vessels (Figure 21.8; see also **Soft tissue neoplasm (1)** and **(2)** clips on DVD). However, using these parameters to distinguish between different types of neoplasia is not possible; therefore, biopsy of the lesion is always required.

Lipoma is the only tumour type which can be distinguished from other forms of neoplasia on ultrasonography. Lipomas are well marginated lesions with smooth margins, homogeneous and mostly isoechoic with the surrounding tissue, with a striated pattern produced by thin parallel hyperechoic lines (Figure 21.9; see also **Lipoma** clip on DVD). They show a very low vascularity. However, lipomas, liposarcomas and infiltrative lipomas can all appear similar, emphasizing the need for tissue sampling. Fatty masses whose margins are difficult to assess ultrasonographically often require CT for pre-surgical planning.

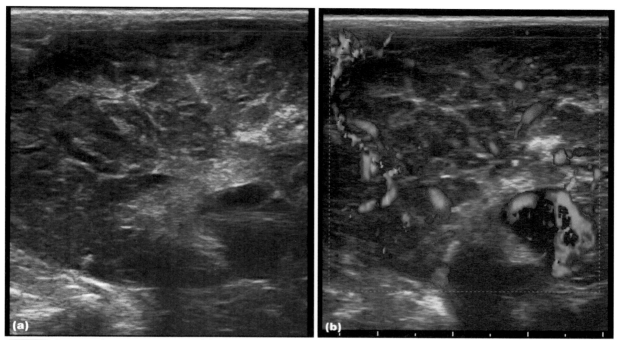

21.8 Large subcutaneous mass of the humeral region, histologically diagnosed as a peripheral nerve sheath tumour. **(a)** The mass is very heterogeneous with irregular hypoechoic and anechoic zones. **(b)** Many of these hypoechoic and anechoic zones represent vessels, as demonstrated on colour Doppler.

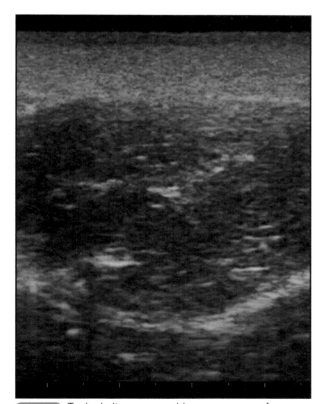

21.9 Typical ultrasonographic appearance of a lipoma. The mass is well marginated with smooth margins, homogeneous and mostly isoechoic with the surrounding tissue. Note also the striated pattern produced by thin parallel hyperechoic lines.

Brachial plexus

The brachial plexus is formed by the contribution of several spinal nerves (sixth, seventh and eighth (sometimes with branches from the fifth) cervical nerves, and first and second thoracic nerves). After exiting the corresponding interverterbal foramina, these nerve roots join one another ventrally toward the axillary region, where the brachial plexus is localized between scapula and the first ribs, close to the axillary artery and vein. The main nerves of the forelimb (suprascapular, subscapular, musculocutaneous, axillary, ulnar, median and radial) originate from the brachial plexus. The ultrasonographic anatomy of these nervous structures has been described in the dog. The scanning technique and ultrasonographic features are detailed in Figures 21.10 and 21.11.

Neoplasia

Neoplasia affecting the brachial plexus is mainly represented by peripheral nerve sheath tumours. Less frequent tumours are sarcomas arising from other soft tissues of the region and metastatic lesions. Ultrasonography of the brachial plexus region can be useful in dogs with unexplained forelimb lameness. Peripheral nerve sheath tumours increase the size of the brachial plexus roots, producing homogeneous, hypoechoic, tubular masses, extending between the vessels and deviating their course. They are typically poorly vascularized lesions. Doppler examination is useful to differentiate these lesions from elongated vascular structures.

Recumbency	Probe position	Beam orientation	View	Features
Lateral – shoulder pulled caudally (area of interest in non-dependent position)	Lateral aspect of the neck at the level of the C5–6, C6–7 and C7–T1 intervertebral foramina	Longitudinal view: aligned perpendicular to the vertebral column with a mild (10–20 degree) ventrocaudal inclination Transverse view: rotate probe 90 degrees from position for longitudinal view	Longitudinal and transverse views of the ventral branches of the sixth, seventh and eighth cervical spinal nerves	Close to the intervertebral foramina: single, round, hypoechoic structure surrounded by a hyperechoic rim (transverse view; Figure 21.11a); single, tubular, hypoechoic band located dorsally to the artery and vein (longitudinal view; Figure 21.11b). More distally, each nerve is formed by multiple small components (Figure 21.11c)
	Aligned parallel to the lateral aspect of the first rib	Mildly caudal	Transverse view showing the multiple branches of the brachial plexus	Multiple small, round, hypoechoic structures surrounded by a hyperechoic rim
	Thoracic inlet window; parasagittal plane with the probe placed between the sternum and the shoulder	Caudal	Transverse view of the brachial plexus close to the axillary artery and vein	Multiple small, round, hypoechoic structures surrounded by a hyperechoic rim (Figure 21.11d)
Dorsal – limb abducted	In the axilla	Dorsal (for both longitudinal and transverse views)	Transverse view of the branches of the brachial plexus (musculocutaneous, median and ulnar nerves) close to the axillary artery and vein	Multiple small, round, hypoechoic structures surrounded by a hyperechoic rim (Figure 21.11e)
Lateral – flexed contralateral leg (area of interest in dependent position)	Medial aspect of the mid-humerus, then exploring the region from the axilla to the elbow	Transverse to the humerus (rotation of 90 degrees)	Transverse and longitudinal views of the musculocutaneous, median and ulnar nerves	Musculocutaneous nerve cranial to the brachial artery. Median and ulnar nerves between the brachial artery and vein
	Mediocaudal aspect of the mid-humerus	Transverse to the humerus	Transverse view of the radial nerve	Cluster of small, round, hypoechoic structures surrounded by a hyperechoic rim
Lateral (area of interest in non-dependent position	Lateral aspect of the distal humerus	Transverse to the humerus	Transverse view of the superficial branch of the radial nerve	Very small, round, hypoechoic structures

21.10 Scanning techniques and ultrasonographic features of the canine brachial plexus.

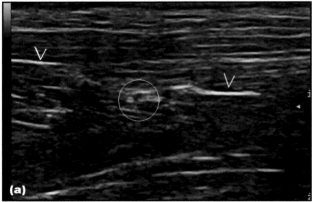
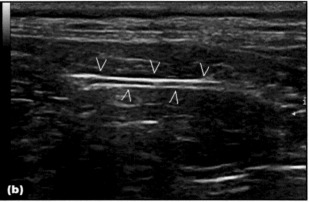

21.11 Ultrasonograms of the lateral aspect of the neck, thoracic inlet and axillary region. The ventral branches of the sixth, seventh and eighth cervical spinal nerves contributing to the brachial plexus, and the major nerve components of the plexus can be identified with ultrasonography. **(a)** Transverse view of the sixth spinal nerve at the level of the intervertebral foramina. The nerve appears as a hypoechoic round structure of 1–2 mm diameter surrounded by a hyperechoic rim (circle). The hyperechoic interfaces produced by the transverse processes of the fifth and sixth vertebrae (arrowheads) are also visible. **(b)** Rotation of the probe through 90 degrees in a mild ventrocaudal direction enables the nerve to be seen in a longitudinal view. The nerve is seen as an elongated hypoechoic band (arrowheads). (continues) ▶

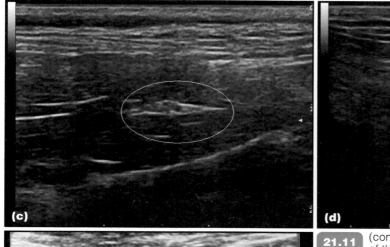

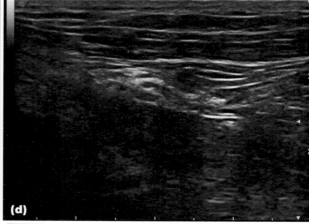

21.11 (continued) Ultrasonograms of the lateral aspect of the neck, thoracic inlet and axillary region. The ventral branches of the sixth, seventh and eighth cervical spinal nerves contributing to the brachial plexus, and the major nerve components of the plexus can be identified with ultrasonography. **(c)** In a more distal position, the nerve appears to be formed by multiple adjacent branches (circle). **(d)** Brachial plexus as seen from a thoracic inlet window. The probe is aligned longitudinally between the sternum and the scapula. Multiple round, hypoechoic, nerve roots are visible. The axillary vein and artery are located close to the nerves but are not visible in this image. **(e)** Brachial plexus as seen from an axillary window. Multiple small nerve roots (arrowed) are located close to the axillary artery (a) and vein (v).

Axillary lymphadenomegaly is another important differential diagnosis. Enlarged lymph nodes have an oval/round shape, more defined border and typical hilar vascularization. Although ultrasonography is able to show peripheral nerve sheath tumours (Figure 21.12; see also **Nerve sheath tumour in the brachial plexus** clip on DVD) located in the axilla, the complete extent of these masses can be underestimated, especially if the lesion extends into the vertebral canal. CT or magnetic resonance imaging (MRI) is therefore required for full evaluation of the lesion and spinal cord for the complete staging of the tumour.

Ultrasound-guided biopsy is indicated if an axillary mass is seen. Ultrasound-guided injection of a small quantity of anaesthetic around the nerve roots has been shown to be a simple and precise procedure in dogs for performing regional nerve blocks.

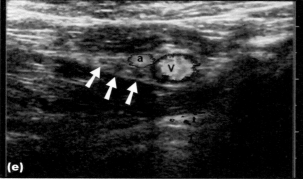

21.12 Nerve sheath tumour of the brachial plexus. The tumour increases the size of the nerve root, producing a homogeneous, hypoechoic, tubular mass, which follows the path of the nerve.

References and further reading

Bagshaw HS, Larenza MP and Seiler GS (2009) A technique for ultrasound-guided paravertebral brachial plexus injections in dogs. *Veterinary Radiology and Ultrasound* **6,** 649–654

De Bulnes AG, Fernandez PG, Aguirre AMM and De la Muela MS (1998) Ultrasonographic imaging of canine mammary tumours. *Veterinary Record* **143,** 687–689

Della Santa D, Rossi F, Carlucci F, Vignoli M and Kircher P (2008) Ultrasound-guided retrieval of plant awns. *Veterinary Radiology and Ultrasound* **49,** 484–486

Diana A, Preziosi R, Guglielmini C *et al.* (2004) High-frequency ultrasonography of the skin of clinically normal dogs. *American Journal of Veterinary Research* **65,** 1625–1630

Gnudi G, Volta A, Bonazzi M, Gazzola M and Bertoni G (2005) Ultrasonographic features of grass awn migration in the dog. *Veterinary Radiology and Ultrasound* **46,** 423–426

Guilherme S and Benigni L (2008) Ultrasonographic anatomy of the brachial plexus and major nerves of the canine thoracic limb. *Veterinary Radiology and Ultrasound* **49,** 577–583

Loh ZHK, Allan GS, Nicoll RG and Hunt GB (2009) Ultrasonographic characteristics of soft tissue tumours in dogs. *Australian Veterinary Journal* **87,** 323–329

Nyman HT, Kristensen AT, Lee MH, Martinussen T and McEvoy FJ (2006) Characterization of canine superficial tumors using gray-scale B mode, color flow mapping, and spectral Doppler ultrasonography – a multivariate study. *Veterinary Radiology and Ultrasound* **47,** 192–198

Nyman HT, Nielsen OL, McEvoy FJ *et al.* (2006) Comparison of B-mode and Doppler ultrasonographic findings with histologic features of benign and malignant mammary tumors in dogs. *American Journal of Veterinary Research* **67**, 985–991

Payan-Carreira R and Martins-Bessa AC (2008) Ultrasonographic assessment of the feline mammary gland. *Journal of Feline Medicine and Surgery* **10**, 466–471

Rose S, Long C, Knipe M and Hornof B (2005) Ultrasonographic evaluation of brachial plexus tumors in five dogs. *Veterinary Radiology and Ultrasound* **46**, 514–517

Trasch K, Wehrend A and Bostedt H (2007) Ultrasonographic description of canine mastitis. *Veterinary Radiology and Ultrasonography* **48**, 580–584

Volta A, Bonazi M, Gnudi G, Gazzola M and Bertoni G (2006) Ultrasonographic features of canine lipoma. *Veterinary Radiology and Ultrasound* **47**, 589–591

Video extras

- Abdominal wall injury (1)
- Abdominal wall injury (2)
- Abscess
- Foreign body (1)
- Foreign body (2)
- Lactating mammary gland
- Lipoma
- Mammary cysts
- Nerve sheath tumour in the brachial plexus
- Soft tissue neoplasm (1)
- Soft tissue neoplasm (2)

Access via QR code or bsavalibrary.com/ultrasound_21

Index

Index

Index

acoustic windows *23*
artefacts *9*, 158–9
comparison with radiography/CT 155–6
indications 155
normal appearance 157–8
patient preparation 157
sampling 163
technique 157
Urine jet *158* ●
Urinoma 122
Urolithiasis 115–17 ●
Uterine stump granuloma *176*
Uterine torsion 174
Uterus
   abnormalities 175–6
   acoustic windows *23*
   comparison with radiography/CT 172
   indications 172
   normal appearance 173 ●
   patient preparation/positioning 172
   pregnancy 173–4 ●
   technique 172–3
Uveitis 185

Vaginal mass *176*
Vascular disease
   abdominal 82–3
   hepatic 96–8
   (see also specific conditions)
Vena cava
   caudal
      abnormalities 82, *96, 97, 153* ●
      normal appearance *77, 78*
Ventricular septal defects 53–5 ●
Vitreal degeneration 187

Wound healing 210